OBSTETRICS

EIGHTH EDITION

by Ten Teachers

OBSTETRICS | 20th EDITION

by Ten Teachers

Edited by

Louise C Kenny MBChB (Hons), MRCOG, PhD

Professor of Obstetrics and Gynaecology

University College Cork

Cork, Ireland

and

Director

The Irish Centre for Fetal and Neonatal Translational Research (INFANT)

Cork, Ireland

Jenny E Myers BMBS, BMedSci (Hons), MRCOG, PhD

NIHR Clinician Scientist and Honorary Consultant in Obstetrics

Maternal & Fetal Health Research Centre

University of Manchester

Manchester, UK

CRC Press
Taylor & Francis Group
Boca Raton London New York

CRC Press is an imprint of the
Taylor & Francis Group, an **informa** business

CRC Press
Taylor & Francis Group
6000 Broken Sound Parkway NW, Suite 300
Boca Raton, FL 33487-2742

© 2017 by Taylor & Francis Group, LLC
CRC Press is an imprint of Taylor & Francis Group, an Informa business

No claim to original U.S. Government works

Printed on acid-free paper by Ashford Colour Press Ltd.

International Standard Book Number-13: 978-1-4987-4439-3 (Pack – Book and Ebook)
International Standard Book Number-13: 978-1-4987-4460-7 (Paperback; restricted territorial availability)

Visit the Taylor & Francis Web site at
http://www.taylorandfrancis.com

and the CRC Press Web site at
http://www.crcpress.com

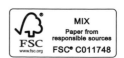

Dedication

This book is dedicated to my sons, Conor and Eamon (LCK)

And to my children Owen and Bethan (JEM)

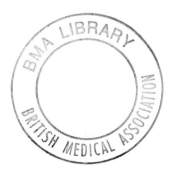

Contents

Preface

Obstetrics by Ten Teachers is an iconic text. First published as *Midwifery by Ten Teachers* in 1917 under the editorship of Comyns Berkley (Obstetric and Gynaecological Surgeon to the Middlesex Hospital), the book is now in its 20th edition and has reached a landmark centenary, cementing its place as one of the oldest, most respected and most popular English language texts on the subject.

As editors who were once students and readers of this textbook, we fully appreciate the responsibility of revising a much-loved classic. Befitting of the next century, the book has been almost completely rewritten by 'Ten Teachers', all internationally renowned experts in their fields and all intimately involved in the delivery of both undergraduate and postgraduate teaching in the UK and Ireland, to reflect the current undergraduate curriculum. This volume has been edited carefully to ensure consistency of structure, style and level of detail, in common with those of its sister text *Gynaecology by Ten Teachers*. The books can therefore be used together or independently as required.

The aim of the book as detailed in the preface of the first edition, published 100 years ago, still pertains today:

This book is frankly written for students preparing for their final examination and in the hope that it will be useful to them afterwards and to others who have passed beyond the stage of examination.

Thus, while the 20th edition is written for medical students, we hope that the text retains its relevance for trainee obstetricians, general practitioners, midwives and other health care professionals with an interest in the field. Furthermore, in line with the popularity of this book elsewhere in the world and reflecting the fact that in 2017, the global burden of maternal morbidity and mortality is greatest in low resource settings, the 20th edition includes a global health perspective throughout.

It has been a privilege and an honour to be the editors of this textbook as it reaches this important milestone; we echo a century of previous editors in hoping that this book will enthuse a new generation of doctors to become obstetricians and work to make pregnancy and childbirth an even safer and more fulfilling experience.

Louise C Kenny
Jenny E Myers
2017

Contributors

Lucy C Chappell MB BChir, MRCOG, PhD
NIHR Research Professor of Obstetrics
King's College London
London, UK

Anna L David MB ChB (Hons), FRCOG, PhD
Professor and Consultant in Obstetrics and
    Maternal Fetal Medicine and Head of Research
Institute for Women's Health
University College London
London, UK

Mark R Johnson MBBS, MRCP, MRCOG, PhD
Professor of Clinical Obstetrics
Imperial College School of Medicine
Chelsea and Westminster Hospital
London, UK

Louise C Kenny MBChB (Hons), MRCOG, PhD
Professor of Obstetrics and Gynaecology
University College Cork
and
Director
The Irish Centre for Fetal and Neonatal
    Translational Research (INFANT)
Cork, Ireland

Fergus McCarthy MBBCh, BAO Dip, MSc, MRCPI,
    MRCOG, PhD
Academic Clinical Lecturer
King's College London
London, UK

Deirdre J Murphy MSc, MD, FRCOG
Professor of Obstetrics and Head of Department
Trinity College Dublin
and
Coombe Women & Infants University Hospital
Dublin, Ireland

Jenny E Myers BMBS, BMedSci(Hons),
    MRCOG, PhD
NIHR Clinician Scientist and Honorary Consultant
    in Obstetrics
Maternal & Fetal Health Research Centre
University of Manchester
Manchester, UK

Mark A Turner BSc, MBChB (Hons), DRCOG,
    MRCP(UK), MRCPCH, PhD
Senior Lecturer in Neonatology
University of Liverpool
and
Honorary Consultant Neonatologist
Liverpool Women's NHS Foundation Trust
Liverpool, UK

Andrew D Weeks MB ChB, MD, DCH, FRCOG
Professor of International Maternal Health
University of Liverpool
and
Honorary Consultant Obstetrician
Liverpool Women's NHS Foundation Trust
Liverpool, UK

David J Williams MB BS, PhD, FRCP
Obstetric Physician
Institute for Women's Health
University College London
London, UK

Abbreviations

AA	arachidonic acid/arterioarterial	CLD	chronic lung disease (of prematurity)
AABR	automated auditory brainstem response	CMV	cytomegalovirus
AC	abdominal circumference	CNS	central nervous system
ACE	angiotensin-converting enzyme	COX	cyclooxygenase
aCL	anticardiolipin antibody	CP	cerebral palsy
ACOG	American College of Obstetricians and Gynecologists	CPAP	continuous positive airways pressure
		CPD	cephalopelvic disproportion
ACR	American College of Rheumatology	CPR	cardiopulmonary resuscitation
ACTH	adrenocorticotrophic hormone	CRH	corticotrophin-releasing hormone
AED	antiepilepsy drug	CRL	crown–rump length
AFI	amniotic fluid index	CRM	clinical risk management
AFP	alpha-fetoprotein	CRP	C-reactive protein
AIDS	acquired immunodeficiency syndrome	CRS	congenital rubella syndrome
ALT	alanine aminotransferase	CSE	combined spinal–epidural
AMP	adenyl monophospate	CSF	cerebrospinal fluid
ANA	antinuclear antibody	CT	computed tomography
ANNP	advanced neonatal nurse practitioner	CTG	cardiotocograph
aOR	adjusted odds ratio	CTPA	computed tomography pulmonary angiogram
A–P	anterior–posterior		
APH	antepartum haemorrhage	CVP	central venous pressure
APS	antiphospholipid syndrome	CVS	chorion villus sampling
ARM	artificial rupture of membranes	D&C	dilation and curettage
ART	antiretroviral therapy	DAT	direct antiglobulin testing
AS	aortic stenosis	DDAVP	desmopressin
AT	antithrombin	DDH	developmental dysplasia of the hip
AV	arteriovenous	DMD	Duchenne's muscular dystrophy/ disease-modifying drug
AZT	azidothymidine, also known as zidovudine (ZDV)		
		DMSA	dimercaptosuccinic acid
BCG	bacillus Calmette-Guérin	DNA	deoxyribonucleic acid
BMI	body mass index	DV	ductus venosus
BPD	biparietal diameter	DVT	deep vein thrombosis
bpm	beats per minute	ECG	electrocardiogram
BPP	biophysical profile	ECV	external cephalic version
BV	bacterial vaginosis	EDD	estimated date of delivery
CAP	contraction-associated protein	(a)EEG	(amplitude integrated) electroencephalography
CB	cerebellum		
CF	cystic fibrosis	EF	ejection fraction
CFM	cerebral function monitoring	EFM	electronic fetal monitoring
CHAOS	congenital high airways obstruction syndrome	EFW	estimated fetal weight
		EIA	enzyme immunoassay
CKD	chronic kidney disease	ELISA	enzyme-linked immunosorbant assay

EMQ	extended matching question		HDFN	haemolytic disease of the fetus and newborn
EON	examination of the newborn		HELLP	haemolysis, elevated liver enzymes and low platelets
ERCS	elective repeat caesarean section			
ESBL	extended spectrum β-lactamase		HIE	hypoxic-ischaemic encephalopathy
ETT	endotracheal tube			
EUA	examination under anaesthesia		HIV	human immunodeficiency virus
FBC	full blood count		HSV	herpes simplex virus
FBM	fetal breathing movement		HZ	herpes zoster
FBS	fetal scalp blood sampling		IAP	intrapartum antibiotic prophylaxis
FDA	Food and Drug Administration		IBD	inflammatory bowel disease
FEV$_1$	forced expiratory volume in 1 second		Ig	immunoglobulin
ffDNA	free fetal deoxyribonucleic acid		IGF	insulin-like growth factor
fFN	fetal fibronectin		IL	interleukin
FGF(R)	fibroblast growth factor (receptor)		IMV	intermittent mandatory ventilation
FGM	female genital mutilation		INR	international normalized ratio
FGR	fetal growth restriction		IOL	induction of labour
FHR	fetal heart rate		IQ	intelligence quotient
FISH	fluorescent *in situ* hybridization		ITP	immune thrombocytopaenic purpura
FL	femur length		IVA	isovaleric acidaemia
FOQ	Family Origin Questionnaire		IVC	inferior vena cava
FRC	functional residual capacity		IVF	*in vitro* fertilization
FSE	fetal scalp electrode		IVH	intraventricular haemorrhage
FTA-abs	fluorescent treponemal antibody-absorbed (test)		LA	lupus anticoagulant
			LFT	liver function test
FVS	fetal varicella syndrome		LLETZ	large loop excision of the transformation zone
GA1	glutaric aciduria type 1			
GBS	group B streptococcus		LMP	last menstrual period
GCS	Glasgow coma score		LMWH	low-molecular-weight heparin
GDM	gestational diabetes		MAP	mean arterial pressure
GFR	glomerular filtration rate		MCA	middle cerebral artery
GGT	gamma-glutamyl transpeptidase		MCADD	medium-chain acyl-CoA dehydrogenase deficiency
GnRH	gonadotrophin-releasing hormone			
GP	general practitioner		M, C and S	microscopy, culture and sensitivity
GTN	glyceryl trinitrate		MCV	mean corpuscular volume
GUM	genitourinary medicine		MEOWS	Modified Early Obstetric Warning System
HAART	highly active antiretroviral therapy			
Hb	haemoglobin		MI	myocardial infarction
HBA1C	glycosated haemoglobin		MMR	mumps, measles, rubella
HBcAb	hepatitis B core antibody		MoM	multiples of median
HbF	fetal haemoglobin		MRI	magnetic resonance imaging
HBsAb	hepatitis B surface antibody		MROP	manual removal of placenta
HBsAg	hepatitis B surface antigen		MRSA	methicillin-resistant *Staphylococcus aureus*
HbSS	homozygous sickle cell disease			
HBV	hepatitis B virus		MS	multiple sclerosis
HC	head circumference		MSLC	Maternity Services Liaison Committee
hCG	human chorionic gonadotrophin			
HCU	homocystinuria		MSU	mid-stream urine specimen
HCV	hepatitis C virus		MSUD	maple syrup urine disease

MVP	maximum vertical pool		PTH	parathyroid hormone
NCT	National Childbirth Trust		PTL	preterm labour
NEC	necrotizing enterocolitis		PTU	propylthiouracil
NFκB	nuclear factor kappa B		PVL	periventricular leukomalacia
NHS	National Health Service		RA	rheumatoid arthritis
NICE	National Institute for Health and Care Excellence		RCM	Royal College of Midwives
			RCOG	Royal College of Obstetricians and Gynaecologists
NICU	Neonatal Intensive Care Unit		RCT	randomized controlled trial
NIPT	non-invasive prenatal testing		RDS	respiratory distress syndrome
NO	nitrous oxide		REM	rapid eye movement
NSAID	non-steroidal anti-inflammatory drug		RI	resistance index
NT	nuchal translucency		RNA	ribonucleic acid
NTD	neural tube defect		ROP	retinopathy of prematurity
OA	occipito-anterior		RPR	rapid plasma reagin (test)
OASI	obstetric anal sphincter injuries		SBA	single best answer
OFD	occipitofrontal diameter		SCD	sickle cell disease
OGTT	oral glucose tolerance test		SDLD	surfactant deficient lung disease
OP	occipito-posterior		SFH	symphysis–fundal height
OT	occipito-transverse		SGA	small for gestational age
OT(R)(-A)	oxytocin (receptor) (antagonist)		SIDS	sudden infant death syndrome
OTC	over-the-counter		SLE	systemic lupus erythematosus
OVD	operative vaginal delivery		SROM	spontaneous rupture of the membranes
PAPP-A	pregnancy-associated plasma protein-A		SSRI	selective serotonin reuptake inhibitor
PBC	primary biliary cirrhosis		(f)T4 (free)	thyroxine
PCA	patient-controlled analgesic device		TAMBA	Twins and Multiple Birth Association
PCR	polymerase chain reaction		TAPS	twin anaemia–polycythemia sequence
PDA	patent ductus arteriosus		TB	tuberculosis
PE	pulmonary embolism		TENS	transcutaneous electrical nerve stimulation
PEP	polymorphic eruption of pregnancy		TFT	thyroid function test
PF	pruritic folliculitis		TNF	tumor necrosis factor
PG	prostaglandin/pemphigoid gestationis		TOF	tracheo-oesophageal fistula
PGDH	15-hydroxyprostaglandin dehydrogenase		TOLAC	trial of labour after caesarean
PH	pulmonary hypertension		TPHA	*T. pallidum* haemagglutination assay
PI	pulsatility index		TRH	thyrotrophin-releasing hormone
PIE	pulmonary interstitial emphysema		TSH	thyroid-stimulating hormone
PKU	phenylketonuria		TTN	transient tachypnoea of the newborn
PlGF	placental growth factor		TTTS	twin-to-twin transfusion syndrome
PMA	postmenstrual age		UDCA	ursodeoxycholic acid
PPH	postpartum haemorrhage		uE3	unconjugated oestriol
PPROM	preterm premature rupture of membranes		UFH	unfractionated heparin
			UTI	urinary tract infection
PR	progesterone receptor		VA	venoarterial
PROM	preterm rupture of membranes		VACTERL	vertebral, anal, cardiac, tracheal, (o)esophageal, renal and limb
PT	prothrombin time			
PTCA	percutaneous transluminal coronary angioplasty		VBAC	vaginal birth after caesarean
PTD	preterm delivery			

VDRL	Venereal Diseases Research Laboratory	VZIG	varicella zoster immunoglobulin
VEGF	vascular endothelial growth factor	VZV	varicella zoster virus
V/Q	ventilation perfusion	WHO	World Health Organization
VTE	venous thromboembolism	ZDV	zidovudine, also known as azidothymidine (AZT)
VV	venovenous		
VWF	von Willebrand factor	ZIG	zoster immunoglobulin

Video resources

Chapter 1   **Obstetric History and Examination**

Video 1.1   How to measure blood pressure in pregnancy:
http://www.routledgetextbooks.com/textbooks/tenteachers/obstetricsv1.1.php

Video 1.2   Examination of the pregnant abdomen:
http://www.routledgetextbooks.com/textbooks/tenteachers/obstetricsv1.2.php

Video 1.3   Symphysis–fundal height (SFH) measurement:
http://www.routledgetextbooks.com/textbooks/tenteachers/obstetricsv1.3.php

Chapter 5   **Prenatal diagnosis**

Video 5.1   Chorionic villus sampling:
http://www.routledgetextbooks.com/textbooks/tenteachers/obstetricsv5.1.php

Video 5.2   Amniocentesis:
http://www.routledgetextbooks.com/textbooks/tenteachers/obstetricsv5.2.php

Chapter 6   **Antenatal obstetric complications**

Video 6.1   External cephalic version (ECV):
http://www.routledgetextbooks.com/textbooks/tenteachers/obstetricsv6.1.php

Video 6.2   Animation of the mechanism of rhesus sensitization and fetal red cell destruction:
http://www.routledgetextbooks.com/textbooks/tenteachers/obstetricsv6.2.php

Chapter 7   **Multiple pregnancy**

Video 7.1   Ultrasound scan of dichorionic and monochorionic twin pregnancies:
http://www.routledgetextbooks.com/textbooks/tenteachers/obstetricsv7.1.php

Chapter 12   **Labour: normal and abnormal**

Video 12.1   The mechanism of a spontaneous vaginal delivery:
http://www.routledgetextbooks.com/textbooks/tenteachers/obstetricsv12.1.php

Chapter 13   Operative delivery

Video 13.1   Repair of an episiotomy/second-degree perineal tear:
                http://www.routledgetextbooks.com/textbooks/tenteachers/obstetricsv13.1.php

Video 13.2   Operative vacuum delivery:
                http://www.routledgetextbooks.com/textbooks/tenteachers/obstetricsv13.2.php

Video 13.3   Operative forceps delivery:
                http://www.routledgetextbooks.com/textbooks/tenteachers/obstetricsv13.3.php

Video 13.4   Caesarean section delivery:
                http://www.routledgetextbooks.com/textbooks/tenteachers/obstetricsv13.4.php

You can access the video clips that are referenced above and in the text directly via the ebook that accompanies this print edition: follow the instructions printed on the inside the front cover. From the ebook click on the list above or use the links from the chapters, indicated in the text by the video icon:

In addition, the videos and images from this book can be accessed via the companion website that accompanies this textbook www.routledge.com/cw/kenny where you will also find resources for the sister volume, *Gynaecology by Ten Teachers, 20th Edition*. Additional video clips and still images will be added to this library over time.

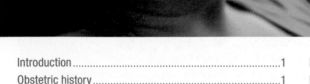

Obstetric history and examination

LOUISE C KENNY AND JENNY E MYERS

CHAPTER 1

LEARNING OBJECTIVES

- To understand the principles of taking an obstetric history.
- To understand the key components of an obstetric examination.
- How to perform an appropriate obstetric examination.

Introduction

Taking a history and performing an obstetric examination are different compared with the history and examination in other specialities. The main difference is that the patient is normally a healthy woman undergoing a normal life event. Antenatal care is designed to support this normal physiological process and to detect early signs of complications. The type of questions asked during the history change with gestation, as does the purpose and nature of the examination. The history will often cover physiology, pathology and psychology and must always be sought with care and sensitivity.

Obstetric history

Introduction

When meeting a patient for the first time, always introduce yourself; tell the patient who you are and why you have come to see them. Make sure that the patient is seated comfortably. Some women will wish another person to be present, even just to take a history, and this wish should be respected.

The questions asked must be tailored to the purpose of the visit. At a booking visit, the history must be thorough and meticulously recorded. Once this baseline information is established, there is no need to go over this information at every visit. All women attend for routine antenatal visits (usually performed by the midwife or general practitioner [GP]) and occasionally women attend for a specific reason or because a complication has developed.

Some areas of the obstetric history cover subjects that are intensely private. In occasional cases there may be events recorded in the notes that are not known by other family members, such as previous terminations of pregnancy. It is vital to be aware of and sensitive to each individual situation.

Dating the pregnancy

Pregnancy has been historically dated from the last menstrual period (LMP), not the date of conception. The median duration of pregnancy is 280 days (40 weeks) and this gives the estimated date of delivery (EDD). This assumes that:

- The cycle length is 28 days.
- Ovulation occurs generally on the 14th day of the cycle.
- The cycle was a normal cycle (i.e. not straight after stopping the oral contraceptive pill or soon after a previous pregnancy).

The EDD is calculated by taking the date of the LMP, counting forward by 9 months and adding 7 days. If the cycle is longer than 28 days, add the difference between the cycle length and 28 to compensate.

In most antenatal clinics, there are pregnancy calculators (wheels) that do this for you (**Figure 1.1**). Pregnancy-calculating wheels do differ a little and may give dates that are a day or two different from those previously calculated. There is also an extensive range of pregnancy calculator Apps for smartphones available to download for free (**Figure 1.2**). However, almost all women who undergo antenatal care in the UK will have an ultrasound scan in the late first trimester or early second trimester. The purposes of this scan are to establish dates, to ensure that the pregnancy is ongoing and to determine the number of fetuses. If performed before 20 weeks, the ultrasound scan can be used for dating the pregnancy. After this time, the variability in growth rates of different fetuses makes it unsuitable for use in defining dates. It has been shown that ultrasound-defined dates are more accurate than those based on a certain LMP. This may be because the actual time

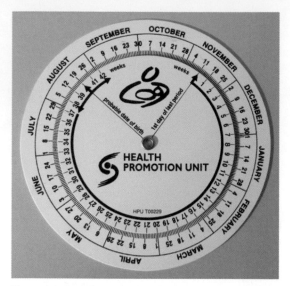

Figure 1.1 Gestation calendar wheel.

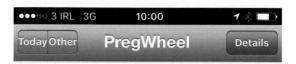

Estimated Date of Delivery:

Mon, May 9, 2016

Estimated Gestational Age on 03/04/2016:

34 6/7 weeks

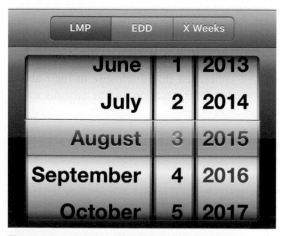

Figure 1.2 Gestation calendar App on a smartphone. (Courtesy of Dr Andrew Yu, Yale University.)

of ovulation in any cycle is much less fixed than was previously thought. Therefore, the National Institute for Health and Care Excellence (NICE) guideline on Antenatal Care recommends that that pregnancy dates are set only by ultrasound using the crown–rump measurement between 10 weeks 0 days and 13 weeks 6 days, and the head circumference from 14 to 20 weeks. Regardless of the date of the LMP this EDD is used.

It is important to define the EDD at the booking visit, as accurate dating is important in later pregnancy for assessing fetal growth. In addition, accurate dating reduces the risk of premature elective deliveries, such as induction of labour for postmature pregnancies and elective caesarean sections.

Social history

The social history requires considerable sensitivity, but it is a vitally important part of the obstetric history as social circumstances can have a dramatic influence on pregnancy outcome. The most recent report from the UK, Confidential Enquiries into Maternal Deaths and Morbidity (2009–12) echoes previous reports and details that maternal mortality is higher amongst older women, those living in the most deprived areas and amongst women from some ethnic minority groups. Importantly, one-third of women who experience domestic violence are hit for the first time while pregnant and women are known to be at higher risk of domestic abuse, leading to homicide when pregnant or postpartum. Women who are experiencing domestic abuse, may be at higher risk of abuse during pregnancy and of adverse pregnancy outcome, because they may be prevented from attending antenatal appointments, may be concerned that disclosure of their abuse may worsen their situation and be anxious about the reaction of health professionals.

Enquiring about domestic violence is extremely difficult. It is recommended that all women are seen on their own at least once during pregnancy, so that they can discuss this, if needed, away from an abusive partner. This is not always easy to accomplish. If you happen to be the person with whom this information is shared, you must ensure that it is passed on to the relevant team, as this may be the only opportunity the woman has to disclose it. Sometimes, younger women find medical students and young doctors much easier to talk to. Be aware of this.

Smoking, alcohol and drug intake also form part of the social history. Smoking causes a reduction in birthweight in a dose-dependent way. It also increases the risk of miscarriage, stillbirth and neonatal death. There are interventions that can be offered to women who are still smoking in pregnancy (see Chapter 3, Normal fetal development and growth and Chapter 6, Antenatal obstetric complications).

Complete abstinence from alcohol is advised, as the safety of alcohol is not proven. However, alcohol is probably not harmful in small amounts (less than one drink per day). Binge drinking is particularly harmful and can lead to a constellation of features in the baby known as fetal alcohol syndrome (see Chapter 3, Normal fetal development and growth and Chapter 6, Antenatal obstetric complications).

Enquiring about recreational drug taking is more difficult. Approximately 0.5–1% of women continue to take recreational drugs during pregnancy. Be careful not to make assumptions. During the booking visit, the midwife should enquire directly about drug taking. If it is seen as part of the long list of routine questions asked at this visit, it is perceived as less threatening. However, sometimes this information comes to light at other times. Cocaine and crack cocaine are the most harmful of the recreational drugs taken, but all have some effects on the pregnancy, and all have financial implications (see Chapter 6, Antenatal obstetric complications).

By the time you have finished your history and examination you should know the following facts that are important in the social history:

- Whether the patient is single or in a relationship and what sort of support she has at home.
- Generally whether there is a stable income coming into the house.
- What sort of housing the patient occupies (e.g. a flat with lots of stairs and no lift may be problematic).
- Whether the woman works and for how long she is planning to work during the pregnancy.
- Whether the woman smokes/drinks or uses drugs.
- If there are any other features that may be important.

Previous obstetric history

Past obstetric history is one of the most important areas for establishing risk in the current pregnancy. It is helpful to list the pregnancies in date order and to discover what the outcome was in each pregnancy.

The features that are likely to have impact on future pregnancies include:

- Recurrent miscarriage (increased risk of miscarriage, fetal growth restriction [FGR]).
- Preterm delivery (increased risk of preterm delivery).
- Early-onset pre-eclampsia (increased risk of pre-eclampsia/FGR).
- Abruption (increased risk of recurrence).
- Congenital abnormality (recurrence risk depends on type of abnormality).
- Macrosomic baby (may be related to gestational diabetes).
- FGR (increased recurrence).
- Unexplained stillbirth (increased risk of gestational diabetes).

The method of delivery for any previous births must be recorded, as this can have implications for planning in the current pregnancy, particularly if there has been a previous caesarean section, difficult vaginal delivery, postpartum haemorrhage or significant perineal trauma.

The shorthand for describing the number of previous pregnancies can be confusing: *gravidity* is the total number of pregnancies regardless of how they ended, *parity* is the number of live births at any gestation or stillbirths after 24 weeks. In terms of parity, twins count as 2. Therefore, a woman at 12 weeks in her first pregnancy who has never had a pregnancy before is gravida 1, para 0. If she delivers twins and comes back next time at 12 weeks, she will be gravida 2, para 2 (twins). A woman who has had six miscarriages with only one live baby born at 32 weeks and is pregnant again will be gravida 8, para 1. Sometimes, this shorthand is also used to describe the number of pregnancies that did not result in live birth or stillbirth after 24 weeks. The last case would thus be defined as para 1+6.

However, when presenting a history, it is much easier to describe exactly what has happened: for example, 'Mrs Jones is in her eighth pregnancy. She has had six miscarriages at gestations of 8–12 weeks and one spontaneous delivery of a live baby boy at 32 weeks. Baby Tom is now 2 years old and healthy.'

Past gynaecological history

The regularity of periods used to be important in dating pregnancy (as above). Women with very long cycles may have a condition known as polycystic ovarian syndrome. This is a complex endocrine condition and its relevance here is that some women with this condition have increased insulin resistance and a higher risk for the development of gestational diabetes.

Contraceptive history can be relevant if conception has occurred soon after stopping the combined oral contraceptive pill or depot progesterone preparations, as again, this makes dating by LMP more difficult. Also, some women will conceive with an intrauterine device still *in situ*. This carries an increase in the risk of miscarriage.

Previous episodes of pelvic inflammatory disease increase the risk for ectopic pregnancy. This is only of relevance in early pregnancy. However, it is important to establish that any infections have been adequately treated and that the partner was also treated.

The date of the last cervical smear should be noted. Every year a small number of women are diagnosed as having cervical cancer in pregnancy, and it is recognized that late diagnosis is more common around the time of pregnancy because smears are deferred. If a smear is due, it can be taken in the first trimester. It is important to record that the woman is pregnant, as the cells can be difficult to assess without this knowledge. It is also important that smears are not deferred in women who are at increased risk of cervical disease (e.g. previous cervical smear abnormality or very overdue smear). Gently taking a smear in the first trimester does not cause miscarriage and women should be reassured about this. Remember that if it is deferred at this point, it may be nearly a year before the opportunity arises again. If there has been irregular bleeding, the cervix should at least be examined to ensure that there are no obvious lesions present.

If a woman has undergone treatment for cervical changes, this should be noted. Knife cone biopsy is associated with an increased risk for both cervical incompetence (weakness) and stenosis (leading to preterm delivery and dystocia in labour, respectively). There is probably a very small increase in the risk of preterm birth associated with large loop excision of the transformation zone (LLETZ); however, women who have needed more than one excision are likely to have a much shorter cervix, which does increase the risk for second and early third trimester delivery.

Previous ectopic pregnancy increases the risk of recurrence to 1 in 10. Women who have had an ectopic pregnancy should be offered an early ultrasound scan to establish the site of any future pregnancies.

Recurrent miscarriage may be associated with a number of problems. Antiphospholipid syndrome increases the risk of further pregnancy loss, FGR and pre-eclampsia. Balanced translocations can occasionally lead to congenital abnormality, and cervical incompetence can predispose to late second and early third trimester delivery. Also, women need a great deal of support during pregnancy if they have experienced recurrent pregnancy losses.

Multiple previous first trimester terminations of pregnancy potentially increase the risk of preterm delivery, possibly secondary to cervical weakness. Sometimes, information regarding these must be sensitively recorded. Some women do not wish this to be recorded in their hand-held notes.

Previous gynaecological surgery is important, especially if it involved the uterus, as this can have potential sequelae for delivery. In addition, the presence of pelvic masses such as ovarian cysts and fibroids should be noted. These may impact on delivery and may also pose some problems during pregnancy. Donor egg or sperm use is associated with an increased risk of pre-eclampsia. However, legally, you should not write down in notes that a pregnancy is conceived by *in vitro* fertilization (IVF) or donor egg or sperm unless you have written permission from the patient. It is obviously a difficult area, as there is an increased risk of maternal problems in these pregnancies and therefore the knowledge is important. Generally, if the patient has told you herself that the pregnancy was an assisted conception, it is reasonable to state that in your presentation.

Medical and surgical history

All pre-existing medical disease should be carefully noted and any associated drug history also recorded.

The major pre-existing diseases that impact on pregnancy and their potential effects are shown below (also see Chapter 10, Medical complications of pregnancy).

Previous surgery should be noted. Occasionally, surgery has been performed for conditions that may continue to be a problem during pregnancy, such as Crohn's disease.

Psychiatric history is important to record. These enquiries should include the severity of the illness, care received and clinical presentation, and should be made in a systematic and sensitive way at the antenatal booking visit. If women have had children before, you can ask whether they had problems with depression or 'the blues' after the births of any of them. Women with significant psychiatric problems should be cared for by a multidisciplinary team, including the midwife, GP, hospital consultant and psychiatric team.

Major pre-existing diseases that impact on pregnancy

- Diabetes mellitus: macrosomia, FGR, congenital abnormality, pre-eclampsia, stillbirth, neonatal hypoglycaemia.
- Hypertension: pre-eclampsia.
- Renal disease: worsening renal disease, pre-eclampsia, FGR, preterm delivery.
- Epilepsy: increased fit frequency, congenital abnormality.
- Venous thromboembolic disease: increased risk during pregnancy; if associated thrombophilia, increased risk of thromboembolism and possible increased risk of pre-eclampsia, FGR.
- Human immunodeficiency virus (HIV) infection: risk of mother-to-child transfer if untreated.
- Connective tissue diseases (e.g. systemic lupus erythematosus), pre-eclampsia, FGR.
- Myasthenia gravis/myotonic dystrophy: fetal neurological effects and increased maternal muscular fatigue in labour.

Drug history

It is vital to establish what drugs a woman has been taking for their condition and for what duration.

This includes over-the-counter (OTC) medication and homeopathic/herbal remedies. In some cases, medication needs to be changed in pregnancy. For some women it may be possible to stop their medication completely for some or all of the pregnancy (e.g. mild hypertension). Some women need to know that they must continue their medication (e.g. epilepsy, for which women often reduce their medication for fear of potential fetal effects, with detriment to their own health).

Very few drugs that women of childbearing age take are potentially seriously harmful, but a few are, and it is always necessary to ensure that drug treatment is carefully reviewed. Prepregnancy counselling is advised for women who are taking potentially harmful drugs such as some anticonvulsant drugs.

Family history

Family history is important if it can:

- Impact on the health of the mother in pregnancy or afterwards.
- Have implications for the fetus or baby.

Important areas are a maternal history of a first-degree relative (sibling or parent) with:

- Diabetes (increased risk of gestational diabetes).
- Thromboembolic disease (increased risk of thrombophilia, thrombosis).
- Pre-eclampsia (increased risk of pre-eclampsia).
- Serious psychiatric disorder (increased risk of puerperal psychosis).

For both parents, it is important to know about any family history of babies with congenital abnormality and any potential genetic problems, such as haemoglobinopathies.

Finally, any known allergies should be recorded. If a woman gives a history of allergy, it is important to ask about how this was diagnosed and what sort of problems it causes.

Obstetric examination

While the incidence amongst the obstetric population is small, adherence to the principles of infection reduction is vital. In any clinical setting, arms should be bare from the elbow down. Alcohol gel should be used when moving from one clinical area to another (e.g. between wards), hands should always be washed or gel used before and after any patient contact.

Before moving on to examine the patient, it is important to be aware of the clinical context. The examination should be directed at the presenting problem, if any, and the gestation. For instance, it is generally unnecessary to spend time defining the presentation at 24 weeks' gestation unless the presenting problem is threatened preterm labour.

Maternal weight and height

The measurement of weight and height at the initial examination is important, to identify women who are significantly underweight or overweight. Women with a body mass index (BMI) [weight (kg)/height (m²)] of <20 are at higher risk of fetal growth restriction and increased perinatal mortality. In the obese woman (BMI >30), the risks of gestational diabetes and hypertension are increased. Additionally, fetal assessment, both by palpation and ultrasound, is more difficult. Obesity is also associated with increased birthweight and a higher perinatal mortality rate.

In women of normal weight at booking, and in whom nutrition is of no concern, there is no need to repeat weight measurement in pregnancy.

Blood pressure measurement

Blood pressure measurement is one of the few aspects of antenatal care that is truly beneficial. The first recording of blood pressure should be made as early as possible in pregnancy and thereafter it should be performed at every visit.

Hypertension diagnosed for the first time in early pregnancy (blood pressure >140/90 mmHg on two separate occasions at least 4 hours apart) should prompt a search for underlying causes (i.e. renal, endocrine and collagen-vascular disease). Although 90% of cases will be due to essential hypertension, this is a diagnosis of exclusion and can only be confidently made when other secondary causes have been excluded (see Chapter 9, Hypertensive disorders of pregnancy).

How to measure blood pressure in pregnancy

- Measure the blood pressure with the woman seated or semi-recumbent.
- Use an appropriately sized cuff. Large women will need a larger cuff. Using one too small will over-estimate blood pressure.
- If using an automated device, check it has been validated for use in pregnancy.
- Ensure that manual devices have been recently calibrated.
- Convention is to use Korotkoff V (i.e. disappearance of sounds), as this is more reproducible than Korotkoff IV.
- Deflate the cuff slowly so that you can record the blood pressure to the nearest 2 mmHg.
- Do not round up or down.

▶ VIDEO 1.1

How to measure blood pressure in pregnancy: http://www.routledgetextbooks.com/textbooks/tenteachers/obstetricsv1.1.php

Urinary examination

All women should be offered routine screening for asymptomatic bacteriuria by midstream urine culture early in pregnancy. Identification and treatment of asymptomatic bacteriuria reduces the risk of pyelonephritis. The risk of ascending urinary tract infection in pregnancy is much higher than in the non-pregnant state. Acute pyelonephritis increases the risk of pregnancy loss/premature labour and is associated with considerable maternal morbidity.

At repeat visits, urinalysis using automated reagent strip readers should be performed. If there is any proteinuria, a thorough evaluation with regard to a diagnosis of pre-eclampsia should be undertaken.

General medical examination

In fit and healthy women presenting for a routine visit there is little benefit in a full formal physical examination. However, when a woman presents with a problem, or in women in certain at-risk groups, there may be a need to undertake a much more thorough physical examination.

Cardiovascular examination

Routine auscultation for maternal heart sounds in asymptomatic women with no cardiac history is unnecessary. However, if a woman has previously lived in an area where rheumatic heart disease is prevalent and/or has a known history of heart murmur or heart disease, she should undergo cardiovascular examination during pregnancy.

Breast examination

Formal breast examination is not necessary. Women should, however, be encouraged to perform self-examination at regular intervals.

Examination of the pregnant abdomen

This is a critical part of routine antenatal care and is an essential skill to learn as a medical student. Always have a chaperone with you to perform this examination and before starting, ask about pain and areas of tenderness.

To examine the abdomen of a pregnant woman, place her in a semi-recumbent position on a couch or bed. In late pregnancy women should never lie completely flat; the semi-prone position or a left lateral tilt will avoid aortocaval compression. The abdomen should be exposed from just below the breasts to the symphysis fundus.

▶ VIDEO 1.2

Examination of the pregnant abdomen: http://www.routledgetextbooks.com/textbooks/tenteachers/obstetricsv1.2.php

Inspection

- Assess the shape of the uterus and note any asymmetry.
- Look for fetal movements.
- Note any signs of pregnancy such as striae gravidarum (stretch marks) or linea nigra (the faint brown line running from the umbilicus to the symphysis pubis).
- Look for scars. The common areas to find scars are:
  - suprapubic (caesarean section, laparotomy for ectopic pregnancy or ovarian masses);
  - sub-umbilical (laparoscopy);
  - right iliac fossa (appendicectomy);
  - right upper quadrant (cholycystectomy).

Palpation

The purpose of palpating the pregnant abdomen is to assess:

- The number of babies.
- The size of the baby.
- The lie of the baby.
- The presentation of the baby.
- Whether the baby is engaged.

Symphysis–fundal height measurement

Symphysis–fundal height (SFH) should be measured and recorded at each antenatal appointment from 24 weeks' gestation. Most UK hospitals now use customized SFH charts, which are generated at the first antenatal visit and are customized to each individual, taking into account the height, weight, ethnicity and parity of the woman (**Figure 1.3**). Using two standard deviations of the mean, it is possible to define the 10th and 90th centile values and these are normally marked on the chart.

Feel carefully for the top of the fundus and for the upper border of the symphysis pubis. Place the tape measure on the symphysis pubis and, using a tape measure with the centimetre marks face down, measure to the top of the fundus. Turn the tape measure over and read the measurement. Plot the measurement on an SFH chart. The mean fundal height measures approximately 20 cm at 20 weeks and increases by 1 cm per week so that at 36 weeks the fundal height should be approximately 36 cm. However, the value of customized charts is that they are more sensitive and specific and serial measurements are of greater value in detecting growth trends than one-off measurements.

A large SFH raises the possibility of:

- A multiple pregnancy.
- Macrosomia.
- Polyhydramnios.

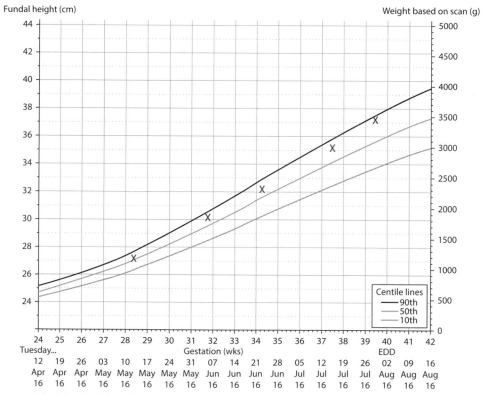

Figure 1.3 A customized symphysis–fundal height chart illustrating the 10th, 50th and 90th centiles and normal fetal growth. (Courtesy of Perinatal Institute.)

A small SFH raises the possibility of:

- FGR.
- Oligohydramnios.

 VIDEO 1.3

Symphysis–fundal height (SFH) measurement: http://www.routledgetextbooks.com/textbooks/tenteachers/obstetricsv1.3.php

Fetal lie, presentation and engagement

After measuring the SFH, next palpate to count the number of fetal poles (**Figure 1.4**). A pole is a head or a bottom. If you can feel one or two, it is likely to be a singleton pregnancy. If you can feel three or four, a twin pregnancy is likely. Sometimes large fibroids can mimic a fetal pole; remember this if there is a history of fibroids.

Next assess the fetal lie and presentation. This is only necessary in late pregnancy as the likelihood of labour increases (i.e. after 36 weeks in an uncomplicated pregnancy).

If there is a pole over the pelvis, the lie is longitudinal regardless of whether the other pole is lying more to the left or right. An oblique lie is where the leading pole does not lie over the pelvis, but just to one side; a transverse lie is where the fetus lies directly across the abdomen.

Presentation can either be cephalic (head down) or breech (bottom/feet down). Using a two-handed approach and watching the woman's face, gently feel for the presenting part. The head is generally much firmer than the bottom, although even in experienced hands it can sometimes be very difficult to tell. At the same time as feeling for the presenting part, assess whether it is engaged or not. If the whole head is palpable and it is easily movable, the head is likely to be 'free'. This equates to 5/5th palpable and is recorded as 5/5. As the head descends into the pelvis, less can be felt. When the head is no longer movable, it has 'engaged' and only 1/5th or 2/5th will be palpable (**Figure 1.5**). Do not use a one-handed technique, as this is much more uncomfortable for the woman.

It can be helpful to determine the fetal position (i.e. whether the fetal head is occipito-posterior, lateral or anterior) as this will make auscultating the fetal heart beat easier.

Auscultation

If the fetus has been active during your examination and the mother reports that the baby is active, it is not necessary to auscultate the fetal heart. Mothers do like to hear the heart beat though and therefore using a hand-held device can allow the mother to hear the heart beat. If you are using a Pinard stethoscope, position it over the fetal shoulder. Hearing the heart sounds with a Pinard takes a lot of practice. If you cannot hear the fetal heart, never say that you cannot detect a heart beat; always explain that a different method is needed and move on to using a hand-held Doppler device. If you have begun the process of listening to the fetal heart, you must proceed until you are confident that you have heard the heart. With twins, you must be confident that both have been heard.

Pelvic examination

Routine pelvic examination during antenatal visits is not necessary. However, there are circumstances in which a vaginal examination is necessary (in most cases a speculum examination is all that is needed). These include:

- Excessive or offensive discharge.
- Vaginal bleeding (in the known absence of a placenta praevia).
- To perform a cervical smear.
- To confirm potential rupture of membranes.
- To confirm and assess the extent of female genital mutilation (FGM) in women who have been subjected to this.

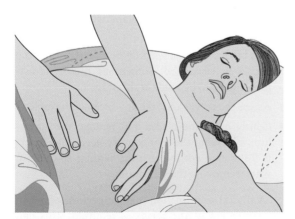

Figure 1.4 Palpation of the gravid abdomen.

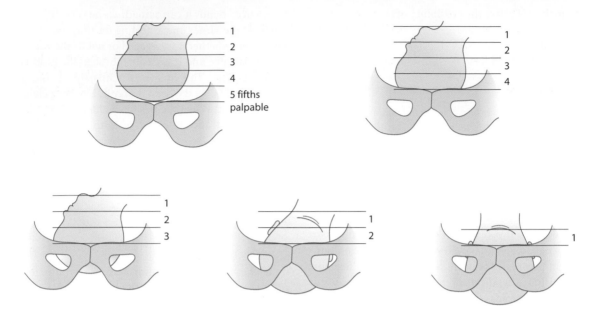

Figure 1.5 Palpation of the fetal head to assess engagement.

Before commencing the examination, consent must be sought and a female chaperone (nurse, midwife, etc. and never a relative) must be present (regardless of the sex of the examiner).

Assemble everything you will need (swabs, etc.) and ensure the light source works. Position the patient semi-recumbent with knees drawn up and ankles together. Ensure that the patient is adequately covered. If performing a speculum examination, a Cusco speculum is usually used (**Figure 1.6**). Select an appropriate size. Proceed as follows:

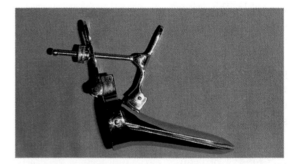

Figure 1.6 A Cusco speculum.

- Wash your hands and put on a pair of gloves.
- If the speculum is metal, warm it slightly under warm water first.
- Apply sterile lubricating gel or cream to the blades of the speculum. Do not use antiseptic cream if taking swabs for bacteriology.
- Gently part the labia.
- Introduce the speculum with the blades in the vertical plane.
- As the speculum is gently introduced, aiming towards the sacral promontory (i.e. slightly downward), rotate the speculum so that it comes

to lie in the horizontal plane with the ratchet uppermost.
- The blades can then slowly be opened until the cervix is visualized. Sometimes minor adjustments need to be made at this stage.
- Assess the cervix and take any necessary samples.
- Gently close the blades and remove the speculum, reversing the manoeuvres needed to insert it. Take care not to catch the vaginal epithelium when removing the speculum.

A digital examination may be performed when an assessment of the cervix is required. This can provide information about the consistency and effacement of the cervix that is not obtainable from a speculum examination.

The contraindications to digital examination are:

- Known placenta praevia or vaginal bleeding when the placental site is unknown and the presenting part unengaged.
- Prelabour rupture of the membranes (increased risk of ascending infection).

The patient should be positioned as before. Examining from the patient's right, two fingers of the gloved right hand are gently introduced into the vagina and advanced until the cervix is palpated. Prior to induction of labour, a full assessment of the Bishop's score can be made (see Chapter 12, Labour: normal and abnormal).

Other aspects of the examination

In women with suspected pre-eclampsia, the reflexes should be assessed. These are most easily checked at the ankle. The presence of more than three beats of clonus is pathological (see Chapter 9, Hypertensive disorders of pregnancy).

Oedema of the extremities affects 80% of term pregnancies and is not a good indicator for pre-eclampsia as it is so common. However, the presence of non-dependent oedema such as facial oedema should be noted.

KEY LEARNING POINTS

- Always introduce yourself and say who you are.
- Make sure you are wearing your identity badge.
- Wash your hands or use alcohol gel.
- Be courteous and gentle.
- Always ensure the patient is comfortable and warm.
- Always have a chaperone present when you examine patients.
- Tailor your history and examination to find the key information you need.
- Adapt to new findings as you go along.
- Present in a clear way.
- Be aware of giving sensitive information in a public setting.

Presentation skills

Part of the art of taking a history and performing an examination is to be able to pass this information on to others in a clear and concise format. It is not necessary to give a full list of negative findings; it is enough to summarize negatives, such as, there is no important medical, surgical or family history of note. Adapt your style of presentation to meet the situation. A very concise presentation is needed for a busy ward round. In an examination, a full and thorough presentation may be required. Be very aware of giving sensitive information in a ward setting where other patients may be within hearing distance. The following template will prove useful for ensuring that you capture all the relevant history.

History template

Demographic details

Name.

Age.

Occupation.

Make a note of ethnic background.

Presenting complaint or reason for attending.

This pregnancy

Gestation, LMP or EDD.

Dates as calculated from ultrasound.

Single/multiple (chorionicity).

Details of the presenting problem (if any) or reason for attendance (such as problems in a previous pregnancy).

What action has been taken?

Is there a plan for the rest of the pregnancy?

What are the patient's main concerns?

Have there been any other problems in this pregnancy?

Has there been any bleeding, contractions or loss of fluid vaginally?

Ultrasound

What scans have been performed?

Why?

Were any problems identified?

Past obstetric history

List the previous pregnancies and their outcomes in order.

Gynaecological history

Periods: regularity.

Contraceptive history.

Previous infections and their treatment.

When was the last cervical smear? Was it normal? Have there ever been any that were abnormal? If yes, what treatment has been undertaken?

Previous gynaecological surgery.

Past medical and surgical history

Relevant medical problems.

Any previous operations: type of anaesthetic used, any complications.

Psychiatric history

Postpartum blues or depression.

Depression unrelated to pregnancy.

Major psychiatric illness.

Family history

Diabetes, hypertension, genetic problems, psychiatric problems, etc.

Social history

Smoking/alcohol/drugs.

Marital status.

Occupation, partner's occupation.

Who is available to help at home?

Are there any housing problems?

Drugs

All medication including OTC medication.

Folate supplementation.

Allergies

To what?

What problems do they cause?

Further reading

National Institute for Health and Care Excellence. Antenatal care. Available at http://www.nice.org.uk/guidance/qs22 (last accessed 01.02.2016).

Saving Lives, Improving Mothers' Care. Surveillance of maternal deaths in the UK 2011–13 and lessons learned to inform maternity care from the UK and Ireland. Confidential Enquiries into Maternal Deaths and Morbidity 2009-13. MBRRACE-UK Available at https://www.npeu.ox.ac.uk/downloads/files/mbrrace-uk/reports/MBRRACE-UK%20Maternal%20Report%202015.pdf (last accessed 23.03.2016).

Antenatal care

FERGUS McCARTHY AND LUCY C CHAPPELL

LEARNING OBJECTIVES

- To understand the principles of routine antenatal care.
- To be aware of the rationale for, and purpose of, clinical investigations during each trimester.

- To differentiate normal pregnancy symptoms from potential underlying pathology.

Overview

Every year in England and Wales approximately 700,000 babies are delivered. The majority of these women are healthy low-risk women with no pre-existing medical problems and have spontaneous vaginal deliveries. A minority will have pre-existing medical conditions that may be affected by pregnancy or may affect the course of pregnancy and require specialist input. The purpose of antenatal care is to optimize pregnancy outcomes for women and their babies through providing support and reassurance to low-risk women and by stratifying care, allowing those at high risk of adverse pregnancy events to receive specialized care in a timely manner.

This chapter provides information on best practice for baseline care of all pregnancies and comprehensive information on the antenatal care of the healthy woman with an uncomplicated singleton pregnancy.

It provides evidence-based information on baseline investigations that are performed and indications for referral to specialist care.

The development of antenatal care

Modern maternity care has evolved over more than 100 years. Many of the changes have been driven by political and consumer pressure and a recognition of the need to align appropriate care to optimal outcomes. Antenatal care continues to evolve with the ongoing publication of good quality research directed at optimizing perinatal outcomes for women and their babies, but the scope and delivery of antenatal care varies widely across the globe, with maternal mortality rates varying substantially between low- and high-income countries. In 2016, approximately 830 women die every day from preventable causes related to pregnancy and childbirth; 99% of all these maternal deaths occur in low-income countries.

History of maternity care in the UK

In 1929, the government in the UK released a document that stated a minimum standard for antenatal care that was so prescriptive in its recommendations that until very recently it was practised in many regions, despite the lack of research to demonstrate effectiveness. The National Health Service Act 1946 came into effect on 5 July 1948 and created the National Health Service (NHS) in England and Wales. The introduction of the NHS provided for maternity services to be available to all without cost. As part of these arrangements, a specified fee was paid to the general practitioner (GP) depending on whether he or she was on the obstetric list (undertaking pregnancy care). This encouraged a large number of GPs to take an interest in maternity care, reversing the previous trend to leave this work to midwives.

Antenatal care became perceived as beneficial, acceptable and available for all. This was reinforced by the finding that the perinatal death rate seemed to be inversely proportional to the number of antenatal visits. In 1963, the first perinatal mortality study showed that the perinatal mortality rate was lowest for those women attending between 10 and 24 times in pregnancy. This failed to take into account prematurity and poor education as reasons for decreased visits and increased mortality. However, antenatal care became established, and with increased professional contact came the drive to continue to improve outcomes, with an emphasis on decreasing maternal and perinatal mortality.

The development and introduction of ultrasound to antenatal care late in the 1960s had a considerable influence on antenatal care, initially limited to confirming multifetal pregnancies, but later being used increasingly for detection of fetal anomalies. This new intervention became quickly established but limited evidence exists supporting its routine regular use. The move towards hospital deliveries began in the early 1950s. At this time, with limited hospital maternity facilities, 1 in 3 were planned home deliveries. The Cranbrook Report in 1959 recommended sufficient hospital maternity beds for 70% of all deliveries to take place in hospital, and the subsequent Peel Report (1970) recommended that a bed should be available for every woman to deliver in hospital if she so wished.

Obstetricians were not alone in the movement towards hospital deliveries. Women themselves were pushing to at least be allowed the choice to deliver in hospital. By 1972, only 1 in 10 deliveries were planned for home, and the publication of the Social Services Committee report in the Short Report (1980) led to further centralization of hospital delivery. It made a number of recommendations. Among these were:

- An increasing number of women should be delivered in large units; selection of women should be improved for smaller consultant units and isolated GP units and home deliveries should be phased out further.

- It should be mandatory that all pregnant women be seen at least twice by a consultant obstetrician – preferably as soon as possible after the first visit to the GP in early pregnancy and again in late pregnancy.

This and subsequent reports including UK government reports in 1982, 1984 and 1985, 'Birth to Five' (Department of Health, 2005) and the 2012/13 Choice Framework (Department of Health, 2012) led to a policy of increasing centralization of units for delivery and, consequently, maternity care.

The gradual decline in maternal and perinatal mortality was thought to be due in greater part to hospital deliveries, although proof for this was lacking. Indeed, the decline in perinatal mortality was least in those years when hospitalization increased the most. As other new interventions became available and were increasingly used, such as continuous fetal monitoring and induction of labour, a change in practice began to establish these as the norm for most women, without robust evaluation of their impact through randomized controlled trials or other high-quality research methodology. In England and Wales between 1966 and 1974, the induction rate rose from 12.7% to 38.9%. During the 1980s, with increasing consumer awareness, the unquestioning acceptance of unproven technologies was challenged. Women, led by groups such as the National Childbirth Trust (NCT), began to question not only the need for any intervention but also the need to come to the hospital at all. The professional bodies also began to question the effectiveness of antenatal care.

The government set up an expert committee to review policy on maternity care and to make recommendations. This committee produced the document Changing Childbirth (Department of Health, Report of the Expert Maternity Group, 1993), which provided purchasers and providers with a number of action points aiming to improve choice, information and continuity for all women. It outlined a number of indicators of success to be achieved within 5 years:

- The carriage of hand-held notes by women.
- Midwifery-led care in 30% of pregnancies.
- A known midwife at delivery in 75% of cases.
- A reduction in the number of antenatal visits for low-risk mothers.

This landmark report provided a new impetus to examine the provision of maternity care in the UK and enshrined choice as a concept in maternity care.

More recently, government documents on maternity care such as Maternity Matters (2007) aimed to address inequalities in maternity care provision and uptake; it enables commissioners to assess maternity care in their area and to ensure that safe and effective care is available to all women. Maternity care now centres on increased choices for women and empowerment of couples, including birth at home or in a stand-alone midwifery unit. The most recent Maternity Review (2016) emphasized the following principles:

- Personalized woman-centred care.
- Continuity of carer.
- Better postnatal and perinatal mental health care.
- A fairer payment system for different types of care.
- Safer care, with multiprofessional working and training and measurement of performance using routinely collected data

Overview of antenatal care

The aims of antenatal care are:

- To optimize pregnancy outcomes for women and babies.

- To prevent, detect and manage those factors that adversely affect the health of mother and baby.
- To provide advice, reassurance, education and support for the woman and her family.
- To deal with the 'minor ailments' of pregnancy.
- To provide general health screening.

Antenatal care aims to make the woman the focus. Women should be treated with kindness and dignity at all times, and due respect given to personal, cultural and religious beliefs. Services should be readily accessible and there should be continuity of care. There is a need for high-quality, culturally appropriate, verbal and written information on which women can base their choices, through a truly informed decision-making process, which is led by them.

In the UK and many countries worldwide, maternity care for an individual woman is provided by a community-based team of midwives and family practitioners (such as GPs), a hospital consultant team or a combination of the two. Some women have complex pregnancies and in these instances a hospital-based obstetric team leads their antenatal care and they are said to have consultant care. Many more women have pregnancies where there are no overtly complicating factors and these women usually have community-based care and are said to be under midwifery care. A further group have risk factors identified at booking, for example previous caesarean section, which mandate clinical input by obstetricians but where the majority of routine care can still be provided by the community team. This is referred to as shared care.

Advice, reassurance and education

Pregnancy is a time of great uncertainty and stress and this is compounded by the many physical changes experienced by the woman during her pregnancy. Common symptoms include nausea, heartburn, constipation, shortness of breath, dizziness, swelling, backache, abdominal discomfort and headaches. Generally, these reflect physiological adaptations to pregnancy but may become extremely debilitating for the pregnant woman. Occasionally they will represent the first presentation of a more serious problem.

Information regarding smoking, alcohol consumption and the use of drugs (both legal and illegal) during pregnancy is extremely important. In some populations almost one-third of women smoke during pregnancy, despite its association with fetal growth restriction, preterm labour, placental abruption and intrauterine fetal death. A major role of antenatal care is to help women limit these harmful behaviours during pregnancy, for example by inclusion in smoking cessation programmes. Alcohol or illegal substance misuse may require more specialized skills from support services including perinatal mental health teams. The information given should be of high quality and evidence based. It should be provided in a manner appropriate to the woman and in different formats (e.g. written information) where appropriate and possible.

Parentcraft education is the term often used to describe formal group discussion of issues relating to pregnancy, labour and delivery and care of the newborn. These sessions offer an opportunity for couples to meet others in the same situation and help to establish a network of social contacts that may be useful after the delivery. They may include a tour of the maternity department, the aim of which is to lessen anxiety and increase the sense of maternal control surrounding delivery.

First trimester

When a woman becomes pregnant one of the first interactions with the health services is known as the booking visit. At this point, or shortly afterwards, a midwife will take a detailed history, examine the woman and perform a series of routine investigations (with the woman's consent) in order that appropriate care can be offered. If risk factors are identified that may potentially impact on the pregnancy outcome, the midwife will access specialized services on behalf of the woman. This may mean referral to a hospital consultant obstetric clinic or other specialist services as appropriate. Medical or psychosocial issues raised at the booking visit may need to be explored in some depth.

Body mass index and weight assessment

Height and weight should be measured at the booking visit, body mass index (BMI) calculated and assessed and women counselled accordingly. If the BMI is more than 35 kg/m^2, it is recommended that the woman is reviewed by an obstetric consultant or other healthcare professional who can provide appropriate advice on the increased pregnancy risks (*Table 2.1*) and interventions to minimize excessive gestational weight gain. The Institute of Medicine have guidelines on recommended weight increase in pregnancy. For normal weight women (BMI 18.5–24.9 kg/m^2) the recommended total weight gain in pregnancy is 11–16 kg (25–35 lb); for overweight women (BMI 25–29.9 kg/m^2) 7–11 kg (15–25 lb); and for obese (≥30 kg/m^2) women 5–9 kg (11–20 lb).

Women with raised BMI should be counselled regarding appropriate weight in pregnancy and counselled regarding the risks. In general, the risks increase as BMI rises.

General pregnancy dietary advice

The Royal College of Obstetricians and Gynaecologists (RCOG) provides the following dietary advice for optimal weight control in pregnancy:

- Do not eat for two; maintain your normal portion size and try and avoid snacks.
- Eat fibre-rich foods such as oats, beans, lentils, grains, seeds, fruit and vegetables as well as whole grain bread, brown rice and pasta.
- Base your meals on starchy foods such as potatoes, bread, rice and pasta, choosing whole grain where possible.
- Restrict intake of fried food, drinks and confectionary high in added sugars, and other foods high in fat and sugar.
- Eat at least five portions of a variety of fruit and vegetables each day.
- Dieting in pregnancy is not recommended but controlling weight gain in pregnancy is advocated.

It may be difficult for pregnant women to make these changes to their diets for the first time in their adult life, and further work is needed to determine how to enable pregnant women to follow this guidance.

General exercise advice

Aerobic and strength conditioning exercise in pregnancy is considered safe and beneficial. It may help

Table 2.1 Maternal and neonatal complications associated with increased BMI in pregnancy

Maternal	Fetal
Antenatal	
Difficulty accurately assessing growth and anatomy of fetus	Increased congenital malformations; if BMI >40 kg/m^2, risk of neural tube defects is three times that of a woman with a BMI <30 kg/m^2 If BMI >30 kg/m^2, high-dose folic acid (5 mg once daily) is recommended prepregnancy and for first 12 weeks' gestation
Increased risk of GDM: three times more likely to develop GDM than women whose BMI <30 kg/m^2	Macrosomia and associated complications
Hypertensive disorders of pregnancy: increased risk of chronic hypertension, gestational hypertension and pre-eclampsia	Fetal growth restriction and associated complications
Increased risk of VTE	
	Miscarriage; overall miscarriage risk is 20%, which increases to 1 in 4 (25%) if BMI >30 kg/m^2
	Stillbirth: doubling of stillbirth risk from 0.5% to 1 in 100 (1%)
Intrapartum	
Difficulty with analgesia (epidurals and spinal) and general anaesthesia if needed	
Difficulty with monitoring in labour	
Increased instrumental delivery rate	
Increased caesarean section rate	
	Macrosomia and shoulder dystocia: risk of macrosomia (neonatal weight >4 kg) increases from 7% to 14% compared to women with a BMI of between 20 and 30 kg/m^2
Postnatal	
VTE risk	
Wound breakdown and infection	
Postnatal depression	
	Increased risk of childhood obesity and diabetes in later life

BMI, body mass index; GDM, gestational diabetes; VTE, venous thromboembolism.

recovery following delivery, reduce back and pelvic pain during pregnancy and contribute to overall wellness. The aim of exercise during pregnancy is to stay fit, rather than to reach peak fitness. Contact sports should be avoided and if the pregnant woman has any coexisting medical conditions, a more tailored exercise programme may be needed. However, there are very few pregnant women for whom some exercise is not appropriate and health care professionals can encourage women to maintain walking, swimming and other forms of non-contact exercise. Pelvic floor exercises during pregnancy and immediately after birth may reduce the risk of urinary and faecal incontinence in the future. Following delivery, generally it is safe to resume exercise gradually as soon as the woman feels ready.

The RCOG provides modified heart rate target zones for exercise in pregnancy. These are age dependent and are as follows: women <20 years of age: target range 140–155 beats per minute (bpm); 20–29 years of age: 135–150 bpm; 30–39 years of age: 130–145 bpm; and >40 years of age: 125–140 bpm.

Breastfeeding education

Breastfeeding protects against diarrhoea and common childhood illnesses such as pneumonia, and may also have longer-term health benefits for the mother and child, such as reducing the risk of obesity later in life. Breastfeeding has also been associated with a higher intelligence quotient (IQ) in children, although it is not clear whether this is a result of confounding. The World Health Organization (WHO) recommends initiation of breastfeeding within an hour of birth, exclusive breastfeeding for the first 6 months of life and continued breastfeeding beyond 6 months and at least up to 2 years of age. Although evidence for interventions to promote breastfeeding are limited, a recent systematic review demonstrated that the greatest improvements in initiation and continuation of breastfeeding were seen when education was provided concurrently across the various settings including home, community and the health system. Baby-friendly hospital support in the health system was the most effective intervention to improve rates of any breastfeeding. As a result, early education in pregnancy about breastfeeding is advocated to improve uptake and engage pregnant women with breastfeeding services to allow them to be fully prepared.

Options for pregnancy care

Following the booking visit and assessment of potential risks a woman may discuss their expectations for the pregnancy and discuss where they would like to receive their antenatal care and deliver their baby. Provided that there are no contraindications to midwifery-led care (such as medical comorbidities or previous obstetric complications that may warrant consultant-led care), the options available for delivery include:

- Home birth: according to the Birthplace Study, in England and Wales approximately 2% of women opt to deliver at home, cared for by a midwife. The advantages of home birth include familiar surroundings, no interruption of labour to go to hospital, no separation from other children or the woman's partner during or after birth, continuity of care and reduced interventions. The disadvantages are that 45% of first time mothers (and 12% of multiparous mothers) planning home birth are transferred to hospital and a poor perinatal outcome occurs in approximately twice as many first time home birth mothers compared with first time mothers delivering in hospital (9.3 vs. 5.3 adverse perinatal events/1,000 births; adjusted odds ratio 1.75, 95% confidence intervals 1.07–2.86). Other disadvantages include limited analgesic options (e.g. no epidurals are available).

- Midwifery units or birth centres: these may be stand-alone where they are located on a separate site to hospital birth centres or adjacent to hospitals ('co-located') with access to obstetric, neonatal and anaesthetic care. Advantages of midwifery units may include continuity of care, fewer interventions and convenience of location. Disadvantages include transfer out to a hospital birth centre (40% nulliparous women and 10% of multiparous women) and limited access to certain analgesic options. There was no difference in the risk of adverse perinatal outcomes between midwifery units and hospital units (4.5 adverse perinatal events/1,000 births in freestanding midwifery unit vs. 4.7 events/1,000 in alongside midwifery unit vs. 5.3 events/1,000 in obstetric unit).

- Hospital birth centre: in hospital birth centres midwives continue to provide care during labour but doctors are available should the need arise. There is direct access to obstetricians, anaesthetists and neonatologists. Disadvantages include lack of continuity of care and a greater likelihood of intervention (compared to midwifery units and home birth).

Antenatal urine tests

Asymptomatic bacteriuria is associated with increased risk of preterm delivery and the development of pyelonephritis during pregnancy. A midstream specimen of urine (MSU) should be sent for culture and sensitivity at the booking visit to screen for asymptomatic bacteriuria. Urinalysis is performed every antenatal visit. Urine is screened for protein (to detect renal disease or pre-eclampsia), persistent glycosuria (to detect pre-existing diabetes or gestational diabetes [GDM]) and nitrites (to detect urinary tract infections). If nitrites are detected on urine dipstick testing, a MSU is sent for microscopy, culture and sensitivity to detect asymptomatic bacteria and appropriate treatment initiated if a positive culture is identified.

Blood pressure assessment

Blood pressure falls by a small amount (a few mmHg) in the first trimester and increases to pre-pregnancy levels by the end of the second trimester. First trimester blood pressure assessment also allows the detection of previously unrecognized chronic hypertension; this enables early initiation of treatment including antihypertensive agents (to reduce episodes of severe hypertension in the mother) and low-dose aspirin, which improves maternal (reduced pre-eclampsia) and fetal (decreased perinatal mortality) outcomes in women with chronic hypertension.

Booking tests in pregnancy

Table 2.2 lists the booking tests often performed at the booking visit.

Full blood count

Full blood count (FBC) measurement allows identification of women with anaemia, to allow early initiation of treatment. Anaemia in pregnancy is defined as a haemoglobin (Hb) <110 g/l in first trimester, <105 g/l in second and third trimesters and <100 g/l in the postpartum period. The detection of anaemia should prompt examination of the mean cell volume to identify likely iron deficiency anaemia (microcytic anaemia) or folate or vitamin B12 deficiency (macrocytic anaemia). Further investigations may include B12, folate or iron (ferritin) studies. Appropriate treatment should be initiated.

In accordance with the British Society for Haematology recommendations for anaemic women in pregnancy, a trial of oral iron should be considered as the first-line management option, with an increment demonstrated at 2 weeks confirming a positive response. Women with known haemoglobinopathy should have serum ferritin checked and offered oral supplements if their ferritin level is <30 µg/l.

A FBC also allows the identification of low platelets, which may rarely represent *de-novo* immune thrombocytopaenic purpura. Gestational thrombocytopaenia (a fall in platelet count in pregnancy) rarely presents in the first trimester and is more commonly detected beyond 28 weeks' gestation. Hence a low platelet count in the first trimester warrants further investigation and haematological input; in many settings the threshold for referral is <100 × 10⁹/l but individual maternity units may set their own criteria. A baseline platelet count is also useful later in pregnancy if there are concerns regarding conditions such as pre-eclampsia or haemolysis, elevated liver enzymes and low platelets (HELLP) syndrome, which may present with thrombocytopaenia.

Blood group

A blood group is checked at booking to identify rhesus D-negative women so that they may be informed regarding the risks of rhesus isoimmunization and sensitization from a rhesus D-positive fetus. Anti-D is administered to rhesus D-negative women in instances of potential sensitizing events such as

Table 2.2 Summary of booking investigations

Investigation	Indication
FBC	Haemoglobin, platelet count, mean cell volume
MSU	Asymptomatic bacteriuria
Blood group and antibody screen	Rhesus status and atypical antibodies
Haemoglobinopathy screening	Screening is based on the FOQ and blood test results
Infection screen	Hepatitis B, syphilis, HIV, (and rubella status)
Dating scan and first trimester screening	Accurate pregnancy dating with provision of risk assessment for trisomy 21, 18 and 13 and identification of major congenital anomalies

FBC, full blood count; FOQ, Family Origin Questionnaire; HIV, human immunodeficiency virus; MSU, mid-stream urine.

postchorionic villous sampling, amniocentesis or trauma to the maternal abdomen.

The British Committee for Standards in Haematology recommends that following potentially sensitizing events, anti-D immunoglobulin should be administered as soon as possible and always within 72 hours of the event. In pregnancies less than 12 weeks' gestation, anti-D immunoglobulin prophylaxis is only indicated following ectopic pregnancy, molar pregnancy, therapeutic termination of pregnancy and in cases of uterine bleeding where this is repeated, heavy or associated with abdominal pain. The minimum dose of anti-D should be 250 IU and a test for feto-maternal haemorrhage is not required. For potentially sensitizing events between 12 and 20 weeks' gestation, a minimum dose of 250 IU should be administered within 72 hours of the event and a test for feto-maternal haemorrhage is not required. Women who are rhesus D negative are now offered prophylactic anti-D administration at 28 weeks' gestation. Antenatal anti-D immunoglobulin prophylaxis using either a single large dose at 28 weeks' gestation or two doses, given at 28 and 34 weeks' gestation, achieves a significant reduction in the incidence of maternal sensitization to rhesus D due to occult sensitizing events. Rhesus D-negative women also receive anti-D postpartum once a baby is confirmed as being rhesus D positive on testing of a cord blood sample.

Assessment of blood group in all pregnant women at 28 weeks' gestation also identifies those with other atypical antibodies so that appropriate monitoring can be put in place. Newer techniques such as non-invasive prenatal testing of maternal blood for fetal rhesus status (determined by analysis of cell-free fetal deoxyribonucleic acid [cffDNA]) may limit the need for anti-D prophylaxis to mothers whose fetuses are known to be rhesus D positive. This is considered more reliable than testing a partner's blood group due to biological paternity not always being that of the assumed partner. For further details, see Chapter 6, Antenatal obstetric complications.

Gestational diabetes

Women who have had previous GDM should be offered a glucose tolerance test or random blood glucose in the first trimester, with the aim of detecting pre-existing diabetes that may have developed since a preceding pregnancy.

Thalassaemia

Thalassaemia is a group of inherited blood disorders where the Hb is abnormal as a result of mutations in genes that code Hb. They are inherited in an autosomal recessive pattern. Although the thalassaemias can occur worldwide, the carrier rate is particularly common in people from Southeast Asia, and also affects those of Mediterranean, North African, Middle Eastern, Indian and Asian origin. A mutation that affects the alpha chain causes alpha-thalassaemia and beta-thalassaemia occurs as a result of a mutation in the beta chain. The alpha chains are produced by four genes, two on each chromosome 16, inherited as pairs. The severity of the condition depends on how many of those genes have been altered. If one gene is mutated, women are asymptomatic. If women carry two mutations (alpha-thalassaemia trait) they may have mild anaemia. Haemoglobin H disease occurs when an individual carries three mutated genes and will lead to chronic anaemia that requires regular blood transfusion. Alpha-thalassaemia major occurs when all four genes are mutated and is associated with a high incidence of intrauterine death.

There are only two beta genes, one each on chromosome 11. The beta-thalassaemia phenotype can range from moderate to severe. Beta-thalassaemia major occurs when both beta genes are affected and affected individuals will require blood transfusions for the rest of their life. Beta-thalassaemia intermedia is the milder form of the condition and is non-transfusion dependent. Screening for thalassaemia in the UK is offered to all pregnant women at booking visit using the Family Origin Questionnaire (FOQ) and/or FBC results; those at high risk of having an affected fetus should be then referred to a fetal medicine unit to discuss the option of invasive confirmatory testing.

Sickle cell screen

Similar to the other haemoglobinopathies, certain ethnic groups are at higher risk of carrying sickle cell trait. The carrier rate for sickle cell trait (HbAS) is approximately 1 in 10 among Afro-Caribbean people but as high as 1 in 4 in people from West Africa. The carrier frequency for haemoglobin C trait (HbAC) is approximately 1 in 30 but up to 1 in 6 in some groups (e.g. Ghanaians). HbSS (homozygous sickle cell disease) is the most serious form of the disease and these patients have chronic haemolytic anaemia and suffer from sickle cell crisis, which may be precipitated by infection. Women can also have the combination of HbS and another ß-globin variant such as HbSC. These individuals have slightly milder features than seen in HbSS but are still at risk of sickle cell crises. Partners of women with sickle cell disease or trait are offered screening early in pregnancy with the option of invasive testing to detect an affected fetus if both parents are carriers.

First trimester infection screen

Rubella

For many years maternal immunity to rubella has been tested at booking visits in most countries. The national organization Public Health England has recently stopped routine testing for rubella (from April 2016) on the grounds that rubella infection levels in the UK are so low they are defined as eliminated by the WHO. Rubella infection in pregnancy is now very rare; the mumps, measles, rubella (MMR) immunization programme has demonstrated that over 90% children aged up to 2 years had received at least one mumps, measles and rubella vaccination. As the screening test used can potentially give inaccurate results and cause unnecessary stress among women, the screening programme has been stopped.

The majority of pregnant women are rubella immune and no further action is required. In instances where a woman is found not to be immune, she is advised to avoid contact with individuals known to be currently infected, and offered the combined MMR vaccination following delivery (see Chapter 11, Perinatal infections).

Syphilis

Syphilis is a sexually transmitted disease caused by transmission of *Treponema pallidum*, a spirochaete bacterium. In pregnancy it may cause miscarriage or stillbirth and can cause active disease in newborn infants if contracted antenatally. Between 2011 and 2012, there were 2,978 cases of syphilis diagnosed in the UK. Although diagnosis is rare in pregnancy, due to the increasing incidence of the disease and the fact that it may be safely treated with penicillin in pregnancy, women continue to be routinely screened for syphilis in pregnancy (see Chapter 11, Perinatal infections).

Hepatitis B

Hepatitis screening is performed in pregnancy to reduce infant infection; without preventive measures 90% of babies born to mothers with hepatitis B will contract the virus and develop chronic infection, which is associated with liver failure, cirrhosis and hepatocellular carcinoma. If a baby is born to a woman with active hepatitis B, then the infant should receive hepatitis B vaccine and one dose of hepatitis B immune globulin within the first 12 hours of life. This confers over 95% protection against chronic hepatitis B infection. The infant will need require additional doses of hepatitis B vaccine at 1 and 6 months of age. The test for screening for hepatitis B involves detection of hepatitis B surface antibody (HBsAb or anti-HBs). Detection of the antibody implies immunity to hepatitis B. Hepatitis B surface antigen (HBsAg) indicates the presence of hepatitis B in the blood. Hepatitis B core antibody (HBcAb or anti-HBc) indicates that a person may have been exposed to the hepatitis B virus (see Chapter 11, Perinatal infections).

Hepatitis C

The National Institute for Health and Care Excellence (NICE) currently recommends that pregnant women should not be offered routine screening for hepatitis C virus because there is insufficient evidence to support its clinical and cost effectiveness. Screening for hepatitis C may be offered to women considered to be at high risk; this includes current or previous intravenous drug use and hepatitis B and/or human immunodeficiency virus (HIV) infection. The risk of transmitting the virus from mother to child is approximately 5%, but this increases significantly up to 36% if there is coinfection with HIV. Screening is performed by examining for hepatitis C virus immunoglobulin (Ig) G antibodies (see Chapter 11, Perinatal infections).

HIV

The estimated HIV prevalence among pregnant women in the UK is 2 per 1,000. With appropriate interventions risk of transmission to the neonate is as low as 0.1%. Interventions to minimize vertical transmission include initiation of antiretroviral therapy (ART) by 24 weeks' gestation if naive to ART, planned elective caesarean section for those with viral load ≥400 HIV ribonucleic acid (RNA) copies/ml at 36 weeks' gestation and exclusive formula feeding from birth regardless of viral load and ART use. It is recommended that women who decline initial screening should be offered screening again at 28 weeks' gestation.

Ultrasound for first trimester dating and screening

Accurate dating through first trimester ultrasound is key to avoiding issues later in pregnancy such as incorrect identification of growth restriction and inadvertent induction of labour for postdates pregnancy. First trimester ultrasound also enables early identification of multifetal pregnancies, screening for trisomies and examination of the fetus for gross anomalies such as anencephaly and cystic hygromas. The dating scan and first trimester screening is best performed between 11+3 and 13+6 weeks' gestation, when the crown–rump length (CRL) measures between 45 and 84 mm. From 14 and 20 weeks' gestation the head circumference is used to date the pregnancy.

Beyond 20 weeks' gestation, the impact of genes and environmental factors can cause variability in fetal size. Dating a pregnancy by ultrasound scan therefore becomes progressively less accurate as the gestation advances. This is just one of the potential problems of 'late booking'.

First trimester screening currently involves:

- Measurement of nuchal translucency (NT). The median and 95th centile for NT is 1.2 mm and 2.1 mm with a CRL of 45 mm, and 1.9 mm and 2.7 mm for a CRL of 84 mm.
- Measurement of maternal free human chorionic gonadotrophin (β-hCG) and pregnancy-associated plasma protein-A (PAPP-A). In trisomy 21 pregnancies the concentration of free β-hCG is higher (around two multiples of median; MoM) and the concentration of PAPP-A is lower (approximately 0.5 MoM).
- Maternal age.

Using an algorithm based on the above criteria the detection rate for trisomy 21 is approximately 90%. The false-positive rate can be reduced to 3% by additionally examining the nasal bone, ductus venosus flow and tricuspid flow and this gives a detection rate of approximately 95%. Screening may also be performed in the second trimester between 14 and 20 weeks' gestation and consists exclusively of risk prediction using maternal biomarkers. The quadruple test measures maternal alpha-fetoprotein (AFP), hCG, unconjugated oestriol (uE3) and inhibin A and has an 80% detection with a 5% false-positive rate. Newer technologies including non-invasive prenatal testing are now available with reported sensitivities for detection of Down's syndrome of more than 99% with a screen-positive rate of <0.2%. These are discussed further in Chapter 5, Prenatal diagnosis.

Identification of high-risk women

Women at high risk of developing pre-eclampsia

NICE currently recommends that women considered to be at high risk of pre-eclampsia should have low-dose aspirin (75 mg) treatment initiated early in pregnancy until delivery. Women considered to be high risk include:

- Hypertensive disease during a previous pregnancy.
- Chronic kidney disease.
- Autoimmune disease such as systemic lupus erythematosus or antiphospholipid syndrome.
- Type 1 or type 2 diabetes.
- Chronic hypertension.

Furthermore, women with two or more moderate risk factors for pre-eclampsia are also recommended to commence aspirin early in pregnancy until delivery. Moderate risk factors for the development of pre-eclampsia include:

- Primiparity.
- Advanced maternal age (>40 years).
- Pregnancy interval of more than 10 years.
- BMI $\geq$35 kg/m^2 at booking visit.
- Family history of pre-eclampsia.
- Multifetal pregnancy.

All women should be screened at every antenatal visit for pre-eclampsia by measurement of blood pressure and urinalysis for protein.

Women at high risk of preterm birth

Women considered to be at high risk of preterm birth include those with previous preterm birth, late miscarriage, multifetal pregnancies and cervical surgery such as previous cone biopsy. These women may be offered serial cervical length screening with or without the use of fetal fibronectin to detect increased risk of preterm birth. Note: no agreed screening protocol for preterm birth is available.

Fetal growth restriction

NICE guidelines recommend that symphysis–fundal height (SFH) measurements should be performed at every antenatal appointment from 24 weeks' gestation. Concerns that fetal growth may be slow, or has stopped altogether, should prompt ultrasound scanning. There is no consensus on the recommended 'routine' use of ultrasound in pregnancy. The majority of units offer dating scans (at end of first trimester) and anomaly scans (at around 20–22 weeks' gestation) but no further growth assessment unless clinically indicated. Some units offer an additional third trimester growth scan but this is still being evaluated in research studies.

Vitamin D deficiency

The RCOG advises that there are no data to support routine screening for vitamin D deficiency in pregnancy in terms of health benefits or cost effectiveness. Women thought to be at increased risk of vitamin D deficiency on the basis of skin colour or coverage, obesity, risk of pre-eclampsia or gastroenterological conditions limiting fat absorption may be screened, but this testing is expensive. Daily vitamin D supplementation with oral cholecalciferol or ergocalciferol is safe in pregnancy. NICE guidance states that all pregnant and breastfeeding women should be advised to take 10 µg of vitamin D supplements daily. Severe vitamin D deficiency in pregnancy results in increased risk of neonatal rickets.

Second trimester care

Anomaly scan

Between 20 and 22 weeks' gestation it is recommended that fetal anatomy be assessed. This is a detailed structural scan aimed at detecting conditions such as spina bifida, major congenital anomalies, diaphragmatic hernia and renal agenesis. Prenatal diagnosis is covered in detail in Chapter 5.

Gestational diabetes mellitus

Universal screening for GDM is available in some countries including the USA and Australia. However, NICE advocates risk-based screening in the UK. GDM is diagnosed if a woman has a fasting plasma glucose level of 5.6 mmol/l or above, or a 2-hour plasma glucose level of 7.8 mmol/l or above.

Risk factors for the development of GDM include women with previous gestational diabetes, previous macrosomia ($\geq$4.5 kg), raised BMI ($\geq$30 kg/m^2), first-degree relative with diabetes or women of Asian, black Caribbean or Middle Eastern origin. If risk factors are present, the woman should be offered a 2-hour 75 g oral glucose tolerance test (OGTT) at 24–28 weeks' gestation. Women with a previous history of GDM should have an oral glucose tolerance test at 16–18 weeks' gestation. The test should be repeated at 24–28 weeks of pregnancy.

Governance of maternity care

Many clinical, political and consumer bodies now contribute to optimizing care for women in pregnancy. These include the following.

NICE

NICE has evaluated maternity care in great detail and continues to publish many important guidelines relating to different aspects of pregnancy, covering antenatal, intrapartum and postnatal care. These provide the benchmark by which Trusts are judged in their ability to provide care. The process of guideline development is rigorous and stakeholders are consulted at each stage of development. The guidelines are available through the NICE website (www.nice.org.uk) and provide the framework for standards of care within England and Wales.

National Screening Committee

Screening has formed a part of antenatal care since its inception. The National Screening Committee is responsible for developing standards and strategies for the implementation of these. The National Screening Committee has unified and progressed standards for all aspects of antenatal screening across the UK. The provision of national standards means that new tests are critically evaluated before being offered to populations. Conditions for which screening is currently not recommended, such as group B streptococcus carriage, are regularly reviewed against current evidence. The National Screening Committee recently recommended the cessation of testing for rubella immunity.

RCOG

The RCOG has many roles. These include developing national guidelines (not covered by the above bodies), setting standards for the provision of care, training and revalidation, audit and research. The RCOG publishes a large number of guidelines pertinent to pregnancy with patient information leaflets to accompany many of these. They are reviewed 3-yearly and are accessible to all on the college website (www.rcog.org.uk). The RCOG works in partnership with other colleges such as the Royal College of Midwives (RCM) to set standards for maternity care. These standards provide important drivers to organizations such as the Clinical Negligence Scheme for Trusts in setting standards for levels of care and performance by hospitals.

Consumer groups

As well as providing support and advice for women, often at times of great need, consumer groups allow women to have a louder voice in the planning and provision of maternity care. National consumer groups such as the NCT have representatives on many influential panels, such as the National Screening Committee and RCOG working groups. At a local level, each hospital should have a Maternity Services Liaison Committee (MSLC). When these committees work well, they can provide essential consumer input into service delivery at a local level.

 KEY LEARNING POINTS

- Antenatal care improves pregnancy outcomes and a variety of models exist.
- There are key visits during the pregnancy when essential investigations or decisions are taken regarding antenatal care and delivery.
- Antenatal care should be seen as an opportunity for education, reassurance and screening for potential problems.
- Continued efforts should be made to improve the access to antenatal care for disadvantaged and minority groups.

Further reading

BCSH guideline for the use of anti-D immunoglobulin for the prevention of haemolytic disease of the fetus and newborn. Available at http://onlinelibrary. wiley.com/doi/10.1111/tme.12091/epdf (last accessed 02.02.2016).

British HIV Association guidelines for the management of HIV infection is available at http://www.bhiva. org/documents/Guidelines/Pregnancy/2012/BHIVA-Pregnancy-guidelines-update-2014.pdf.

Fetal anomaly screening programme. https://www. gov.uk/government/uploads/system/uploads/ attachment_data/file/421650/FASP_Standards_ April_2015_final_2_.pdf.

Infectious Diseases in Pregnancy Screening (IDPS) Programme. UK National Screening Committee. September 2010. https://www.gov.uk/government/ uploads/system/uploads/attachment_data/file/384721/ IDPS_programme_standards_Revised_Final.pdf.

National Institute for Health and Care Excellence. Antenatal care. Available at http://www.nice.org.uk/ guidance/qs22.

Royal College of Obstetricians and Gynaecologists Clinical Guidelines. https://www.rcog.org.uk/ guidelines.

Self assessment

CASE HISTORY

Mrs Singh, a 39-year-old woman originally from Pakistan, is approximately 8 weeks' gestation and attends a booking visit with her community midwife, who fills out her client-held records. This is Mrs Singh's fourth pregnancy, having had two normal deliveries following by a caesarean section for a transverse lie. The previous babies' weights were 2.30 kg, 2.40 kg and 2.35 kg, all born at 39 weeks' gestation. Mrs Singh's booking blood pressure is 140/95 mmHg and her BMI is 37.

Identify the key issues raised and prepare a plan for management during the pregnancy.

ANSWER

Mrs Singh is originally from Pakistan, although she has been a UK citizen for many years. This makes a language problem less likely. However, there is no record that a thalassaemia screen has ever been performed. This is important because thalassaemia trait (carrier status) might contribute to maternal anaemia. Furthermore, if the father of this baby is also a carrier, the child will have a 1 in 4 chance of having thalassaemia. It is reassuring that all the children are fit and well, but this does not exclude the possibility that they are both carriers.

Mrs Singh is 39 years old. This slightly increases the risks of pregnancy complications including pre-eclampsia, but, more significantly, it is associated with an increase in the risk of certain fetal chromosomal abnormalities, principally Down's syndrome. The decision to undergo screening and invasive testing is a personal one, often influenced by cultural and religious beliefs, but an offer of screening should be made to all women.

Mrs Singh likely has chronic hypertension (possibly related to her body weight) but is not currently on medication. Mrs Singh should be commenced on 75 mg aspirin to reduce the risk of pre-eclampsia. She should also be assessed further for consideration of starting an antihypertensive agent.

Mrs Singh's children have all been of low birthweight. It is difficult to determine whether they were constitutionally (genetically) small, but healthy, or whether they were pathologically small (i.e. growth restricted). Serial ultrasound scans should be performed as surveillance for fetal growth restriction.

Mrs Singh has a raised BMI; this increases her risks of anaesthetic complications (such as failure to intubate or successfully site a spinal anaesthetic) and also her risks of developing GDM. An OGTT will be recommended at 28 weeks' gestation to screen for this.

Finally, the mode of delivery after a previous caesarean section requires discussion. The transverse lie was probably secondary to uterine laxity, but this would need to be confirmed by obtaining the previous pregnancy notes. The options for mode of delivery (vaginal birth after caesarean 'VBAC' vs. elective repeat caesarean section 'ERCS') will need to be discussed. Malpresentation at term may occur again.

In conclusion, Mrs Singh has a number of factors that increase the risk of complications in this pregnancy. Shared care under a hospital consultant would be the appropriate form of antenatal care.

EMQ

A Quadruple test.

B Anatomy scan.

C OGTT.

D FBC.

E Ferritin.

F MSU.

G Cervical length and fetal fibronectin.

H Sickle cell testing.

I Refer to fetal medicine unit.

J Observe the pregnant woman.

K 75 mg aspirin.

For each description, choose the SINGLE most appropriate answer from the list of options. Each option may be used once, more than once or not at all.

1 You review a pregnant woman at booking visit who previously was delivered at 32 weeks' gestation for severe pre-eclampsia.

2 A woman attends your clinic following first trimester screening that has shown the fetus to have a 1 in 25 risk of trisomy 21.

3 A woman attends for booking visit having had previous GDM.

4 A woman attends your booking clinic at 18 weeks' gestation. She recently discovered she was pregnant and is concerned about trisomy 21.

ANSWERS

1K This woman is at high risk of recurrence of pre-eclampsia and should be commenced on low-dose aspirin.

2I Following high-risk screening the woman should be counselled regarding the availability of invasive testing to rule out trisomy 21, with referral to a fetal medicine unit.

3C This woman is at high risk of GDM but also of pre-existing diabetes. Therefore she should be offered an early OGTT and a repeat test at 26–28 weeks' gestation if the first one is negative.

4A The best screening option in the second trimester is the quadruple test.

SBA QUESTIONS

Choose the single best answer.

1 According to NICE, which of the following is NOT a risk factor for screening for GDM?

A Previous GDM.

B Previous macrosomia (≥4.5 kg).

C Maternal raised BMI (≥30 kg/m^2).

D European descent.

ANSWER

D Women with a raised BMI, a history of GDM or a history of macrosomia in a previous pregnancy are at increased risk of GDM. Certain ethnic groups, particularly women from South Asia and South East Asia are at high risk from GDM when compared to women of European descent.

2 According to NICE, which of the following is NOT a high risk factor for developing pre-eclampsia?

A Chronic kidney disease.

B Autoimmune disease such as systemic lupus erythematosus or antiphospholipid syndrome.

C Thyroid disease.

D Chronic hypertension.

ANSWER

C Women considered to be at high risk of pre-eclampsia include:

- Hypertensive disease during a previous pregnancy.
- Chronic kidney disease.
- Autoimmune disease such as systemic lupus erythematosus or antiphospholipid syndrome.
- Type 1 or type 2 diabetes.
- Chronic hypertension.

Thyroid disease is not a risk factor for the development of pre-eclampsia.

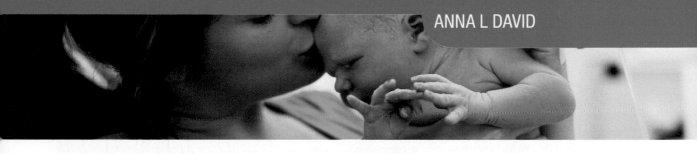

Normal fetal development and growth

CHAPTER 3

ANNA L DAVID

LEARNING OBJECTIVES

- To understand that fetal growth and birthweight are important determinants of immediate neonatal health and long-term adult health.

- To appreciate the fetal, maternal and placental factors that affect fetal growth and development.

- To be familiar with the fetal circulation, the specific shunts that ensure that the best oxygenated blood from the placenta is delivered to the fetal brain, and to appreciate how the fetal circulation transitions at birth to an adult circulation.

- To be aware of normal development of fetal organs during pregnancy, how fetal structural abnormalities arise and what effects they have on the fetus and neonate.

- To recognize the importance of normal amniotic fluid physiology to fetal growth and development.

Introduction

An understanding of normal development, growth and maturation is important for understanding the complications that may arise in pregnancy and for the neonate. For example, an understanding of the development of the lungs will explain why preterm infants are at risk of respiratory distress syndrome and term infants are not, and why bowel protruding into the umbilical cord at 10 weeks' gestation is normal and is not diagnosed as an omphalocele (exomphalos).

This chapter provides an overview of the development, growth and maturation of the main body organs and systems in the human fetus and the implications of disordered growth.

Fetal growth

Fetal growth and the eventual weight of the fetus at birth are important not only for the immediate health of the neonate but also for the long-term health of the adult, and even into the next generation. The thrifty phenotype (Barker) hypothesis says that reduced fetal growth is strongly associated with a number of chronic conditions later in life. This increased susceptibility results from adaptations made by the fetus in an environment limited in its supply of nutrients. These chronic conditions include coronary heart disease, stroke, diabetes and hypertension.

Fetal size can be assessed antenatally in two ways, either externally by using a tape measure to assess the uterine size from the superior edge of the pubic symphysis to the uterine fundus (symphysis–fundal height [SFH] measurement) or using ultrasound to measure specific parts of the fetus and then calculating the estimated fetal weight (EFW) using equations such as those described by Hadlock (see Chapter 4, Assessment of fetal wellbeing). The fetal size is described in terms of its size for gestational age and is presented on centile charts. Centile charts can be designed for a population.

Figure 3.1 shows the EFW centile chart for two fetuses. Fetus A has an EFW that is growing normally along the 75th centile. Fetus B is small and has suboptimal fetal growth; the EFW starts below the 5th centile and becomes progressively further away from the normal centiles as gestation advances.

More recently, customized centile charts have been developed as illustrated in Figure 1.2, Chapter 1, Obstetric history and examination, that take into consideration factors that are known to affect fetal growth such as maternal height, weight, parity, ethnicity and fetal sex.

A fetus that is less than the 10th centile is described as being small for gestational age (SGA) (**Figure 3.1** Fetus B). This is a statistical concept designed to categorize on size but not necessarily on outcome. An SGA fetus may be constitutionally small; in other words their growth potential was

reached and they were destined to be that small. Many fetuses that are SGA, however, have failed to reach their full growth potential, a condition called fetal growth restriction (FGR). FGR is associated with a significant increased risk of perinatal morbidity and mortality. Growth-restricted fetuses are more likely to suffer intrauterine hypoxia/asphyxia and, as a consequence, be stillborn or demonstrate signs and symptoms of hypoxic-ischaemic encephalopathy (HIE), including seizures and multiorgan damage or failure in the neonatal period. Other complications to which these growth-restricted babies are more prone include neonatal hypothermia, hypoglycaemia, infection and necrotizing enterocolitis. In the medium term, cerebral palsy is more prevalent and it is now recognized from large epidemiological studies that low birthweight infants are more likely to develop hypertension, cardiovascular disease (ischaemic heart disease and stroke) and diabetes in adult life, indicating that the impact of FGR is long lasting. One challenge in obstetric practice is to recognize potentially small fetuses, and then, from this group, to identify those that are 'small and healthy' and those that are 'small and unhealthy'. Interventions to deliver the growth-restricted fetuses early from the intrauterine environment may improve outcome. It is important to note, however, that not all growth-restricted fetuses are SGA, in that while their birthweight is

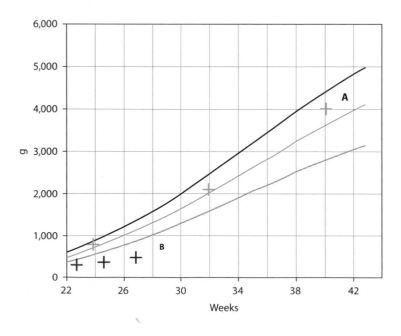

Figure 3.1 Population centile chart for estimated fetal weight by ultrasound measurements. Fetus (**A**) has normal growth; fetus (**B**) has suboptimal growth.

within the normal range for gestation (above the 10th centile) they still may have failed to reach their full growth potential. Detecting these fetuses is even more difficult than identification of the small growth-restricted fetus.

Determinants of fetal growth and birthweight

Determinants of fetal growth and birthweight are multifactorial. They reflect the influence of the natural growth potential of the fetus dictated largely by the fetal genome and epigenome, but also by the intrauterine environment that is influenced by both maternal and placental factors. The ultimate birthweight is therefore the result of the interaction between the fetus and the maternal uterine environment. Fetal growth is dependent on adequate delivery to, and transfer of nutrients and oxygen across, the placenta, which relies on appropriate maternal nutrition and placental perfusion. Factors affecting these are discussed below and in Chapter 9, Hypertensive disorders of pregnancy). Other factors are important in determining fetal growth and include, for example, fetal hormones that affect the metabolic rate, growth of tissues and maturation of individual organs. In particular, insulin-like growth factors (IGFs) coordinate a precise and orderly increase in growth throughout late gestation. Insulin and thyroxine (T4) are required through late gestation to ensure appropriate growth in normal and adverse nutritional circumstances. Fetal hyperinsulinaemia, which occurs in association with maternal diabetes mellitus when maternal glycaemic control is suboptimal, results in fetal macrosomia with, in particular, excessive fat deposition. This leads to complications such as late stillbirth, shoulder dystocia and neonatal hypoglycaemia.

Other factors relate to fetal, maternal and placental influences.

Fetal influences

Genetic

It is recognized that fetal genome plays a significant role in determining fetal size. Obvious and sometimes severe FGR is seen in fetuses with chromosomal defects such as the trisomies, particularly of chromosomes 13 (Patau's syndrome) and 18 (Edward's syndrome). Less severe FGR is common in trisomy 21 (Down's syndrome). The other genetic influence is fetal sex, with slightly greater birthweights in males.

Epigenetic

Increasingly it is recognized that epigenetic changes plays a role in determining fetal size. Epigenetic changes are modifications of deoxyribonucleic acid (DNA), which occur without any alteration in the underlying DNA sequence and can control whether a gene is turned on or off and how much of a particular message is made. Genomic imprinting is an epigenetic process that silences one parental allele, resulting in monoallelic expression. Emerging evidence shows that genes that are paternally expressed promote fetal growth, whereas maternally expressed genes suppress growth.

Infection

Although relatively uncommon in the UK, infection has been implicated in FGR, particularly rubella, cytomegalovirus, *Toxoplasma* and syphilis (discussed in further detail in Chapter 11, Perinatal infections). When faced with a fetus that is found to be very small on ultrasound measurement (for example EFW less than the 5th centile for gestational age), it is common to test the maternal blood for antibodies to these infections. The results are then compared with samples taken at booking (see Chapter 2, Antenatal care) to determine if the mother has evidence of seroconversion during pregnancy, which would suggest an acute infection.

Maternal influences
Physiological influences

In normal pregnancy, maternal physiological influences on birthweight include maternal height, prepregnancy weight, age and ethnic group. Heavier and taller mothers tend to have bigger babies and certain ethnic groups lighter babies (e.g. South Asian and Afro-Caribbean). Parity is also an influence with increasing parity being associated with increased birthweight. Age influences relate to the association with age and parity (i.e. older mothers are more likely to be parous). In older women, however, the increased risk of chromosomal abnormalities and maternal disease, for example hypertension, lead to lower birthweights. Teenage pregnancy is also associated with FGR.

Behavioural

Maternal behavioural influences are also important with smoking, alcohol and recreational drug use all associated with reduced fetal growth and birthweight. Babies born to mothers who smoke during pregnancy deliver babies up to 300 g lighter than non-smoking mothers. This effect may be through toxins, for example carbon monoxide, or vascular effects on the uteroplacental circulation. Stopping smoking, even partway through pregnancy, can lead to increased birthweight. Alcohol crosses the placenta and a dose-related effect has been noted, with up to 500 g reduction in birthweight, along with other anomalies occurring in women who drink heavily (two drinks per day), such as developmental delay. The use of recreational drugs is often associated with smoking and alcohol use but there is evidence to suggest that heroin is independently associated with a reduction in birthweight. Cocaine use is associated with spontaneous preterm birth, low birthweight and small head circumference. Placental abruption is associated with cigarette smoking and use of recreational drugs such as cocaine.

Chronic disease

Chronic maternal disease may restrict fetal growth. Such diseases are largely those that affect placental function or result in maternal hypoxia. Conditions include hypertension (essential or secondary to renal disease) and lung or cardiac conditions (cystic fibrosis, cyanotic heart disease). Hypertension can lead to placental infarction that impairs its function. Maternal thrombophilia can also result in placental thrombosis and infarction.

Placental influences

Normal placental development and function from early pregnancy is key to ensuring that the fetus receives adequate oxygen and nutrients from the mother. Placental insufficiency occurs when there is inadequate transfer of nutrients and oxygen across the placenta to the fetus. It can be due to poor maternal uterine artery blood flow, a thicker placental trophoblast barrier and/or abnormal fetus villous development. Placental infarction secondary to the

maternal chronic conditions discussed above or acute premature separation as in placental abruption can impair this transfer and hence fetal growth. Recurrent bleeding from the placenta (antepartum haemorrhage) can, over time, compromise placental function, leading to poor fetal growth in the latter part of pregnancy. FGR is discussed further in Chapter 9, Hypertensive disorders of pregnancy.

Fetal development

Cardiovascular system and the fetal circulation

The fetal circulation is quite different from that of the adult (**Figure 3.2**). The fetal circulation is characterized by four shunts that ensure that the oxygenated blood from the placenta is delivered to the fetal brain. These shunts are the:

- Umbilical circulation.
- Ductus venosus.
- Foramen ovale.
- Ductus arteriosus.

The umbilical circulation carries fetal blood to and from the placenta for gas and nutrient exchange. The umbilical arteries arise from the caudal end of the dorsal fetal aorta and carry deoxygenated blood from the fetus to the placenta. Normally two umbilical arteries are present, but a single umbilical artery is relatively common (approximately 0.5% of fetuses) and can be associated with reduced fetal growth velocity and some congenital anomalies. Oxygenated blood is returned to the fetus via the umbilical vein to the fetal liver. A small proportion of blood oxygenates the liver but the bulk passes through the ductus venosus bypassing the liver and joins the inferior vena cava (IVC) as it enters the right atrium. The ductus venosus is a narrow vessel and high blood velocities are generated within it. This streaming of the ductus venosus blood, together with a membranous valve in the right atrium (the crista dividens), prevents mixing of the well-oxygenated blood from the ductus venosus with the desaturated blood of the IVC. The ductus venosus stream passes across the right atrium through a physiological defect in the atrial septum called the foramen ovale, to the

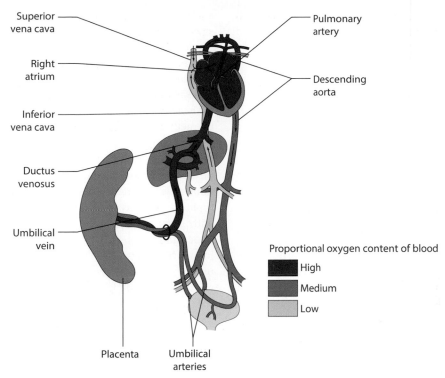

Figure 3.2 Diagrammatic representation of fetal circulation. (Adapted from Harrington K, Campbell S. *A Colour Atlas of Doppler Ultrasonography in Obstetrics*, London: Arnold, 1995.)

left atrium. From here, the blood passes through the mitral valve to the left ventricle and hence to the aorta. About 50% of the blood goes to the head and upper extremities, providing high levels of oxygen to supply the fetal heart, upper thorax and brain; the remainder passes down the aorta to mix with blood of reduced oxygen saturation from the right ventricle. Deoxygenated blood returning from the fetal head and lower body flows through the right atrium and ventricle and into the pulmonary artery, after which it bypasses the lungs to enter the descending aorta via the ductus arteriosus that connects the two vessels. Only a small portion of blood from the right ventricle passes to the lungs, as they are not functional. By this means, the desaturated blood from the right ventricle passes down the aorta to enter the umbilical arterial circulation and be returned to the placenta for reoxygenation.

Prior to birth, the ductus ateriosus remains patent due to the production of prostaglandin E2 and prostacyclin, which act as local vasodilators. Premature closure of the ductus arteriosus has been reported with the administration of cyclooxygenase inhibitors. At birth, the cessation of umbilical blood flow causes cessation of flow in the ductus venosus, a fall in pressure in the right atrium and closure of the foramen ovale. Ventilation of the lungs opens the pulmonary circulation, with a rapid fall in pulmonary vascular resistance, which dramatically increases the pulmonary circulation. The ductus arteriosus closes functionally within a few days of birth.

Occasionally, this transition from fetal to adult circulation is delayed, usually because the pulmonary vascular resistance fails to fall despite adequate breathing. This delay, termed persistent fetal circulation, results in left-to-right shunting of blood from the aorta through the ductus arteriosus to the lungs. The baby remains cyanosed and can suffer from life-threatening hypoxia. This delay in closure of the ductus arteriosus is most commonly seen in infants born preterm (<37 weeks' gestation). It results in congestion in the pulmonary circulation and a reduction in blood flow to the gastrointestinal tract and brain, and is implicated in the pathogenesis of necrotizing enterocolitis and intraventricular haemorrhage, both of which are complications associated with preterm birth.

Central nervous system

Neural development is one of the earliest systems to begin and one of the last to be completed during pregnancy, generating the most complex structure within the fetus. The early central nervous system (CNS) begins as a simple neural plate that folds to form a groove then tube, open initially at each end. Failure of these opening to close contributes a major class of neural abnormalities called neural tube defects (NTDs) (See Chapter 5, Prenatal diagnosis). Later development of the fetal brain involves elaborate folding of the neurocortex that occurs from the second half of pregnancy. There is a rapid increase in total grey matter in the last trimester that is mainly due to a fourfold increase in cortical grey matter.

Respiratory system

The lung first appears as an outgrowth from the primitive foregut at about 3–4 weeks postconception and by 4–7 weeks epithelial tube branches and vascular connections are forming. By 20 weeks the conductive airway tree and parallel vascular tree is well developed. By 26 weeks, with further development of the airway and vascular tree, type I and II epithelial cells are beginning to differentiate. Pulmonary surfactant, a complex mixture of phospholipids and proteins that reduces surface tension at the air–liquid interface of the alveolus, is produced by the type II cells starting from about 30 weeks. Dilatation of the gas exchanging airspaces, alveolar formation and maturation of the surfactant system continues between this time and delivery at term. The fetal lung is filled with fluid, the production of which starts in early gestation and ends in the early stages of labour. At birth, the production of this fluid ceases and the fluid present is absorbed. Adrenaline, to which the pulmonary epithelium becomes increasingly sensitive towards term, appears to play a major role in this process. With the clearance of the fluid and with the onset of breathing, the resistance in the vascular bed falls and results in an increase in pulmonary blood flow. A consequent increased pressure in the left atrium leads to closure of the foramen ovale.

Pulmonary surfactant prevents the collapse of small alveoli during expiration by lowering surface tension. The predominant phospholipid in surfactant (80% of the total) is phosphatidylcholine (lecithin), the production of which is enhanced by cortisol, growth restriction and prolonged rupture of the membranes, and is delayed in maternal diabetes mellitus. Inadequate amounts of surfactant result in poor lung expansion and poor gas exchange. In infants delivering preterm, prior to the maturation of the surfactant system, this results in a condition known as respiratory distress syndrome (RDS). It typically presents within the first few hours of life with signs of respiratory distress, including tachypnoea and cyanosis. It occurs in more than 80% of infants born between 23 and 27 weeks, falling to 10% of infants born between 34 and 36 weeks. Acute complications include hypoxia and asphyxia, intraventricular haemorrhage and necrotizing enterocolitis. The incidence and severity of RDS can be reduced by administering steroids antenatally to mothers at risk of preterm delivery. The steroids cross the placenta and stimulate the premature release of stored fetal pulmonary surfactant in the fetal alveoli.

Numerous, but intermittent, fetal breathing movements occur *in utero*, especially during rapid eye movement (REM) sleep. By opposing lung recoil, fetal breathing movements (FBM) help to maintain the high level of lung expansion that is now known to be essential for normal growth and structural maturation of the fetal lungs. During 'apnoeic' periods between successive episodes of FBM, active laryngeal constriction has the effect of opposing lung recoil by resisting the escape of lung liquid via the trachea. The prolonged absence or impairment of FBM is likely to result in a reduced mean level of lung expansion that can lead to hypoplasia of the lungs. An adequate amniotic fluid volume is also necessary for normal lung maturation. Oligohydramnios (reduced amniotic fluid volume), decreased intrathoracic space (e.g. diaphragmatic hernia) or chest wall deformities can result in pulmonary hypoplasia, which leads to progressive respiratory failure from birth.

Alimentary system

The primitive gut is present by the end of the fourth week, having been formed by folding of the embryo in both craniocaudal and lateral directions, with the resulting inclusion of the dorsal aspect of the yolk sac into the intraembryonic coelom. The primitive gut consists of three parts, the foregut, midgut and hindgut, and is suspended by a mesentery through which the blood supply, lymphatics and nerves reach the gut parenchyma. The foregut endoderm gives rise to the oesophagus, stomach, proximal half of the duodenum, liver and pancreas. The midgut endoderm gives rise to the distal half of the duodenum, jejunum, ileum, caecum, appendix, ascending colon and the transverse colon. The hindgut endoderm develops into the descending colon, sigmoid colon and the rectum.

Between 5 and 6 weeks, probably due to the lack of space in the abdominal cavity as a consequence of the rapidly enlarging liver and elongation of the intestine, the midgut is extruded into the umbilical cord as a physiological hernia. While herniated into the umbilical cord, the gut undergoes rotation prior to re-entering the abdominal cavity by 12 weeks of gestation. Failure of the gut to re-enter the abdominal cavity results in the development of an omphalocele (otherwise called an exomphalos) and this condition is associated with chromosomal anomaly (**Figure 3.3**).

Other malformations include those that result from failure of the normal rotation of the gut, fistulae and atresias. Malrotation anomalies can result in volvulus and bowel obstruction. Atresias exist when there is a segment of bowel in which the lumen is not patent and most commonly occur in the upper gastrointestinal tract (i.e. the oesophagus or duodenum). As the fetus continually swallows amniotic fluid, any obstruction that prevents fetal swallowing or passage of amniotic fluid along the gut will result in the development of polyhydramnios (excess amniotic fluid). Gastrointestinal fistulae can also occur, the most common being a tracheo-oesophageal fistula (TOF) (**Figure 3.4**), in which a connection exists between the distal end of the oesophagus and the trachea. Without surgical intervention the neonate can develop complications after birth as breathing causes air to pass from the trachea to the oesophagus and stomach, and feeding results in swallowed milk and stomach acid passing into the lungs. Some babies with TOF also have other congenital anomalies. This is known as VACTERL (vertebral, anal, cardiac, tracheal, (o)esophageal, renal and limb).

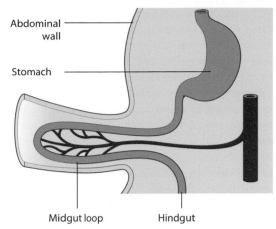

Figure 3.3 Midgut herniation.

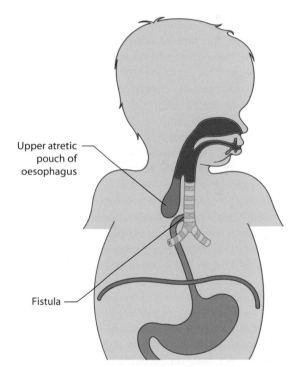

Figure 3.4 Tracheo-oesophageal fistula.

Peristalsis in the intestine occurs from the second trimester. The large bowel is filled with meconium at term. Defecation *in utero*, and hence meconium in the amniotic fluid, is associated with post-term pregnancies and fetal hypoxia. Aspiration of meconium-stained liquor by the fetus at birth can result in meconium aspiration syndrome and respiratory distress.

In the last trimester of pregnancy while body water content gradually diminishes, glycogen and fat stores increase about fivefold. Preterm infants have virtually no fat and a severely reduced ability to withstand starvation. This is aggravated by an incompletely developed alimentary system, and may manifest in a poor and unsustained suck, uncoordinated swallowing mechanism, delayed gastric emptying and poor absorption of carbohydrates, fat and other nutrients. Growth-restricted fetuses also have reduced glycogen stores and are therefore more prone to hypoglycaemia within the early neonatal period.

Liver, pancreas and gall bladder

The pancreas, liver and epithelial lining of the biliary tree derive from the endoderm of the foregut. The liver and biliary tree appear late in the third week or early in the fourth week as the hepatic diverticulum, which is an outgrowth of the ventral wall of the distal foregut. The larger portion of this diverticulum gives rise to the parenchymal cells (hepatocytes) and the hepatic ducts, while the smaller portion gives rise to the gall bladder.

By the sixth week, the fetal liver performs haematopoiesis. This peaks at 12–16 weeks and continues until approximately 36 weeks.

In utero, the normal metabolic functions of the liver are performed by the placenta. For example, unconjugated bilirubin from haemoglobin breakdown is actively transported from the fetus to the mother, with only a small proportion being conjugated in the liver and secreted in the bile (the mechanism after birth). The fetal liver also differs from the adult organ in many processes; for example, the fetal liver has a reduced ability to conjugate bilirubin because of relative deficiencies in the necessary enzymes such as glucuronyl transferase. After birth, the loss of the placental route of excretion of unconjugated bilirubin, in the presence of reduced conjugation, particularly in the premature infant, may result in transient unconjugated hyperbilirubinaemia or physiological jaundice of the newborn.

Glycogen is stored within the liver in small quantities from the first trimester, but storage is maximal in the third trimester, with abundant stores being present at term. Growth-restricted and premature infants have deficient glycogen stores; this renders them prone to neonatal hypoglycaemia.

Kidney and urinary tract

The kidney, recognized in its permanent final form (metanephric kidney), is preceded by the development and subsequent regression of two primitive forms; the pronephros and mesonephros. The pronephros originates at about 3 weeks in a ridge that forms on either side of the midline in the embryo, known as the nephrogenic ridge. In this region, epithelial cells arrange themselves in a series of tubules and join laterally with the pronephric duct. The pronephros is non-functional in mammals.

Each pronephric duct grows towards the tail of the embryo. As it does so it induces intermediate mesoderm in the thoracolumbar area to become epithelial tubules called mesonephric tubules. The pronephros degenerates while the mesonephric (Wolffian) duct extends towards the most caudal end of the embryo, ultimately attaching to the cloaca.

During the fifth week of gestation the ureteric bud develops as an out-pouching from the Wolffian duct. This bud grows towards the head of the embryo and into the intermediate mesoderm and as it does so it branches to form the collecting duct system (ureter, pelvis, calyces and collecting ducts) of the kidney and induces the formation of the renal secretory system (glomeruli, convoluted tubes, loops of Henle). Subsequently the lower portions of the nephric duct will migrate caudally (downward) and connect with the bladder, thereby forming the ureters. As the fetus develops, the torso elongates and the kidneys rotate and migrate upwards within the abdomen, which causes the length of the ureters to increase.

Failure of the normal migration of the kidney upwards can result in a pelvic kidney, where it remains in the pelvic area. Abnormal development of the collecting duct system can result in duplications such as duplex kidneys. The most common sites of congenital urinary tract obstructive uropathies are at the pyelouretic junction, the vesicoureteric junction or as a consequence of posterior urethral valves, an obstructing membrane in the posterior male urethra (**Figure 3.5**). Severe obstruction *in utero* can lead to hydronephrosis and renal interstitial fibrosis.

In humans, all of the branches of the ureteric bud and the nephronic units have been formed by 32–36 weeks' gestation. However, these structures are not yet mature, and the maturation of the excretory and

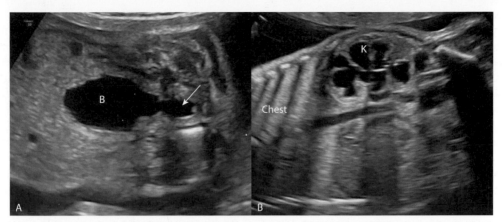

Figure 3.5 Posterior urethral valves. **(A)** The typical 'keyhole' sign in the fetal bladder (B), where the dilated upper posterior urethra is indicated (white arrow); **(B)** dilatation of the collecting system of the fetal kidney (K).

concentrating ability of the fetal kidneys is gradual and continues after birth. In the preterm infant this may lead to abnormal water, glucose, sodium or acid–base homeostasis.

As fetal urine forms much of the amniotic fluid, renal agenesis will result in severe reduction (oligohydramnios) or absence of amniotic fluid (anhydramios). Babies born with bilateral renal agenesis (Potter's syndrome), which is associated with other features such as widely spaced eyes, small jaw and low set ears, results that are secondary to oligohydramnios, do not pass urine and usually die either as a consequence of 'renal failure' or pulmonary hypoplasia, again secondary to severe oligohydramnios.

Skin and homeostasis

Fetal skin protects and facilitates homeostasis. The skin and its appendages (nails, hair) develop from the ectodermal and mesodermal germ layers. The epidermis develops from the surface ectoderm; the dermis and the hypodermis, which attaches the dermis of the skin to underlying tissues, both develop from mesenchymal cells in the mesoderm.

By the fourth week following conception, a single-cell layer of ectoderm surrounds the embryo. At about 6 weeks this ectodermal layer differentiates into an outer periderm and an inner basal layer. The periderm eventually sloughs as the vernix, a creamy protective coat that covers the skin of the fetus. The basal layer produces the epidermis and the glands, nails and hair follicles.

Over the ensuing weeks, the epithelium becomes stratified and by 16–20 weeks all layers of the epidermis are developed and each layer assumes a structure characteristic of the adult. Preterm babies have no vernix and thin skin; this allows a proportionately large amount of insensible water loss. Thermal control in cool, ambient temperatures is limited by a large surface-to-body weight ratio and poor thermal insulation. Heat may be conserved by peripheral vasoconstriction and can be generated by brown fat catabolism, but this is deficient in preterm or growth-restricted babies because of the small amount of subcutaneous fat and immaturity of vascular tone regulation in the former. The response to warm ambient temperatures is also poor and can result in overheating of the infant.

Hair follicles begin to develop as hair buds between 12 and 16 weeks from the basal layer of the epidermis. By 24 weeks the hair follicles produce delicate fetal hair called lanugo, first on the head and then on other parts of the body. This lanugo is usually shed before birth.

Blood and immune system

Red blood cells and immune effector cells are derived from pluripotent haematopoietic cells, first noted in the blood islands of the yolk sac. By 8 weeks the yolk sac is replaced by the liver as the source of these cells and by 20 weeks almost all of these cells are produced by the bone marrow.

The development of the thymus and the secondary lymphoid organs is a highly ordered process that undergoes a rapid expansion in the first trimester of pregnancy and appears to be largely finished by the time of birth. T-cell precursors transit to the thymus by 9 weeks of gestation and mature naïve and memory αβ T cells are readily found by 12–14 weeks in spleen and lymph nodes; circulating mature T cells are present by 16 weeks of gestation. In the second trimester, the fetal tissues have an increased frequency of regulatory T cells, more than at any other time in fetal, neonatal or adult development, and this is important for the induction of specific tolerance. Complement proteins are present by the middle of the second trimester and reach 50% of adult levels at term. Lymphoid precursor cells develop into B-lymphocytes, detected in the fetal liver at 8 weeks of gestation and appear in fetal blood circulation by 12 weeks of gestation. They undergo subsequent functional maturation in secondary lymphoid tissue (e.g. lymph nodes and spleen). Immunoglobulin somatic hypermutation and class switch recombination occur already during intrauterine life, although much of the immunoglobulin (Ig) G in the fetus originates from the maternal circulation and crosses the placenta to provide passive immunity to the fetus and neonate. The fetus normally produces only small amounts of IgM and IgA, which do not cross the placenta. Detection of IgM/IgA in the newborn, without IgG, is indicative of fetal infection.

Most haemoglobin in the fetus is fetal haemoglobin (HbF), which has two gamma-chains (alpha-2, gamma-2). This differs from the adult haemoglobins HbA and HbA2, which have two beta-chains (alpha-2, beta-2) and two delta-chains (alpha-2, delta-2), respectively. Ninety percent of fetal haemoglobin is HbF between 10 and 28 weeks gestation. From 28 to 34 weeks, a switch to HbA occurs, and at term the ratio of HbF to HbA is 80:20; by 6 months of age, only 1% of haemoglobin is HbF. A key feature of HbF is a higher affinity for oxygen than HbA. This, in association with a higher haemoglobin concentration (at birth, the mean capillary haemoglobin is 18 g/dl), enhances transfer of oxygen across the placenta.

Abnormal haemoglobin production results in thalassaemia. The thalassaemias are a group of genetic haematological disorders characterized by reduced or absent production of one or more of the globin chains of haemoglobin. Beta-thalassaemia results from reduced or absent production of the beta-globin chains. As the switch from HbF to HbA described above occurs, the absent or insufficient beta-globin chains shorten red cell survival, with destruction of these cells within the bone marrow and spleen. Beta-thalassaemia major results from the inheritance of two abnormal beta genes; without treatment, this leads to severe anaemia, FGR, poor musculoskeletal development and skin pigmentation due to increased iron absorption. In the severest form of alpha-thalassaemia, in which no alpha-globin chains are produced, severe fetal anaemia occurs with cardiac failure, hepatosplenomegaly and generalized oedema. The infants are stillborn or die shortly after birth.

Endocrine system

Major components of the hypothalamic–pituitary axis are in place by 12 weeks gestation. Thyrotrophin-releasing hormone (TRH) and gonadotrophin-releasing hormone (GnRH) have been identified in the fetal hypothalamus by the end of the first trimester. Testosterone produced by the interstitial cells of the testis is also synthesized in the first trimester of pregnancy and increases to 17–21 weeks, which mirrors the differentiation of the male urogenital tract. Growth hormone is similarly present from early pregnancy and detectable in the circulation from 12 weeks. The thyroid gland produces T4 from 10 to 12 weeks. Growth-restricted fetuses exist in a state of relative hypothyroidism, which may be a compensatory measure to decrease metabolic rate and oxygen consumption.

Behavioural states

From conception, the fetus follows a developmental path with milestones that continue into childhood. The first activity is the beating of the fetal heart followed by fetal movements at 7–8 weeks. These start as just discernable movements and graduate through startles to movements of arms and legs, breathing movements and by 12 weeks yawning, sucking and swallowing. This means that in the first trimester of pregnancy the fetus exhibits movements that are observed after birth. Further maturation does not add new movements but a change in respect of combinations of movements and activity that reflect fetal behavioural states. In the second trimester, for example, cycles of absence or presence of movements change, meaning that periods over which body movements are absent increase.

Four fetal behavioural states have been described, annotated 1F–4F. 1F is quiescence, 2F is characterized by frequent and periodic gross body movements with eye movements, 3F no gross body movements but eye movements and 4F vigorous continual activity again with eye movements. 1F is similar to quiet or non-REM sleep in the neonate, 2F to REM sleep, 3F to quiet wakefulness and 4F active wakefulness. An understanding of fetal behaviour can assist in assessing fetal condition and wellbeing.

Amniotic fluid

By 12 weeks' gestation, the amnion comes into contact with the inner surface of the chorion and the two membranes become adherent, but never intimately fuse. Neither the amnion nor the chorion contains vessels or nerves, but both do contain a significant quantity of phospholipids as well as enzymes involved in phospholipid hydrolysis. Choriodecidual function is thought to play a pivotal role in the initiation of labour through the production of prostaglandins E2 and F2a.

The amniotic fluid is initially secreted by the amnion, but by the 10th week it is mainly a transudate of the fetal serum via the skin and umbilical cord.

From 16 weeks' gestation, the fetal skin becomes impermeable to water and the net increase in amniotic fluid is through a small imbalance between the contributions of fluid through the kidneys and lung fluids and removal by fetal swallowing. The amniotic fluid contains growth factors as well as multipotent stem cells, the function of which at present is unknown. Amniotic fluid volume increases progressively (10 weeks: 30 ml; 20 weeks: 300 ml; 30 weeks: 600 ml; 38 weeks: 1,000 ml), but from term there is a rapid fall in volume (40 weeks: 800 ml; 42 weeks: 350 ml). The reason for the late reduction has not been explained. The amniotic fluid index is calculated as the total measurement of the deepest pool in the four quadrants of the uterus (**Figure 3.6**).

The function of the amniotic fluid is to:

- Protect the fetus from mechanical injury.
- Permit movement of the fetus while preventing limb contracture.
- Prevent adhesions between fetus and amnion.
- Permit fetal lung development in which there is two-way movement of fluid into the fetal bronchioles; absence of amniotic fluid in the second trimester is associated with pulmonary hypoplasia.

Major alterations in amniotic fluid volume occur when there is reduced contribution of fluid into the amniotic sac in conditions such as renal agenesis, cystic kidneys or FGR; oligohydramnios results.

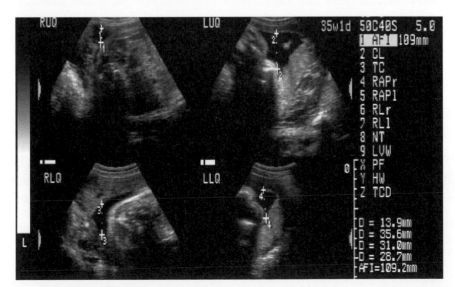

Figure 3.6 Amniotic fluid measurement and normal ranges.

Reduced removal of fluid in conditions such as congenital neuromuscular disorders, anencephaly and oesophageal/duodenal atresia that prevent fetal swallowing is associated with polyhydramnios.

 KEY LEARNING POINTS

- Determinants of birthweight are multifactorial, and reflect the influence of the natural growth potential of the fetus and the intrauterine environment.
- The fetal circulation is quite different from that of the adult. Its distinctive features are:
  - oxygenation occurs in the placenta, not the lungs;
  - the right and left ventricles work in parallel rather than in series;
  - the heart, brain and upper body receive blood from the left ventricle, while the placenta and lower body receive blood from both right and left ventricles.
- Surfactant prevents collapse of small alveoli in the newborn lung during expiration by lowering surface tension. Its production is maximal after 28 weeks.
- RDS is common in babies born prematurely and is associated with surfactant deficiency.
- The fetus requires an effective immune system to resist intrauterine and perinatal infections. Lymphocytes appear from 8 weeks and, by the middle of the second trimester, all phagocytic cells, T and B cells and complement are available to mount a response.
- Fetal skin protects and facilitates homeostasis.
- *In utero*, the normal metabolic functions of the liver are performed by the placenta. The loss of the placental route of excretion of unconjugated bilirubin, in the face of conjugating enzyme deficiencies, particularly in the premature infant, may result in transient unconjugated hyperbilirubinaemia or physiological jaundice of the newborn.
- Growth-restricted and premature infants have deficient glycogen stores; this renders them prone to neonatal hypoglycaemia.
- The function of the amniotic fluid is to:
  - protect the fetus from mechanical injury;
  - permit movement of the fetus while preventing limb contracture;
  - prevent adhesions between fetus and amnion;
  - permit fetal lung development in which there is two-way movement of fluid into the fetal bronchioles; absence of amniotic fluid in the second trimester is associated with pulmonary hypoplasia.

Further reading

Moore KL *et al.* (2015). *The Developing Human: Clinically Oriented Embryology*, 10 Edition. Saunders ISBN-10: 0323313388.

Self assessment

CASE HISTORY 1

A 26-year-old is admitted to the labour ward at 32 weeks' gestation. She gives a history suggestive of preterm rupture of membranes and is experiencing uterine contractions. On abdominal examination the fetus is in cephalic presentation. On vaginal examination, there is clear liquor draining, the cervix is found to be 8 cm dilated and she rapidly goes on to have an uncomplicated vaginal delivery of a male infant weighing 1,650 g. At birth he is intubated because of poor respiratory effort and transferred to the neonatal intensive care unit.

As a premature infant, from which complications is he particularly at risk?

ANSWER

Fetal growth

Deficient glycogen stores in the liver increase the risk of hypoglycaemia. This is compounded by the increased glucose requirements of premature infants.

Cardiovascular system

Patent ductus arteriosus may result in pulmonary congestion, worsening lung disease and decreased blood flow to the gastrointestinal tract and brain. The duct can be closed by administering prostaglandin synthetase inhibitors, for example indomethacin, or by surgical ligation.

Respiratory system

RDS and apnoea of prematurity may lead to hypoxia. The administration of antenatal steroids to the mother reduces the risk and severity of RDS. For maximal benefit to be gained, steroids need to be administered at least 24 hours before delivery. In this case, delivery occurred too rapidly for steroids to be administered. The severity of RDS can also be reduced by giving surfactant via the endotracheal tube used to ventilate the baby.

Fetal blood

Anaemia of prematurity is common because of low iron stores and red cell mass at birth, reduced erythropoiesis and decreased survival of red blood cells. Treatment is by blood transfusion, iron supplementation or, in some cases, the use of erythropoietin.

Immune system

Preterm babies have an increased susceptibility to infection due to impaired cell-mediated immunity and reduced levels of immunoglobulin. Suspected infection should be treated early with antibiotics because deterioration in these premature small infants can be rapid.

Skin and homeostasis

Hypothermia is common in preterm infants secondary to a relatively large body surface area, thin skin, lack of subcutaneous fat and lack of a keratinized epidermal layer of skin. High insensible water losses due to skin immaturity may aggravate dehydration and electrolyte problems secondary to immaturity in renal function (see below). The environment can be controlled by nursing this type of infant in an incubator.

Alimentary system

Necrotizing enterocolitis is an inflammatory condition of the bowel leading to necrosis, and is thought to be secondary to alterations in gut blood flow, hypotension, hypoxia, infection and feeding practices. Feeding problems are common in preterm infants because they have immature suck and swallowing reflexes and gut motility. Parenteral nutrition is usually required in these very premature infants, with gradually increasing volumes of milk given by nasogastric tube.

Liver and gall bladder

Jaundice (hyperbilirubinaemia) secondary to liver immaturity and a shorter half-life of red blood cells is common in premature infants. Treatment with phototherapy is required because premature infants are at greater risk of bilirubin encephalopathy.

Kidney and urinary tract

Immaturity of the kidneys can lead to a poor ability to concentrate or dilute urine. This can result in dehydration and electrolyte disturbances: hypernatraemia and hyponatraemia, hyperkalaemia and metabolic acidosis.

Central nervous system

Periventricular and intraventricular haemorrhages result from bleeding from the immature rich capillary bed of the germinal matrix lining the ventricles. Such haemorrhages are more likely in the presence of hypoxia. Major degrees of haemorrhage can result in hydrocephalus and neurological abnormalities such as cerebral palsy. Periventricular leukomalacia is ischaemic necrosis in the white matter surrounding the lateral ventricles, and commonly leads to cerebral palsy.

CASE HISTORY 2

A 16-year-old is admitted to the labour ward at 38 weeks' gestation. She gives a history suggestive of rupture of membranes with meconium staining and is experiencing uterine contractions. She was seen at 10 weeks' gestation for consideration of termination of pregnancy and had a scan at that time that confirmed her gestational age. She opted to continue with the pregnancy but did not attend for antenatal care. She admitted to smoking 20 cigarettes per day. Abdominal examination shows the fetus is in cephalic presentation. The SFH measurement is 30 cm. Vaginal examination confirms that the cervix is 8 cm dilated. A cardiotocograph demonstrates a baseline fetal heart rate of 170 bpm with persistent variable decelerations for more than 30 minutes, and fetal scalp pH is 7.14 with a base deficit of 12 mmol/l. A category 1 emergency caesarean section is performed and a male infant weighing 1,900 g is delivered within 20 minutes of the decision. Apgar scores are 3 at 1 minute and 8 at 5 minutes. The placental histology confirms patchy hypoplasia of the distal villous tree and a number of villous infarcts suggesting chronic placental pathology. From which complications are such severely growth-restricted infants particularly at risk?

ANSWER

Reduced oxygen supply *in utero* can result in the fetus being stillborn or suffering damage from acute asphyxia. In the latter case, the neonate may demonstrate features of HIE, which may lead to death from multiorgan failure. If the infant survives, neurological damage and cerebral palsy may result. Chronic hypoxia *in utero* can also result in neurological damage without the acute manifestations of HIE. Other consequences of reduced oxygen supply *in utero* include increased haemopoiesis and cardiac failure. Increased haemopoiesis can in turn result in coagulopathy, polycythaemia and jaundice in the newborn. Neonatal hypothermia and hypoglycaemia are also more common in this type of infant and result from reduced body fat and glycogen stores. Both of these conditions, if untreated, can lead to increased mortality and neurological damage.

Reduced supply of amino acids *in utero* can impair immune function, increasing the risk of infection in the newborn.

Growth-restricted babies are also at increased risk of chronic diseases such as coronary heart disease, stroke, hypertension and non-insulin-dependent diabetes in adulthood. This is thought to be because the fetal adaptation to undernutrition *in utero* results in the permanent resetting of homeostatic mechanisms, and this leads to later disease.

CASE HISTORY 3

A 24 year old nulliparous woman had a detailed fetal anomaly ultrasound scan at 20 weeks' gestation. This showed reduced amniotic fluid index (2 cm) and an enlarged, thick-walled bladder and a dilated urethra with a 'keyhole' sign, bilateral hydroureternephrosis (dilated ureter and renal pelvis) and bilateral echogenic kidneys. The fetus was a male. There were no other fetal structural abnormalities. The findings at the dating scan at 12 weeks had been apparently normal. She had no family or personal history of renal problems. What is the likely diagnosis and what is the prognosis?

ANSWER

The likely diagnosis is posterior urethral valves, which is the most common congenital cause of bladder outflow obstruction in male neonates. This occurs in 1 in 5,000 live male births and is caused by an obstructing membrane in the posterior male urethra as a result of abnormal *in utero* development. The differential diagnosis includes urethral atresia and bilateral vesicoureteric reflux. The majority of cases are suspected prenatally and referred to specialist centres at birth.

Early prenatal diagnosis (before 24 weeks' gestation), ultrasound evidence of echogenic renal parenchyma and reduced amniotic fluid volume have been identified as predictors of a poor prognosis, as in this case. Prenatal interventions such as percutaneous ultrasound-guided vesicocentesis (drainage of the bladder) can be used to relieve the obstruction temporarily. Ultrasound-guided placement of a vesicoamniotic shunt (between the bladder and the amniotic cavity) seems to improve perinatal survival. Whether this treatment or conservative management is used, however, the surviving children have a high rate of end-stage renal failure requiring dialysis and transplantation. The condition accounts for 25–30% of paediatric renal transplantations in the UK.

CASE HISTORY 4

A 30-year-old multiparous woman is referred to the Fetal Medicine Unit because the midwife is concerned about the size of the uterus during a routine antenatal check at 30 weeks' gestation. The SFH measures 38 cm. Down's syndrome screening by the combined test gave a low risk (1 in 20,000). On ultrasound examination, the fetal measurements are on the 80th centile. There is increased amniotic fluid with a single deepest pool of 8.97 cm (normal range <8 cm) and amniotic fluid index 35 cm (normal range <25 cm). Fetal movements and fetal umbilical artery and middle cerebral artery Doppler measurements are normal. In the transverse fetal abdominal views there was a double bubble seen on the left side of the abdomen (**Figure 3.7**). There were no other abnormalities detectable; in particular, the fetal face was normal. The placenta was anterior high and had a normal structural appearance.

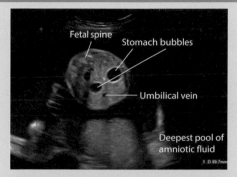

Figure 3.7 Ultrasound image showing the 'double bubble' appearance and polyhydramnios associated with duodenal atresia.

What is the most likely diagnosis and what are the differential diagnoses? What is the optimum management for the rest of the pregnancy and at birth?

ANSWER

Polyhydramnios occurs in approximately 1–1.5% of pregnancies. This is a case of mild polyhydramnios (single deepest pool of liquor 8–11 cm). An underlying disease is only found in 17% of cases in mild polyhydramnios. In contrast, an underlying disease is detected in 91% of cases in moderate (12–15 cm) to severe polyhydramnios (>15 cm). The most likely diagnosis is duodenal atresia, the congenital absence or complete closure of a portion of the lumen of the duodenum, which occurs in 1:2,500–5,000 live births. In 25–40% of cases there is associated trisomy 21 (Down's syndrome). The differential diagnosis includes:

- An obstructive structural malformation that prevents fetal swallowing (e.g. facial cleft or congenital high airways obstruction syndrome [CHAOS]) or prevents passage of amniotic fluid along the gut (e.g. oesophageal atresia).

- Congenital problems that prevent normal swallowing function (e.g. neurological structural problems such as anencephaly or neuromuscular disorders such as myotonic dystrophy).
- Fetal anaemia (e.g. due to Rh incompatibility, or virus infection such as with parvovirus B19); usually there are other associated findings such as pleural effusion or ascites.
- Multiple pregnancies; particularly those with a monochorionic placenta.
- Maternal diabetes.

Management of a case of polyhydramnios includes a detailed fetal anomaly scan to observe fetal movements and structures, counselling about the risk of trisomy 21 and an offer of fetal karyotyping by amniocentesis, glucose tolerance test for maternal diabetes and a maternal antibody blood test for virus infections.

In this case the patient declined amniocentesis. She was seen antenatally by the paediatric surgeons to discuss surgical management postnatally. She was counselled about the risk of spontaneous preterm labour, preterm premature rupture of the membranes, abnormal fetal presentation and cord prolapse in labour. She was monitored by scan every 2 weeks; the amniotic fluid index remained the same and she had only mild uterine activity. She did not require amnioreduction (amniocentesis to drain off excessive fluid). She presented in labour at 36 weeks' gestation with the fetus in cephalic presentation and had a normal vaginal delivery. The neonate weighing 3.7 kg was born with good Apgar scores and he was transferred to the neonatal intensive care unit for monitoring. At 1 day of age he underwent laparoscopic duodenostomy for duodenal atresia and had a good recovery.

EMQ

The factors or diagnoses below may be associated with abnormal fetal growth and development.

A Gestational diabetes.

B Maternal cocaine abuse.

C Maternal BMI of 43.

D Parvovirus infection.

E Maternal chronic kidney disease.

F Early-onset pre-eclampsia.

For each description, choose the SINGLE most appropriate answer from the list of options. Each option may be used once, more than once or not at all.

1 A woman at 36 weeks' gestation whose fetal abdominal circumference has increased from her anomaly scan to be above the 95th centile, but whose fetal head circumference has maintained on the 50th centile since her anomaly scan.

2 A woman at 32 weeks' gestation whose fetus is symmetrically small with an EFW on the 5th centile for gestation.

3 A woman who presents with a placental abruption at 32 weeks' gestation.

4 A woman at 28 weeks' gestation whose fetus is hydropic on ultrasound.

5 A woman at 28 weeks' gestation whose fetus has an EFW over the 95th centile.

6 A woman at 32 weeks' gestation whose fetus has a preserved head circumference on the 25th centile, but whose abdominal circumference and femur length are on the 5th centile.

ANSWERS

1A Gestational diabetes. Gestational diabetes is associated with fetal macrosomia. The abdominal circumference increases, reflecting increased glycogen deposition in the fetal liver and increased abdominal adipose tissue formation, whereas the bony parameters of the fetal head tend to remain within normal limits.

2E Maternal chronic kidney disease. Maternal chronic kidney disease is often associated with maternal chronic hypertension and both conditions, alone or together, are associated with early-onset fetal growth restriction, which is typically characterized by the presence of a symmetrically small fetus from the late second or early third trimester.

3B Maternal cocaine abuse. The rate of abruption in patients who abuse cocaine is significantly increased. Hypertension and increased level of catecholamines, caused by exposure to cocaine and thought to cause acute vasospasm in the uterine blood vessels, leads to placental separation and abruption.

4D Maternal parvovirus infection. Maternal parvovirus infection is usually mild and occasionally subclinical. In the fetus, however, it causes aplastic anaemia that in turn leads to high-output cardiac failure and fetal hydrops.

5C Maternal BMI of 43. Maternal obesity is associated with an increased incidence of gestational diabetes. Even in the absence of gestational diabetes, obese mothers have a significant risk of larger babies.

6F Early-onset pre-eclampsia. Asymmetric fetal growth restriction, characterized by decreased abdominal and long bone measurements but with 'head sparing', is typically caused by uteroplacental insufficiency and this commonly copresents with pre-eclampsia, particularly preterm.

SBA QUESTION

Anhydramnios is associated with which of the following? Choose the single best answer.

A Gestational diabetes.

B Fetal renal agenesis.

C Fetal cleft lip and palate

D Multiple pregnancy.

E Fetal oesophageal atresia.

ANSWER

B Fetal renal agenesis. Polyhydramnios (excessive amniotic fluid) is associated with gestational diabetes, fetal oesophageal atresia (an obstruction that prevents amniotic fluid from passing down the fetal gut) and fetal cleft lip and palate (prevents normal fetal swallowing function). In monochorionic multiple pregnancy there may be oligohydramnios of one twin and polyhydramnios of the cotwin when twin-to-twin transfusion occurs, but anhydramnios is uncommon.

Assessment of fetal wellbeing

ANNA L DAVID

LEARNING OBJECTIVES

- To understand the principles of imaging in obstetrics, its safety and benefits for examining the fetus during gestation.
- To know how ultrasound is used in pregnancy to confirm gestational age, to detect fetal structural abnormalities, to monitor fetal growth and development, to study the placenta and to assess fetal wellbeing.

- To recognize the value of antenatal cardiotocography (CTG) to assess fetal wellbeing and to screen for fetal hypoxia.
- To be aware of the role of Doppler ultrasound to monitor and guide the management of pregnancies at risk of adverse outcomes.

Introduction

Ultrasound is the principal imaging modality used in obstetrics. Indeed, diagnostic ultrasound is used to screen all pregnancies in most high- and middle-income countries. Ultrasound is used to date pregnancies, to monitor growth of the fetus and to identify congenital abnormalities. Colour and spectral Doppler are used to interrogate the uterine, placental and fetal blood vessels, providing information on uteroplacental function and the fetal wellbeing and its circulatory response to hypoxia and anaemia, for example.

Antenatal tests of fetal wellbeing are now principally based on ultrasound techniques and are designed to identify fetuses that are in the early or late stages of fetal hypoxia. Continuous wave Doppler ultrasound is employed in the cardiotocograph (CTG) to provide continuous tracings of the fetal heart rate, the patterns of which alter when the fetus is hypoxic.

Three-dimensional (3D) ultrasound and increasingly magnetic resonance imaging (MRI) are used to provide further information when a fetal abnormality is suspected.

Diagnostic ultrasound in obstetric practice

In 1959, Professor Ian Donald, the Regius Chair of Midwifery at Glasgow University, noted that clear echoes could be obtained from the fetal head using ultrasound. Since the reporting of this initial discovery, the technique of ultrasound has developed into one that now plays an essential role in the care of pregnant women.

The ultrasound technique uses very high frequency sound waves of between 3.5 and 7.0 MHz emitted from a transducer. Transducers can be placed and moved across the maternal abdomen (transabdominal, **Figure 4.1**) or mounted on a probe that can be inserted into the vagina (transvaginal, **Figure 4.2**).

Transvaginal ultrasonography is useful in early pregnancy, for examining the cervix later in pregnancy and for identifying the lower edge of the placenta. It is also useful in early pregnancy in women with significant amounts of abdominal adipose tissue through which abdominal ultrasound waves would need to travel, and hence be attenuated prior to reaching the uterus and its contents, making visualization difficult. In general, however, after 12 weeks' gestation, an abdominal transducer, which is a flat or curvilinear probe with a much wider array, is used. Crystals within the transducer emit a focused ultrasound beam in a series of pulses and then receive the reflected signals from within the uterus between the pulses. The strength of the reflected sound wave depends on the difference in 'acoustic impedance' between adjacent structures. The acoustic impedance of a tissue is related to its density; the greater the difference in acoustic impedance between two adjacent

tissues the more reflective will be their boundary. The returning signals are transformed into visual signals and generate a continuous picture of the moving fetus. Movements such as fetal heart beat and structures in the fetus can be assessed and measurements can be made accurately on the images displayed on the screen. Such measurements enable the assessment of gestational age, size and growth in the fetus. Ultrasound images obtained can also be processed with computer software to produce 3D images and even four-dimensional (4D, moving 3D images), which provide more detail on fetal anatomical structure and the identification of anomalies.

The use of Doppler ultrasound allows the assessment of the velocity of blood within fetal and placental vessels and provides indirect assessment of fetal and placental condition. Doppler ultrasound makes use of the phenomenon of the Doppler frequency shift, where the reflected wave will be at a different frequency from the transmitted one if it interacts with moving structures, such as red blood cells flowing along a blood vessel, with the change in frequency being proportional to the velocity of the blood cells. If the red blood cells are moving towards the beam, the reflected signal will be at a higher frequency than the transmitted one and conversely the reflected beam will be at a lower signal if the flow is away from the beam. In this modality, signals from a particular vessel can be isolated and displayed in graphic form, with the velocity plotted against time. The significance of changes observed in waveform patterns obtained from placental and fetal vessels, and how these observations can be used in clinical practice, will be discussed later in the chapter.

Ultrasound scanning is currently considered to be a safe, non-invasive, accurate and cost-effective investigation in the fetus. There are guidelines that cover the safe use of ultrasound in pregnancy. These include the ALARA (As Low As Reasonably Achievable) principle, a practice mandate adhering to the principle of keeping radiation doses to patients and personnel as low as possible. Examination times are kept as short as is necessary to produce a useful diagnostic result, particularly before 10 weeks' gestation when the embryo may be more sensitive to the effects of thermal and mechanical injury. This chapter will consider the diagnostic use of these techniques in more detail.

The main uses of ultrasonography in pregnancy are in the areas discussed below.

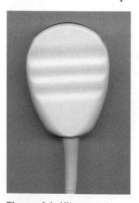

Figure 4.1 Ultrasound probe: abdominal.

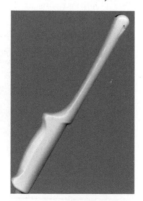

Figure 4.2 Ultrasound probe: transvaginal.

Diagnosis and confirmation of viability in early pregnancy

The gestational sac can be visualized from as early as 4–5 weeks' gestation and the yolk sac at about 5 weeks (**Figure 4.3**). The embryo can be observed and measured at 5–6 weeks' gestation. Beating of the fetal heart can be visualized by about 6 weeks.

Transvaginal ultrasound plays a key role in the diagnosis of disorders of early pregnancy, such as incomplete or missed miscarriage, blighted ovum where no fetus is present (**Figure 4.4**) and ectopic pregnancy. In a missed miscarriage, for example, the fetus can be identified, but with an absent fetal heartbeat. In a blighted ovum (or anembryonic pregnancy), there is a gestation sac present but it is empty because the fetus has failed to develop. An ectopic pregnancy is suspected if, in the presence of a positive pregnancy test, an ultrasound scan does not identify a gestation sac within the uterus, there is an adnexal mass with or without a fetal pole or there is fluid in the pouch of Douglas.

Determination of gestational age and assessment of fetal size and growth

Up to approximately 20 weeks' gestation the range of values around the mean for measurements of fetal length, head size and long bone length is narrow and hence assessment of gestation based on these measures is accurate. The crown–rump length (CRL) is used up to 13 weeks + 6 days, and the head circumference (HC) from 14 to 20 weeks' gestation. The biparietal diameter (BPD) (**Figure 4.5**) and femur length (FL) (**Figure 4.6**) can also be used to determine gestational age. Essentially, the earlier the measurement is made, the more accurate the prediction, and measurements made from an early CRL (accuracy of prediction 6 ± 5 days) will be preferred to a BPD at 20 weeks (accuracy of prediction 6 ± 7 days).

In the latter part of pregnancy, measuring fetal abdominal circumference (AC) (**Figure 4.7**) and HC will allow assessment of the size and growth of the fetus and will assist in the diagnosis and management of fetal growth restriction (FGR). In addition to AC and HC, BPD and FL, when combined in an equation, provide a more accurate estimate

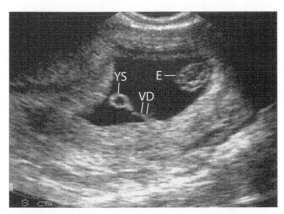

Figure 4.3 Ultrasound sac showing yolk sac (YS) and embryo (E) with the vitelline duct (VD).

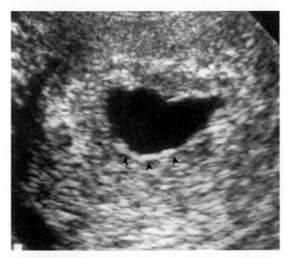

Figure 4.4 Ultrasound image showing empty gestation sac (arrowheads) in a case of blighted ovum.

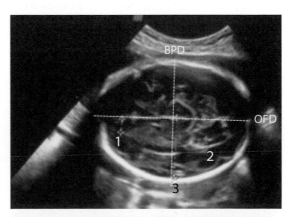

Figure 4.5 Biparietal diameter (BPD). 1, anterior ventricle; 2, posterior ventricle; 3, cerebral hemisphere. OFD, occipitofrontal diameter.

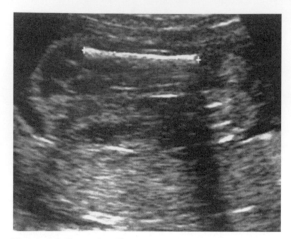

Figure 4.6 Femur length.

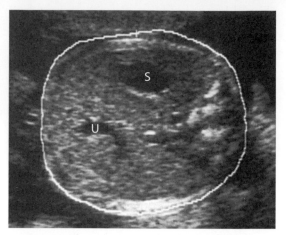

Figure 4.7 Abdominal circumference measurement demonstrating the correct section showing the stomach (S) and the umbilical vein (U).

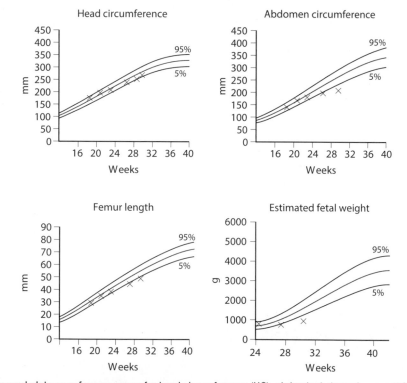

Figure 4.8 Ultrasound plots on reference range for head circumference (HC), abdominal circumference (AC) and estimated fetal weight in a case of early-onset fetal growth restriction (FGR). Note that HC remains above 5th centile while the AC falls below 5th centile. This is a case of asymmetric FGR with head sparing.

of fetal weight (EFW) than any of the parameters taken singly.

In pregnancies at high risk of FGR, serial measurements are plotted on the normal reference range. Growth patterns are helpful in distinguishing between different types of growth restriction (symmetrical and asymmetrical). Asymmetry between head measures (BPD, HC) and AC can be identified in FGR, where a brain-sparing effect will result in a relatively large HC compared with the AC (**Figure 4.8**). The opposite would occur in a diabetic pregnancy, where the abdomen is disproportionately large due to the effects of insulin on the fetal liver and fat stores. Cessation of growth is an ominous sign of placental failure.

Gestational age cannot be accurately calculated by ultrasound after 20 weeks' gestation because of the wider range of normal values of AC and HC around the mean.

Multiple pregnancy

Ultrasound is now the most common way in which multiple pregnancies are identified (**Figure 4.9**). In addition to identifying the presence of more than one fetus, it is used to determine the chorionicity of the pregnancy, which is important in stratifying the risk of particularly pregnancy complications.

Monochorionic twin pregnancies (i.e. those who 'share' a placenta) are associated with an increased risk of pregnancy complications such as twin-to-twin transfusion syndrome and a higher perinatal mortality rate than dichorionic twin pregnancies. It is therefore clinically useful to be able to determine chorionicity early in pregnancy (see Chapter 7, Multiple pregnancy).

The dividing membrane between monochorionic twins is formed by two layers of amnion and in dichorionic twins the dividing membrane consists of two layers of chorion and two of amnion. Dichorionic twin pregnancies therefore have a thicker dividing membrane than monochorionic

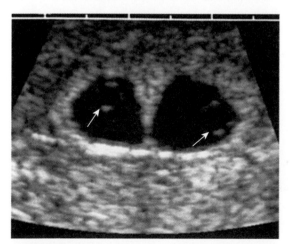

Figure 4.9 Early twin dichorionic pregnancy (arrows); note the 'peaked' inter-twin membrane.

twin pregnancies and this can be perceived qualitatively on ultrasound. Sonographically, dichorionic twin pregnancies in the first trimester of pregnancy have a thick inter-twin separating membrane (septum), flanked on either side by a very thin amnion. This is in contrast to a monochorionic twin pregnancy, which on 2D ultrasound has a very thin inter-twin septum.

Another method of determining chorionicity in the first trimester uses the appearance of the septum at its origin from the placenta. On ultrasound, a tongue of placental tissue is seen within the base of dichorionic membranes and has been termed the 'twin peak' or 'lambda' sign (**Figure 4.9**). The optimal gestation at which to perform such ultrasonic chorionicity determination is 9–10 weeks. Dichorionicity may also be confirmed by the identification of two placental masses and later in pregnancy by the presence of different-sex fetuses.

Ultrasound is also invaluable in the management of twin pregnancy in terms of confirming fetal presentations, which may be difficult on abdominal palpation, evidence of growth restriction, fetal anomaly and the presence of placenta praevia, all of which are more common in this type of pregnancy, and any suggestion of twin-to-twin transfusion syndrome.

Diagnosis of fetal abnormality

Major fetal structural abnormalities occur in 2–3% of pregnancies and many can be diagnosed by an ultrasound scan at around or before 20 weeks' gestation. Increasingly as ultrasound technology improves, these abnormalities are being detected at the first trimester 'dating' scan. Common examples include spina bifida and hydrocephalus, skeletal abnormalities such as achondroplasia, abdominal wall defects such as exomphalos and gastroschisis, cleft lip/palate and congenital cardiac abnormalities (see Chapter 3, Normal fetal development and growth). When a fetal structural abnormality is detected, the woman may be referred to a fetal medicine specialist for further advice about prognosis and management.

Detection rates of between 40 and 90% have been reported at the 20-week 'anomaly' scan. This means that a 'normal scan' is not a guarantee of a normal baby. A number of factors can influence the success of detecting an abnormality. Some are very difficult to visualize or to be absolutely certain about. Some conditions, for example hydrocephalus, may not have been obvious at the time of early scans. Neuronal migration disorders that affect cerebral development may not manifest until the third trimester. Women should be informed of the limitations of routine ultrasound screening and that detection rates vary by the type of fetal anomaly, the woman's body mass index and the position of the unborn baby at the time of the scan. The position of the baby in the uterus will influence visualization of organs such as the heart, face and spine. Repeat scans are sometimes required if visualization is a problem in anticipation that the fetus will be in a more accessible position.

Some obstetric ultrasound findings are considered variants of normal but are noteworthy because they also increase the risk for underlying fetal aneuploidy such as Down's syndrome. These findings are known as 'soft markers' and are considered distinct from fetal structural malformations. Detection of first trimester ultrasonic 'soft' markers for chromosomal abnormalities, such as the absence of fetal nasal bone and an increased fetal nuchal translucency (NT) (the area at the back of the neck), are now in common use to enable detection of fetuses at risk of chromosomal anomalies such as Down's syndrome (see Chapter 5, Prenatal diagnosis). On the routine anomaly scan, detection of an increased nuchal fold (>6 mm) or two or more soft markers should prompt referral to a fetal medicine specialist for advice.

Placental localization

Placenta praevia, a placenta that is inserted wholly or in part into the lower segment of the uterus, can cause life-threatening haemorrhage in pregnancy. Ultrasonography has become indispensible in the localization of the site of the placenta. Ultrasonographic identification of the lower edge of the placenta to exclude or confirm placenta praevia as a cause for antepartum haemorrhage is now a part of routine clinical practice. The transvaginal approach, undertaken with caution, can be helpful in clearly identifying the lower placental edge if it is not seen clearly with an abdominal probe.

At the 20 weeks scan, it is customary to identify women who have a low-lying placenta. At this stage, the lower uterine segment has not yet formed and most low-lying placentas will appear to 'migrate' upwards as the lower segment stretches in the late second and third trimesters. About 15–20% of women have a low-lying placenta at 20 weeks, and only 10% of this group will eventually be shown to have a placenta praevia.

Amniotic fluid assessment

Ultrasound can be used to identify both increased and decreased amniotic fluid volumes. The fetus has a role in the control of the volume of amniotic fluid. It swallows amniotic fluid, absorbs it in the gut and later excretes urine into the amniotic sac. Congenital abnormalities that either structurally or functionally impair the fetus's ability to swallow, for example oesophageal atresia or anencephaly, will result in an increase in amniotic fluid. Congenital abnormalities that result in a failure of urine production or passage, for example renal agenesis and posterior urethral valves, will result in reduced or absent amniotic fluid. FGR can be associated with reduced amniotic fluid because of reduced renal perfusion and hence urine output. Variation from the normal range of amniotic fluid volume calls for a further detailed ultrasound assessment of possible causes.

Assessment of fetal wellbeing

Ultrasound can be used to assess fetal wellbeing by evaluating fetal movements, tone and breathing in the biophysical profile. Doppler ultrasound can be used to assess placental function and identify evidence of blood flow redistribution in the fetus, which is a sign of hypoxia. These aspects of ultrasound use will be discussed later in the chapter.

Measurement of cervical length

Evidence suggests that approximately 50% of women who deliver before 34 weeks' gestation will have a short cervix at the midtrimester of pregnancy. Cervical length is best measured using a transvaginal probe that allows accurate identification of the internal and external os (see Chapter 8, Preterm labour). Current National Institute for Health and Care Excellence (NICE) guidance (NICE Guidelines NG25: Preterm labour and birth) recommends serial cervical length assessment from 16 weeks' gestation in those women with a history of spontaneous preterm birth or midtrimester loss.

Kidney and urinary tract

Ultrasonography is also of value in other obstetric conditions such as:

- Confirmation of intrauterine death.
- Confirmation of fetal presentation in uncertain cases.
- Diagnosis of uterine and pelvic abnormalities during pregnancy, for example fibromyomata and ovarian cysts.

Ultrasound schedule in clinical practice

NICE recommends that all pregnant women should be offered scans at between 10 and 14 weeks' and 18 and 21 weeks' gestation (Antenatal Care for Uncomplicated Pregnancies, 2008). The first trimester scan is principally to determine gestational age, to detect multiple pregnancies and to determine NT as part of screening for Down's syndrome. The 18–21-week scan primarily screens for structural anomalies, giving couples reproductive choice (e.g. termination of pregnancy vs. continuing with the pregnancy) and allowing antenatal care and delivery to be planned, including intrauterine therapy if available. Evidence suggests that routine ultrasound in early pregnancy appears to enable better gestational age assessment, earlier detection of multiple pregnancies and earlier detection of clinically unsuspected fetal malformation at a time when termination of pregnancy is possible. In uncomplicated pregnancies, scans are only performed after this stage in pregnancy if there is a clinical indication, such as concern about fetal growth or wellbeing, discussed later in the chapter. Additional ultrasound examinations, particularly for fetal growth and wellbeing, are offered to women who are identified as needing additional antenatal care (NICE Antenatal Care overview), for example those who had problems during a previous pregnancy or who have pre-existing maternal disease.

Ultrasound in the assessment of fetal wellbeing

Amniotic fluid volume

The amount of amniotic fluid in the uterus is a guide to fetal wellbeing in the third trimester. The influence of congenital abnormalities on amniotic fluid volume in early pregnancy has already been described.

A reduction in amniotic fluid volume is referred to as 'oligohydramnios' and an excess is referred to as 'polyhydramnios'. Definitions of oligohydramnios and polyhydramnios are based on sonographic criteria. Two ultrasound measurement approaches give an indication of amniotic fluid volume. These are maximum vertical pool and amniotic fluid index.

The maximum vertical pool is measured after a general survey of the uterine contents. Measurements of less than 2 cm suggest oligohydramnios, and measurements of greater than 8 cm suggest polyhydramnios.

The amniotic fluid index (AFI) is measured by dividing the uterus into four 'ultrasound' quadrants. A vertical measurement is taken of the deepest pool of fluid that is free of umbilical cord in each quadrant and the results summated. The AFI alters throughout gestation, but in the third trimester it should be between 10 and 25 cm; values below 10 cm indicate a reduced volume and those below 5 cm indicate oligohydramnios, while values above 25 cm indicate polyhydramnios.

Amniotic fluid volume is decreased in FGR as a consequence of redistribution of fetal blood away from the kidneys to vital structures such as the brain and heart, with a consequent reduction in renal perfusion and urine output.

The cardiotocograph

The cardiotocograph (CTG) is a continuous tracing of the fetal heart rate used to assess fetal wellbeing, together with an assessment of uterine activity. Cardiotocography is sometimes called electronic fetal monitoring (EFM). The CTG recording is obtained with the pregnant woman positioned comfortably in a left lateral or semi-recumbent position to avoid compression of the maternal vena cava. Two external transducers are placed on the mother's abdomen, each attached with a belt. One transducer is a pressure-sensitive contraction tocodynometer (stretch gauge) that measures the pressure required to flatten a section of the abdominal wall. This correlates with the internal uterine pressure and indicates if there is any uterine activity (contractions). The second transducer uses ultrasound and the Doppler effect to detect motion of the fetal heart, and measures the interval between successive beats, thereby allowing a continuous assessment of fetal heart rate. Recordings are then made for at least 30 minutes with the output from the CTG machine producing two 'lines' traced onto a running piece of paper, one a tracing of fetal heart rate and a second a tracing of uterine activity. The mother may be given a button to press to record any fetal movements that she has felt. In addition, the CTG machine may record fetal movements detected via the tocodynometer.

Important CTG features

Fetal cardiac behaviour is regulated through the autonomic nervous system and by vasomotor, chemoceptor and baroreceptor mechanisms. Pathological events, such as fetal hypoxia, modify these signals and hence cardiac response including variation in heart rate patterns, which can be detected and recorded in the CTG. Features that are reported from a CTG to define normality and identify abnormality and potential concern for fetal wellbeing include the:

- Baseline rate.
- Baseline variability.
- Accelerations.
- Decelerations.

Each of these is discussed further below. Interpretation of the CTG must be in the context of any risk factors, for example suspected FGR or fetal anaemia, and all features must be considered in order to make a judgment about the likelihood of fetal compromise.

Baseline fetal heart rate

The normal fetal heart rate at term is 110–150 beats per minute (bpm). Higher rates are defined as fetal tachycardia and lower rates as fetal bradycardia. The baseline fetal heart rate falls with advancing gestational age as a result of maturing fetal parasympathetic tone and, prior to term, 160 bpm is taken as the upper limit of normal. The baseline rate is best determined over a period of 5–10 minutes. Fetal tachycardias can be associated with maternal or fetal infection, acute fetal hypoxia, fetal anaemia and drugs such as adrenoceptor agonists, for example ritodrine.

Baseline variability

Under normal physiological conditions, the interval between successive fetal heart beats (beat-to-beat) varies. This is called 'short-term variability' and increases with increasing gestational age. It is not visible on a standard CTG but can be measured with computer-assisted analysis. In addition to these beat-to-beat variations in heart rate, there are longer-term fluctuations in heart rate occurring between two and six times per minute. This is known as 'baseline variability'. Normal baseline variability reflects a normal fetal autonomic nervous system. Baseline variability is considered abnormal when it is less than 10 bpm (**Figure 4.10**). As well as gestational age, baseline variability is modified by fetal sleep states and activity, and also by hypoxia, fetal infection and drugs suppressing the fetal central nervous system, such as opioids, and hypnotics (all of which reduce baseline variability). As fetuses display deep sleep cycles of 20–30 minutes at a time, baseline variability may be normally reduced for this length of time, but should be preceded and followed by a period of normal baseline variability on the CTG trace.

Fetal heart rate accelerations

These are increases in the baseline fetal heart rate of at least 15 bpm, lasting for at least 15 seconds. The presence of two or more accelerations on a 20–30-minute antepartum fetal CTG defines a reactive trace and is indicative of a non-hypoxic fetus (i.e. they are a positive sign of fetal health).

Fetal heart rate decelerations

These are transient reductions in fetal heart rate of 15 bpm or more, lasting for more than 15 seconds. Decelerations can be indicative of fetal hypoxia or

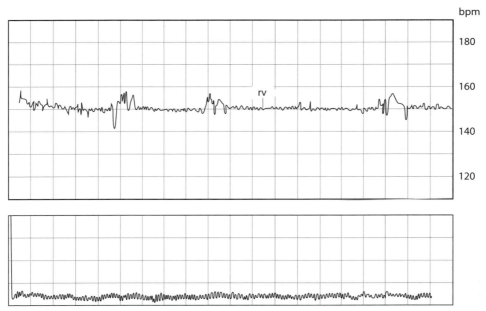

Figure 4.10 A fetal cardiotocograph showing a baseline of 150 bpm but with reduced variability (rv).

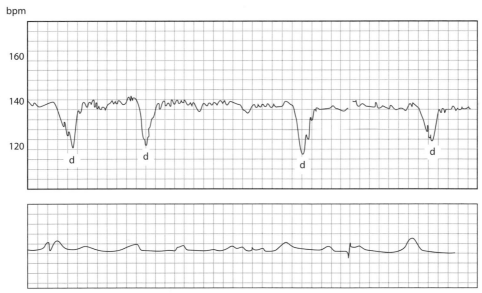

Figure 4.11 An admission cardiotocograph from a term pregnancy. Although the baseline fetal heart rate is normal, there is reduced variability, an absence of fetal heart rate accelerations and multiple decelerations (d). The decelerations were occurring after uterine tightening and are therefore termed 'late'.

umbilical cord compression. There is a higher chance of fetal hypoxia being present if there are additional abnormal features such as reduced variability or baseline tachycardia (**Figure 4.11**).

From the above descriptions, a normal antepartum fetal CTG can therefore be defined as a baseline of 110–150 bpm, with baseline variability exceeding 10 bpm, and with more than one acceleration being seen in a 20–30 minute tracing. Reduced baseline variability, absence of accelerations and the presence of decelerations are all suspicious features. A suspicious CTG must be interpreted within the

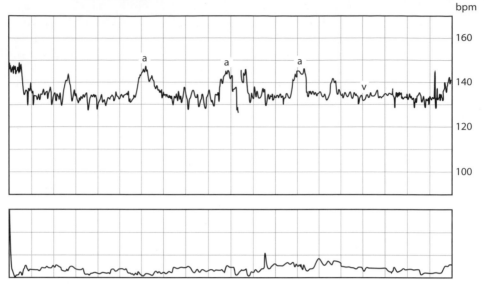

Figure 4.12 A normal fetal cardiotocograph showing a normal rate, normal variability (v) and the presence of several accelerations (a).

clinical context. If many antenatal risk factors have already been identified, a suspicious CTG may warrant delivery of the baby, although where no risk factors exist, a repeated investigation later in the day may be more appropriate (**Figure 4.12**).

The computerized cardiotocograph

Standard CTG has a high intra- and interobserver variability. The basis of fetal CTG is pattern recognition, and this leads to differences in interpretation amongst different clinicians. Computerized CTG interpretation is objective and more consistent than standard CTG interpretation, and there are normal ranges for computerized CTG parameters available throughout gestation. Fetal heart rate variation is the most useful predictor of fetal wellbeing in small for gestational age (SGA) fetuses, and a short-term variation ≤3 ms (within 24 hours of delivery) has been associated with a higher rate of metabolic acidaemia and early neonatal death.

Computerized CTG interpretation packages have been shown to be equal (or superior) to human interpretation in differentiating normal from abnormal outcome. Compared to standard CTG, a Cochrane review found that use of computerized CTG was associated with a reduction in perinatal mortality.

Biophysical profile

In an effort to refine the ability of fetal CTG to identify antenatal hypoxia, investigators have looked at additional fetal parameters such as fetal breathing movements (movements of the fetal chest) (FBMs), gross body movements, flexor tone and accelerations in fetal heart rate related to movements, all of which are reduced or absent when the fetus is hypoxic. A biophysical profile (BPP) (**Figure 4.13**) includes four acute fetal variables: FBMs, fetal gross

Parameter	Score 2	Score 0
Non-stress cardiotocograph	Reactive	Fewer than two accelerations in 40 minutes
Fetal breathing movements	≥30 movements in 30 minutes	Fewer than 30 seconds of fetal breathing in 30 minutes
Fetal body movements	≥3 movements in 30 minutes	Two of fewer gross body movements in 30 minutes
Fetal tone	One episode of limb flexion	No evidence of fetal movement or flexion
Amniotic fluid volume	Large cord-free pocket of fluid over 1 cm	Less than 1cm pocket of fluid

Figure 4.13 Biophysical profile scoring system.

body movement, fetal tone and CTG and amniotic fluid volume. A score of either 2 (normal) or 0 (suboptimal) is assigned to each of the variables, to give an individual fetus a total score of between 0 and 10. A score of 0, 2 or 4 is considered abnormal and a score of 8 or 10 normal. A score of 6 is equivocal and requires repeat within a reasonable timescale (hours) to exclude a period of fetal sleep as a cause.

Early observational studies suggested that delivery at a score of less than 6 was associated with a lower perinatal mortality than in similar high-risk pregnancies in which BPPs were not performed. However, a systematic review of the effectiveness of BPP as a surveillance tool in high-risk pregnancies (five studies, testing 2,974 fetuses) found that the use of BPP was not associated with a reduction in perinatal deaths or Apgar scores <7 at 5 minutes.

There are a number of problems with the BPP that limit its utility. BPPs can be time consuming. Fetuses spend approximately 30% of their time asleep, during which they are not very active and do not exhibit breathing movements. It is therefore necessary to scan them for long enough (at least 30 minutes) to exclude this physiological cause of a poor score. Ultimately, however, by the time a fetus develops an abnormal score prompting delivery, it is likely to already be severely hypoxic. While delivery may reduce the perinatal death rate (death *in utero* or within the first week of life), it may not increase long-term survival and, in particular, survival without significant mental and physical impairment. There is currently insufficient evidence from randomized trials to support the use of BPP as a test of fetal wellbeing in high-risk pregnancies.

Doppler investigation

The principles of Doppler have already been discussed. Waveforms can be obtained from the umbilical and fetal vessels and the maternal uterine artery. Data obtained from the umbilical artery provide indirect information about placenta function, whereas data from the fetal vessels provide information on the fetal response to hypoxia. Doppler insonation of the uterine artery can be used to assess the degree of placental insufficiency (see Chapter 3, Normal fetal development and growth).

Umbilical artery

Waveforms obtained from the umbilical artery provide information on placental resistance to blood flow and hence indirectly placenta 'health' and function. An infarcted placenta secondary to maternal hypertension, for example, will have increased resistance to flow. A normal umbilical arterial waveform is shown in **Figure 4.14**. The plot is obtained using Doppler ultrasound of velocity of blood flow against time and demonstrates forward flow of blood throughout the whole cardiac cycle (i.e. both systole and diastole). A useful analogy to understand the concept of umbilical Doppler and placental resistance is to consider the umbilical artery as a hose carrying water towards a placenta, which in a healthy pregnancy will act like a sponge and in an infarcted placenta will act more like a brick wall. So, with a normal pregnancy, blood will flow through the placenta without difficulty like water from a hose directed at the sponge and will pass straight through the sponge. In a diseased placenta the blood will reflect back from the high resistance placenta like water from a hose being bounced back from the wall at which it is directed. In the normal pregnancy, the normal constant forward flow of blood in diastole will be seen, but in the diseased placenta flow during diastole may be reduced, absent or even reversed (**Figure 4.15**). Reversed end-diastolic flow effectively means that during diastole, there is flow of fetal blood away from the placenta and back to the fetus.

Most studies investigating the value of using this technique in clinical practice have looked at resistance to flow, which is indicated by the diastolic component. A reduced amount of diastolic flow implies high resistance downstream to the vessel being

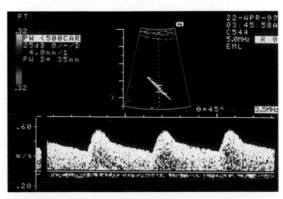

Figure 4.14 Normal umbilical arterial Doppler waveform.

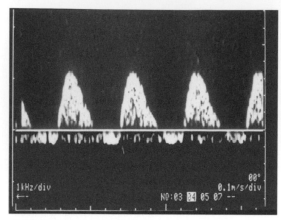

Figure 4.15 Reverse end-diastolic flow in the umbilical artery.

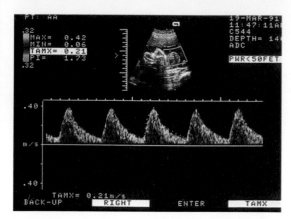

Figure 4.16 Reduced end-diastolic flow in umbilical artery compared to normal in 4.14.

studied and implies low perfusion (**Figure 4.16**). An increased diastolic flow indicates low resistance downstream and implies high perfusion. Doppler indices such as the pulsatility index or the resistance index are useful as they calculate the variability of blood velocity in a vessel, comparing the amount of diastolic flow relative to systolic flow. When these indices are high, there is high resistance to blood flow; when the indices are low, resistance to blood flow is low. Normally, diastolic flow in the umbilical artery increases (i.e. placental resistance falls) throughout gestation. Absent or reversed end-diastolic flow in the umbilical artery is a particularly serious development with a strong correlation with fetal hypoxia and intrauterine death.

An analysis of randomized controlled trials of the use of umbilical Doppler in high-risk pregnancy involving over 10,000 women found that compared to no Doppler ultrasound, the use of Doppler ultrasound in high-risk pregnancy (especially those complicated by hypertension, SGA or FGR) was associated with a reduction in perinatal deaths from 1.7% to 1.2%. There were also fewer inductions of labour and fewer admissions to hospital without reports of adverse effects. The use of Doppler ultrasound in high-risk pregnancies appears therefore to improve a number of obstetric care outcomes and reduces perinatal deaths.

Fetal vessels

Falling oxygen levels in the fetus lead to a redistribution of blood flow to 'essential' organs, such as the brain, heart and adrenal glands, from

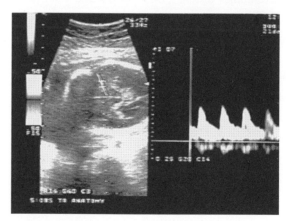

Figure 4.17 Middle cerebral artery Doppler showing increased diastolic flow with possible redistribution to brain in hypoxia.

'non-essential' organs where there is vasoconstriction. Several fetal vessels have been studied, and reflect this 'centralization' of flow, often called cerebral redistribution. As hypoxia increases the pulsatility index in the middle cerebral artery falls, indicating increasing diastolic flow as the cerebral circulation opens up (**Figure 4.17**). At the same time there is increased resistance in the fetal aorta reflecting compensatory vasoconstriction in the fetal body. Absent diastolic flow in the fetal aorta implies fetal acidaemia. Perhaps the most sensitive index of fetal acidaemia and incipient heart failure is demonstrated by increasing pulsatility in the central veins supplying the heart, such as the ductus venosus (DV) and inferior vena cava (IVC). The DV shunts a portion of the umbilical vein blood flow directly to the IVC and thence to the right atrium, allowing oxygenated blood from the placenta to bypass the fetal liver. The DV Doppler flow velocity therefore reflects atrial pressure–volume changes during the cardiac cycle. As FGR worsens there is a direct effect of hypoxia and acidaemia on cardiac function, leading to increased afterload and preload. This leads to a reduced velocity in the DV a-wave owing to increased end-diastolic pressure. A retrograde DV a-wave signifies the onset of overt cardiac compromise (**Figures 4.18, 4.19**), and delivery should be considered as fetal death is imminent.

Measurement of velocity of blood flow in the middle cerebral artery also gives an indicator of the presence of fetal anaemia. When the fetus is anaemic, the peak systolic velocity increases. This technique is particularly useful to assess the severity of Rhesus isoimmunization disease, and in twin-to-twin transfusion syndrome that results in anaemia in the donor twin.

Uterine artery

Doppler studies of the uterine artery during the first and early second trimester may be used to predict pregnancies at risk of adverse outcome, particularly pre-eclampsia. The proposed pathogenic model of pre-eclampsia is one of incomplete physiological invasion of the spiral arteries by the trophoblast, with a resultant increase in uteroplacental vascular resistance (see Chapter 9, Hypertensive disorders of pregnancy). This is reflected in the Doppler waveforms obtained from the maternal uterine artery circulation. Doppler ultrasound studies of the uterine arteries may demonstrate markers of increased resistance to flow including the diastolic 'notch' in the waveform (**Figure 4.20**) in early diastole, thought to result from increased vascular resistance in the uteroplacental vascular bed. High-resistance waveform patterns are associated with adverse outcomes, including pre-eclampsia, FGR and placental abruption. Sixty to seventy per cent of women at 20–24 weeks' gestation with bilateral notched uterine arteries will subsequently develop one or more of these complications. Consequently, such pregnancies will require close monitoring of fetal growth rate and increased surveillance for the possible development of maternal hypertension and proteinuria.

Uterine artery Doppler evaluation at 20–24 weeks' gestation can be used to stratify women with risk factors for a SGA baby, for example smoking, chronic hypertension, diabetes and vascular disease, previous SGA baby or stillbirth. Women with a normal uterine artery pulsatility index and normal waveform may be reassured that there is a low probability of an SGA birth. Serial ultrasound to assess fetal growth and umbilical artery Doppler for fetal wellbeing is recommended if the uterine artery Doppler assessment is abnormal.

Cerebroplacental ratio

The cerebroplacental Doppler ratio is a ratio of the pulsatility indices of the middle cerebral artery and the umbilical artery. It is emerging as an important predictor of adverse pregnancy outcome. Fetuses with an abnormal ratio that are appropriately grown for gestational age or have late-onset

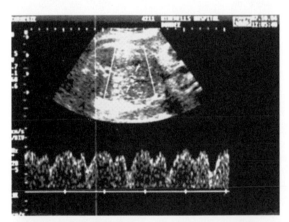

Figure 4.18 Normal ductus venosus Doppler waveform.

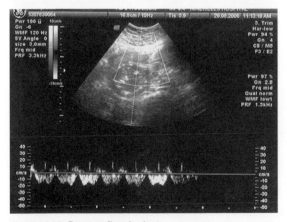

Figure 4.19 Reverse flow in ductus venosus.

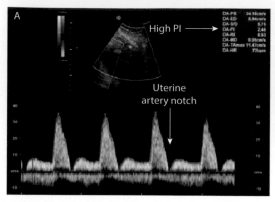 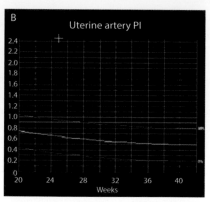

Figure 4.20 (**A**) Uterine artery waveform with diastolic notch, and (**B**) pulsatility index (PI) above 97th centile.

SGA (>34 weeks' gestation) have a higher incidence of abnormal intrapartum CTG requiring emergency caesarean delivery, a lower cord pH and an increased admission rate to neonatal intensive care unit when compared with fetuses with a normal ratio. In fetuses with early-onset SGA (<34 weeks' gestation), an abnormal ratio is associated with a lower birthweight, and an increased rate of adverse neonatal outcome and perinatal death when compared to a normal ratio.

Ultrasound and invasive procedures

Ultrasound is used to guide invasive diagnostic procedures such as amniocentesis, chorion villus sampling and cordocentesis, and therapeutic procedures such as the insertion of fetal bladder shunts or chest drains. If fetoscopy is performed, the endoscope is inserted under ultrasound guidance. This use of ultrasound has greatly reduced the possibility of fetal trauma, as the needle or scope is visualized throughout the procedure and guided with precision to the appropriate place.

3D and 4D ultrasound

3D and 4D ultrasound are mainly used as an adjunct to 2D ultrasound, either to interrogate fetal structures that may be difficult to visualize, such as the corpus callosum or fetal spine, or to demonstrate fetal structural abnormalities to the parents, for example cleft lip and palate.

KEY LEARNING POINTS

The aims of obstetric ultrasound include:
- The early pregnancy scan (11–14 weeks):
  - to confirm fetal viability;
  - to provide an accurate estimation of gestational age;
  - to diagnose multiple gestation, and in particular to determine chorionicity;
  - to identify markers that would indicate an increased risk of fetal chromosome abnormality such as Down's syndrome;
  - to identify fetuses with gross structural abnormalities.
- The 20 week scan (18–22 weeks):
  - to provide an accurate estimation of gestational age if an early scan has not been performed;
  - to carry out a detailed fetal anatomical survey to detect any fetal structural abnormalities or markers for chromosome abnormality;
  - to locate the placenta and identify women who have a low-lying placenta for a repeat scan at 34 weeks to exclude placenta praevia;
  - to estimate the amniotic fluid volume;
  - to perform Doppler ultrasound examination of maternal uterine arteries to screen for adverse pregnancy outcome, for example SGA;
  - to measure cervical length to assess the risk of preterm delivery where women have risk factors for spontaneous preterm birth.
- Ultrasound in the third trimester:
  - to assess fetal growth;
  - to assess fetal wellbeing.

Magnetic resonance imaging

MRI utilizes the effect of powerful magnetic forces on spinning hydrogen protons, which when knocked off their axis by pulsed radio waves, produce radio frequency signals as they return to their basal state. The signals reflect the composition of tissue (i.e. the amount and distribution of hydrogen protons) and thus the images provide significant improvement over ultrasound in tissue characterization. Ultrafast MRI techniques enable images to be acquired in less than 1 second to reduce the detrimental effect of fetal motion on image quality. Such technology has led to increased usage of fetal MRI, which provides multiplanar views, better characterization of anatomic details of, for example, the fetal brain, and information for planning the mode of delivery and airway management at birth. Fetal MRI is also being used to detect cerebral lesions after fetal interventions. For example, fetal brain MRI may be performed a few weeks after laser fetoscopic coagulation of placental anatomoses in twin-to-twin transfusion syndrome, to examine for acute cerebral ischaemic lesions.

Further reading

Alfirevic Z, Neilson JP (1996). Doppler ultrasound for fetal assessment in high risk pregnancies. *Cochrane Database of Systematic Reviews* 4:CD000073.
Lalor JG, Fawole B, Alfirevic Z, Devane D (2008). Biophysical profile for fetal assessment in high risk pregnancies. *Cochrane Database of Systematic Reviews* 1:CD000038.

Self assessment

CASE HISTORY

An 18-year-old in her first pregnancy attends for review at the antenatal clinic at 34 weeks' gestation. Her dates were confirmed by ultrasound at booking (12 weeks). She is a smoker. The midwife measures her fundal height at 30 cm. An ultrasound scan is performed because of the midwife's concern that the fetus is SGA, and the measurements are plotted in **Figure 4.21**.

A Do the ultrasound findings support the clinical diagnosis of SGA?

B What additional features/measures on ultrasound assessment could give an indication of fetal wellbeing?

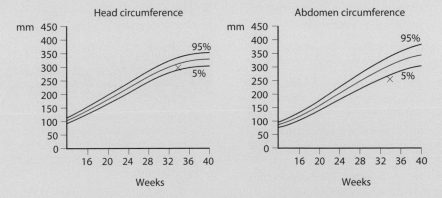

Figure 4.21 Plot of fetal head circumference and fetal abdominal circumference.

ANSWER

A   Yes, because the fetal AC is below the 5th centile for gestation. This finding does not give an indication of the wellbeing of the fetus and is compatible with FGR secondary to placental insufficiency or a healthy, constitutionally small baby.

B

Liquor volume

Amniotic fluid volume is decreased in FGR associated with fetal hypoxia where there may be redistribution of fetal blood flow away from the kidneys to vital structures such as the brain and heart, with a consequent reduction in renal perfusion and urine output.

Doppler ultrasound

Umbilical artery

Waveforms from the umbilical artery provide information on fetoplacental blood flow and placental resistance. Diastolic flow in the umbilical artery increases (i.e. placental resistance falls) throughout gestation. If the resistance index (RI) in the umbilical artery rises above the 95th centile of the normal graph, this implies poor perfusion of the placenta, which may eventually result in fetal hypoxia. Absent or reversed end-diastolic flow in the umbilical artery is a particularly serious development, with a strong correlation with fetal hypoxia and intrauterine death.

Fetal vessels

Falling oxygen levels in the fetus may lead to cerebral redistribution, diverting blood from the fetal body to the brain, heart, adrenals and spleen. The middle cerebral artery will show increasing diastolic flow as hypoxia increases, while a rising resistance in the fetal aorta reflects compensatory vasoconstriction in the fetal body. When diastolic flow is absent in the fetal aorta, this implies fetal acidaemia. Increasing pulsatility in the central veins supplying the heart, such as the DV and IVC, is an indicator of fetal acidaemia and impending heart failure; when late diastolic flow is absent in the ductus venosus, fetal death is imminent.

Cardiotocography

Fetal tachycardia, reduced variability in heart rate, absence of accelerations and presence of decelerations identified on a CTG are associated with fetal hypoxia.

EMQ

These ultrasound investigations may be of use in fetal monitoring.

A   Transvaginal cervical length measurement.
B   Ultrasound assessment of fetal growth.
C   Middle cerebral artery Doppler examination.
D   Uterine artery Doppler examination.
E   CTG.
F   BPP.
G   'Kick chart'.
H   Umbilical artery Doppler.

For each description, choose the SINGLE most appropriate answer from the list of options. Each option may be used once, more than once or not at all.

1   A woman with previous severe pre-eclampsia presents at 22 weeks concerned about her risk of recurrence. Her anomaly scan was normal.

2   A woman at 16 weeks who spontaneously delivered in her last pregnancy at 26 weeks' gestation.

3   A woman at 28 weeks has been exposed to parvovirus and the baby is hydropic.

4   A woman at 36 weeks has a symphysis–fundal height of 32 cm.

5   A woman at 34 weeks has had a growth scan showing that the estimated fetal weight is on the 5th centile for gestation. She presents a week later with reduced fetal movements.

ANSWERS

1D Uterine artery Doppler examination. Uterine artery Doppler will allow the risk of recurrent pre-eclampsia to be estimated.

2A Transvaginal cervical length measurement. If her cervical length is short, her risk of recurrent spontaneous preterm birth may be reduced by interventions such as progesterone or a cervical cerclage.

3C Middle cerebral artery Doppler examination. The hydropic fetus is probably anaemic. This can be confirmed by measurement of the middle cerebral artery peak systolic velocity in the fetus. If it is above the 95th centile for gestational age, this would indicate a very high chance of fetal anaemia. At this gestation an ultrasound-guided fetal cord blood transfusion would be the best treatment rather than delivery. Hydrops will have been diagnosed already on ultrasound. If performed the CTG is likely to be abnormal.

4B Ultrasound assessment of fetal growth. This is the most accurate way to measure fetal size. A CTG will tell us only about immediate fetal wellbeing.

5E CTG. CTG will best inform as to the immediate wellbeing of the fetus. Umbilical artery Doppler would be helpful but is not the first-line test to be done in this situation. Middle cerebral artery Doppler provides information on the fetal response to the presumed placental insufficiency, but alone will not be as useful as a CTG. Assessment of the CPR may also be helpful but not immediately.

SBA QUESTION

Which of the following are not used as indicators of fetal wellbeing beyond 24 weeks of pregnancy? Choose the single best answer.

A CTG.

B Fetal lie.

C Fetal movements.

D FBMs.

E Umbilical artery Dopplers.

ANSWER

B Fetal lie. All of the other parameters are used to indicate fetal wellbeing. CTG is used antenatally to screen for fetal hypoxia. Reduced or absent fetal movements and FBMs are associated with fetal hypoxia. Umbilical artery Doppler ultrasound examination detects the resistance of the placental circulation to perfusion, by measurement of the pulsatility index and assessing the degree of blood flow at the end of fetal diastole.

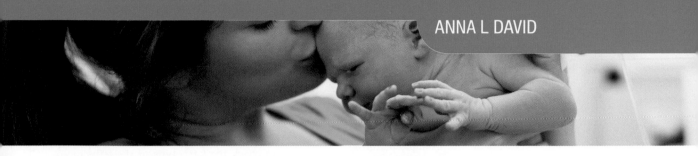

Prenatal diagnosis

ANNA L DAVID

LEARNING OBJECTIVES

- To understand why prenatal diagnosis is performed and what conditions can be tested for in the fetus.
- To be aware of the invasive prenatal diagnostic tests that can be performed, their risks and benefits.
- To appreciate how to appropriately counsel a woman and her partner who are considering having an invasive prenatal diagnostic test.

- To know the various screening tests that are used to predict the risk of a woman having a pregnancy affected by Down's syndrome.
- To learn about newer non-invasive methods of prenatal diagnosis based on measurement of cell-free fetal DNA in the maternal circulation.

Introduction

Prenatal diagnosis is the identification of a disease in the fetus prior to birth. This chapter will discuss why prenatal diagnostic tests may be performed and the types of non-invasive and invasive tests that are available. It will discuss factors that should be taken into consideration prior to offering testing, and emphasizes the importance of good communication with women and multidisciplinary working.

Why is prenatal diagnostic testing performed?

Prenatal diagnosis is usually performed because something leads to the suspicion of disease in the fetus being present. For example:

- Family history – genetic disease with a known recurrence risk.
- Past obstetric history – RhD alloimmunization.

- Serum screening tests – trisomy 21.
- Ultrasound screening – 12 week dating or 20 week anomaly scan.

Prenatal diagnosis frequently follows a prenatal screening test, whether this is simply the history taking at the booking visit or a more formal screening test such as those offered for Down's syndrome, haemoglobinopathies or ultrasound screening.

Attributes of a screening test:

- Relevance – the condition screened for must be relevant and important.
- Effect on management – alternative management options must be available, for example planning therapy or offering termination of an affected pregnancy.
- Sensitivity – the test must have a high detection rate for the condition.
- Specificity – the test must exclude the vast majority who do not have the condition.
- Predictive value – the test must predict accurately who does, and who does not have the condition.
- Affordability – the test should be cheap enough to be cost effective.
- Equity – the test should be available to all.

Classification

Prenatal diagnostic tests can be divided into non-invasive tests and invasive tests. The main non-invasive test is the use of ultrasound scanning to screen for structural fetal abnormalities, such as neural tube defects, gastroschisis, cystic adenomatoid malformation of lung, renal abnormalities (*Table 5.1*).

Maternal blood can be tested for exposure to viruses (viral serology). If a woman has no immunoglobulin (Ig) G or IgM for a particular virus early in pregnancy, but then develops IgM and IgG later in pregnancy, it suggests that she has had a clinical or subclinical infection with that virus earlier during pregnancy. Maternal blood is usually only tested if features on ultrasound are suggestive of infection having occurred, for example hydrops or ventriculomegaly, or if there

is a history of exposure to a particular virus, for example parvovirus.

Cell-free fetal DNA (cffDNA) can be extracted from maternal blood to determine fetal blood group in cases of RhD alloimmunization, to determine the sex of the fetus in X-linked disorders, or to diagnose skeletal dysplasias such as achondroplasia. There is much interest in using next-generation sequencing analysis of cffDNA in maternal blood for non-invasive prenatal diagnosis of aneuploidy and of monogenic disorders such as the haemoglobinopathies.

Amniocentesis and chorion villus sampling (CVS) are the two most common invasive tests and are used to check the karyotype of the fetus or to diagnose single gene disorders. These tests carry a small risk of miscarriage, therefore the risk of being affected by the condition and the seriousness of the condition should be severe enough to warrant taking the risk. Rarely, cordocentesis is used as an invasive diagnostic test.

Frequently, non-invasive tests and invasive tests are used together. The ultrasound scan may diagnose a structural problem in the fetus such as a congenital diaphragmatic hernia, but since congenital diaphragmatic hernias are associated with underlying chromosomal abnormalities, an invasive prenatal diagnostic test would then be offered.

Table 5.1 Examples of conditions and their method of diagnosis

Diagnostic test	Condition
Ultrasound diagnosis	Neural tube defect Gastroschisis Cystic adenomatoid malformation of lung Twin-to-twin transfusion syndrome
Invasive test – CVS or amniocentesis	Down's syndrome Cystic fibrosis Thalassaemia
Invasive test – cordocentesis	Alloimmune thrombocytopaenia
Ultrasound then invasive test	Congenital diaphragmatic hernia Exomphalos Ventriculomegaly Duodenal atresia

CVS, chorion villus sampling.

Invasive testing

Pretest counselling

Invasive tests are most frequently performed to diagnose aneuploidy, for example Down's syndrome or genetic conditions such as cystic fibrosis or thalassaemia. Women choose to have, or not to have, invasive testing. This is an important decision which may have lifelong consequences and therefore must be a decision that is fully informed.

For a clinician to discuss the option of invasive testing in a meaningful way with a woman, the clinician should know:

- The condition suspected and its severity so that the woman can assess the effect that having a child with this disorder would have on her and her family.
- That the history is correct – involvement of colleagues from the Clinical Genetics Department is often invaluable.
- An accurate assessment of the risk of an affected fetus – again colleagues from the Clinical Genetics Department may be helpful.
- That a test is available – sometimes the mutation has not been found.
- What sample is needed, and how it should be processed.
- The accuracy and limitations of the particular laboratory test being performed, including culture failure rates and reporting times.
- Acceptability – some women feel that they cannot accept the small risk of miscarriage.
- Whether it is ethical – some genetic mutations may not carry a significant risk of serious disability for an individual, and yet it is possible to offer prenatal diagnosis for them, for example sickle cell disease.

Prior to the test, the clinician should also discuss with the women what options would be available to her if the test result shows that the fetus is affected with the condition. This is an important part of the decision-making process. There is often little point doing an invasive test if it will not be of benefit to the woman or her baby.

The three options available are usually to:

1 Continue – the information from the test may facilitate plans for care around the time of delivery, or may help the woman and her family prepare for the birth of a baby with a serious condition.
2 Influence the decision to terminate the pregnancy.
3 Terminate, but provide information which may prove useful when counselling about recurrence risks in future pregnancies.

Some women decline invasive testing as they feel that it would not provide them with useful information, and would put them at risk of miscarriage. To ensure informed consent, the clinician needs to be certain that the woman understands the procedure, why it is being offered and the risks, limitations and subsequent management options. The clinician also needs to be sure that the woman is not under duress from others such as her family, community or religious groups. It is good practice to complete a consent form as a formal record that the discussion has taken place.

Invasive prenatal procedures should not be carried out without reviewing available bloodborne virus screening tests such as human immuno-deficiency virus (HIV) and hepatitis. If these are declined or unavailable the woman should be counselled about the potential risk of vertical transmission of infection to the fetus.

Chorion villus sampling (also known as chorion villus biopsy)

Fetal trophoblast cells in the mesenchyme of the villi divide rapidly in the first trimester. A CVS procedure aims to take a sample of these rapidly dividing cells from the developing placenta. This is done either by passing a needle under ultrasound guidance through the abdominal wall and myometrium into the placenta (**Figure 5.1A**), or by passing a fine catheter (or biopsy forceps) through the cervix into the placenta (**Figure 5.1B**).

The woman is scanned initially:

- To confirm that the pregnancy is viable prior to the procedure.
- To ensure that it is a singleton pregnancy (prenatal diagnosis in multiple pregnancy is more complex).
- To confirm gestational age (CVS should not be performed before 10 weeks' gestation).
- To localize the placenta and determine whether a transabdominal or transcervical approach is more appropriate.

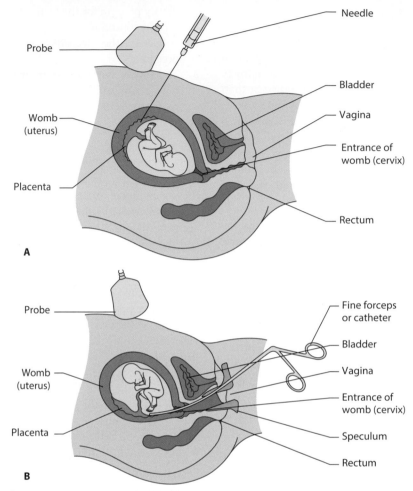

Figure 5.1 A, B: Chorionic villus sampling. (Adapted from the RCOG information leaflet of both approaches.)

▶ **VIDEO 5.1**

Chorionic villus sampling:
http://www.routledgetextbooks.com/textbooks/
tenteachers/obstetricsv5.1.php

Transabdominal procedures are performed more commonly, but they may not be feasible if the uterus is retroverted or the placenta is low on the posterior wall of the uterus.

The additional overall risk of miscarriage from CVS is approximately 2%. This is in addition to the background (natural) risk of miscarriage for a first trimester pregnancy. Many laboratories can provide a result for common aneuploidies (T21, 18, 13, X and Y) within 48 hours for a CVS sample.

Full culture results take approximately 7–10 days and results for genetic disorders take varying amounts of time.

Placental mosaicism is sometimes found. This is the occurrence of two different cell types in the same sample; usually one cell line is normal and one cell line is abnormal. It occurs in approximately 1% of CVS procedures, and this is higher than for amniocentesis. The mosaic pattern may be present in the placenta and not occur in the fetus (confined placental mosaicism). Mosaic results should be discussed with the Clinical Genetics Department to get accurate information on the impact this may have on the fetus. If necessary, another fetal tissue (e.g. amniotic fluid) may need to be sampled to make a definitive diagnosis.

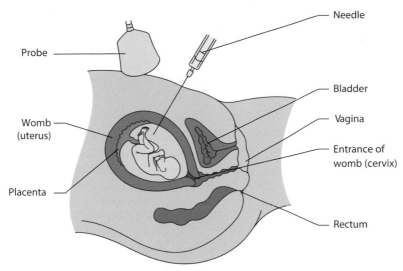

Probe

Needle

Bladder

Vagina

Womb
(uterus)

Entrance of
womb (cervix)

Placenta

Rectum

Figure 5.2 Amniocentesis. (Adapted from the RCOG information leaflet.)

Amniocentesis

Amniotic fluid contains amniocytes and fibroblasts shed from fetal membranes, skin and the fetal genitourinary tract. An amniocentesis procedure takes a sample (15–20 ml) of amniotic fluid that contains these cells. This is done by passing a needle under continuous direct ultrasound control through the abdominal wall and myometrium into the amniotic cavity and aspirating the fluid (**Figure 5.2**).

An initial ultrasound is performed prior to the procedure. The estimated total postamniocentesis pregnancy loss (background and procedure-related loss combined) is 1.9% (95% CI 1.4–2.5) for a procedure performed from 15 weeks of gestation under ultrasound guidance.

Many laboratories can provide a result for common aneuploidies (T21, 18, 13, X and Y) within 48 hours for an amniocentesis sample. Full culture results take approximately 7–10 days and results for genetic disorders take varying amounts of time. This is similar to CVS.

Amniotic fluid may be used to check for fetal viral infections, for example cytomegalovirus. In the past, it was also used for biochemical tests, for example alpha-fetoprotein (AFP) for spina bifida and spectrophotometric tests for RhD haemolytic disease. These have been superseded by ultrasound imaging.

The advantage of CVS over amniocentesis is that it can be performed earlier in pregnancy, at a stage when surgical termination is possible in the event

 VIDEO 5.2

Amniocentesis:
http://www.routledgetextbooks.com/textbooks/
tenteachers/obstetricsv5.2.php

of a 'bad result', and at a stage in pregnancy before a woman has needed to disclose the pregnancy to family, friends and employers. For some genetic disorders, for example haemoglobinopathies, CVS may be preferred over amniocentesis because it provides a larger sample of DNA for rapid polymerase chain reaction (PCR) analysis. However, the additional risk of miscarriage following CVS may be higher than that of amniocentesis carried out after 15 weeks of gestation.

Cordocentesis

Cordocentesis is performed when fetal blood is needed, or when a rapid full culture for karyotype is needed. The most common reason for performing a cordocentesis is for suspected severe fetal anaemia or thrombocytopaenia, with availability of immediate transfusion if confirmed.

A needle is passed under ultrasound guidance through the abdominal wall and myometrium and, most commonly, into the umbilical cord at the point where it inserts into the placenta. This point is chosen because the umbilical cord is fixed and does not move. Cordocentesis can be performed from about 20 weeks'

Table 5.2 Comparison of invasive tests

Test	CVS	Amniocentesis	Cordocentesis
Gestation from which test can be performed	11 weeks	15 weeks	Around 20 weeks
Miscarriage risk	2 per cent	1 per cent	2–5 per cent

CVS, chorion villus sampling.

gestation. The risk of miscarriage varies with indication and position of the placenta (*Table 5.2*).

Care after any invasive test

Following any invasive procedure there should be:

- Accurate labelling of the sample that is checked with the patient.
- Prompt and secure transport of the sample to the appropriate laboratory.
- Documentation of the procedure and any complications in the woman's notes.
- Communication with the referring clinician.
- The woman should be advised to avoid strenuous exercise for the next 24 hours.
- She should be advised that while she may experience some mild abdominal pain, it should be relieved by paracetamol.
- She should be advised that if she has any fever, bleeding, pain not relieved by paracetamol or leakage of fluid vaginally she should seek medical advice, and told how to access this.
- She should be given appropriate contact numbers.
- A process for giving results should be agreed, including who will give the results, how they will be given and when the results are likely to be available.
- If the woman is RhD negative, an appropriate dose of anti-D should be administered (with a Kleihauer test if more than 20 weeks' gestation).
- A plan of ongoing care should be discussed once the results are available.

Down's syndrome and other aneuploidies

In the UK, prenatal diagnosis of Down's syndrome is the most common reason for performing invasive prenatal diagnostic testing. The risk of a fetus having other aneuploidies such as trisomy 13 (Patau's syndrome) and trisomy 18 (Edward's syndrome) may also be indicated when using current Down's syndrome screening tests.

Most prenatal diagnostic tests arise following a 'high-risk' screening test. In the UK, the National Institute for Health and Care Excellence (NICE) has recommended that all women should be offered screening for Down's syndrome as part of their routine antenatal care. It is also recommended that the screening test offered should have at least a 75% detection rate for a 3% false-positive rate.

Several different screening tests are available, but the UK National Screening Committee recommends combined screening in the first trimester. This test involves the combination of an ultrasound scan to measure the nuchal translucency (NT) and the crown–rump length (CRL) from 11+2–14+1 weeks' gestation, and a blood test between 10+0–14+1 weeks' gestation to measure the levels of human chorionic gonadotrophin (hCG) and pregnancy associated plasma protein-A (PAPP-A) in maternal blood.

The NT measurement is the thickness of a collection of fluid under the skin in the nuchal (neck) region of the fetus. Fetuses with Down's syndrome tend to have a thicker NT, hence a thick NT measurement increases the risk of the fetus having Down's syndrome (**Figure 5.3**).

The risk of Down's syndrome increases with maternal age. For each woman, the individual risk can be calculated by taking her age-related risk and then adjusting this up or down based on the measurements obtained for the NT, hCG and PAPP-A. Based on her individual result, the woman can then choose whether to have an invasive test or not.

The UK National Screening Committee recommends the quadruple test (hCG, AFP, unconjugated oestriol and inhibin A) as the screening strategy of choice in the 2nd trimester for women booking later in pregnancy or when it is not possible to measure the NT. The test can be performed between 14+2 and 20+0 weeks' gestation.

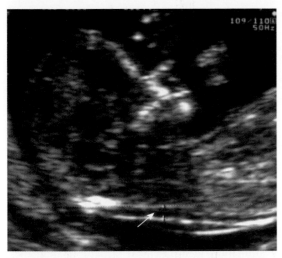

Figure 5.3 Ultrasound image demonstrating the measurement of nuchal translucency (arrow).

Prior to performing the screening test, the woman should be encouraged to consider what action she would take, and how she would feel if she screened positive. It is also important to explain to women that this initial test is simply a screening test and not a diagnostic test. A low-risk result does not rule out the possibility of Down's syndrome completely (even if the result shows a very low risk of 1:10,000, she could be the 1 person in 10,000 who has an affected fetus). With a high-risk result of 1:10, 9 out of 10 or 90% of fetuses would be normal. The diagnostic tests available to her should be explained.

The accuracy of the screening test for Down's syndrome can be refined by adding further markers such as measuring the nasal bone and frontomaxillary nasal angle and looking for the presence of tricuspid regurgitation and at the ductus venosus wave form. These increase the sensitivity of the test and reduce the false-positive rate. However, they are resource intensive, and a prenatal diagnostic test must still be performed to reach a definitive diagnosis.

The use of cffDNA to screen for Down's syndrome and other aneuploidies is rapidly being implemented into clinical practice. Current studies suggest that non-invasive prenatal testing (NIPT) using cffDNA detects around 98% of all babies with Down's, Patau's and Edward's syndrome. NIPT is not diagnostic, however, and it is recommended that women be offered an invasive prenatal diagnostic test to confirm the result.

New developments

Fragments of DNA are released from fetuses and their placenta into the maternal circulation. The concentration of cffDNA increases with gestation from around 10% at 10 weeks of gestation. After delivery, the level of cffDNA drops rapidly and is usually undetectable by the first day after birth. By amplifying the cffDNA using PCR, it makes it possible to check the fetal genotype.

Increasingly, prenatal diagnostic tests are being offered based on this premise. Care must be taken to ensure there is sufficient concentration of cffDNA in the maternal blood (the 'fetal fraction') for the test to be accurate. This may mean that the mother's blood needs to be retested later in pregnancy when the fetal fraction of cell-free DNA is higher. Maternal obesity is associated with a larger blood volume and this may make a conclusive result impossible. Two recent examples of such diagnostic tests are for single gene disorders and to check the fetal blood group.

Fetal single gene disorders

Certain autosomal dominant single gene disorders can now be diagnosed. The test can be offered when the father is known to be affected by the condition, when there is risk of recurrence or where the condition is suspected on ultrasound scan; for example, the autosomal dominant severe skeletal dysplasias such as achondroplasia and thanatophoric dysplasia that are caused by a mutation in the fibroblast growth factor 3 receptor gene (FGFR3). Ultrasound findings such as short long bones (<3rd centile), a small narrow chest with normal head and abdominal measurements can indicate an affected fetus. If the mother is unaffected she will have a normal FGFR3 gene. Where a PCR test on the cell-free DNA in the mother's blood identifies a mutation in the FGFR3 gene, this must have come from the fetus indicating that the fetus is affected. If the PCR test is negative for the FGFR3 mutation the fetus is unaffected. Since an invasive prenatal diagnostic test is not necessary to make the diagnosis, it can be avoided.

Fetal blood group

Similarly, if RhD-positive DNA is amplified from the blood of a RhD-negative woman, this must have come from the fetus (as the mother has no RhD-positive DNA of her own), and the test therefore shows that the fetus is RhD-positive. In RhD-negative women with anti-D antibodies, this test is used to determine the blood group of the fetus, as a RhD-positive fetus is at risk of alloimmune haemolytic disease, whereas a RhD-negative fetus is not at risk. Intensive surveillance can be instituted for the mother of the RhD-positive fetus, and the mother of the RhD-negative fetus can be reassured that problems will not occur. Fetal blood group can be determined from samples taken in the first trimester and testing for the common blood group antigens, including Rhesus and Kell, performed.

Other abnormalities

There is much promising work on a non-invasive diagnostic test for Down's syndrome using cffDNA in the maternal blood. Single-molecule counting methods such as digital PCR are based on the detection of the extra copy of chromosome 21 to distinguish normal cases from trisomy 21 cases. Detecting the different DNA methylation patterns between the maternal and fetal circulating DNA molecules has been proposed as an alternative strategy for the identification of cffDNA sequences. This is based on the ratio of a subset of fetal-specific methylated regions located on chromosome 21 compared with normal cases. These tests have the potential to replace invasive prenatal diagnostic testing for Down's syndrome.

Fetal magnetic resonance imaging (MRI) can improve the analysis of central nervous system abnormalities in the fetus, particularly in the differential diagnosis of ventriculomegaly, where ultrasound may not be able to provide sufficient soft tissue resolution. Currently there are limitations to fetal MRI as it is exquisitely sensitive to fetal motion, although fast imaging techniques have overcome this to some extent. It is hoped that MRI may also provide a better assessment of placental function, which ultrasound is currently unable to provide.

3D and 4D ultrasound has so far had a limited role as a diagnostic tool. Surface rendering can help

in the visualization of cleft lip and palate for parents. Volume rendering allows the volume of an organ, such as the lung for example, to be calculated. 3D can also be used in the presence of ventriculomegaly to detect the intact corpus callosum, a structure that is often difficult to visualize with ultrasound.

Chromosomal microarray analysis is a relatively new technique that identifies chromosomal abnormalities, including submicroscopic abnormalities that are too small to be detected by conventional karyotyping. Like conventional fetal karyotyping, prenatal chromosomal microarray analysis requires direct testing of fetal tissue and thus can be offered only with CVS, amniocentesis or cordocentesis. It is likely to be increasingly offered when ultrasound examination identifies fetal structural anomalies. There is the potential for complex results and detection of clinically uncertain findings that can result in substantial patient anxiety. Comprehensive pretest counselling is therefore recommended.

KEY LEARNING POINTS

- Detailed counselling prior to embarking on any screening or diagnostic tests is extremely important. The woman must understand the potential outcomes, the choices available to her and should be encouraged to consider how the outcome of the test would affect the decisions she made during her pregnancy.

- If a fetal abnormality is diagnosed antenatally, multidisciplinary management is important. This will help to provide the woman with the best information about the likely outcome for her baby, facilitate her decision making and provide appropriate support from experienced professionals at a difficult time.

Further reading

Fetal anomaly screening programme. https://www.gov.uk/government/uploads/system/uploads/attachment_data/file/421650/FASP_Standards_April_2015_final_2_.pdf.

National Institute for Health and Care Excellence. Antenatal care. Available at http://www.nice.org.uk/guidance/qs22.

Self assessment

CASE HISTORY 1

N is a 22-year-old woman living in the North West of England. She found herself unexpectedly pregnant and had not been taking periconceptual folic acid. When she first attended the antenatal clinic an ultrasound scan showed her to be 19 weeks pregnant. The fetus was noted to have an abnormal head shape, the cerebellum was described as banana shaped and a myelomeningocoele was identified in the lumbar region. The fetus had bilateral talipes.

Figure 5.4 shows normal intracranial anatomy imaged in (A) the plane of the thalami to visualize the ventricles and (B) the transcerebellar plane. Note the ovoid head shape and the dumb bell-shaped cerebellum (indicated by white arrow, CB).

Figure 5.5 is a similar plane in Ms N, whose fetus has a neural tube defect. Note the scalloped head shape anteriorly (lemon shaped) marked by the white arrows and the banana-shaped cerebellum marked by the red arrow. Alongside is a section through the brain at the level of the thalami and ventricles indicating bilateral severe ventriculomegaly, marked by the white stars. In each image, A indicates the anterior and P indicates the posterior part of the head.

A How should this patient be managed?
B What is the outlook for the baby/child?
C What options does Ms N have?
D What is the risk of it happening again in a future pregnancy?
E What advice would you give about future pregnancies?

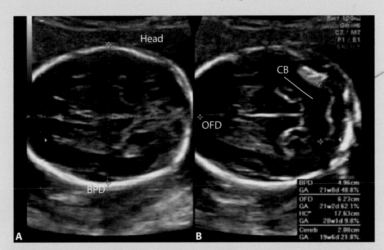

Figure 5.4 Normal cranial anatomy in the transcerebellar plane. Note the ovoid head shape and the dumb bell-shaped cerebellum. BPD, biparietal diameter; CB, cerebellum; OFD occipitofrontal diameter.

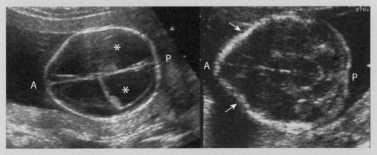

Figure 5.5 is in a similar plane in Ms N, whose fetus has a neural tube defect. Note the scalloped head shape anteriorly (lemon shaped) marked by the white arrows and the banana-shaped cerebellum (red arrow). A, anterior; P, posterior.

ANSWERS

A   A prenatal diagnosis of a neural tube defect has been made on ultrasound scan. Ultrasound scan will detect at least 90% of all neural tube defects. Ms N should be seen by the consultant and the ultrasound findings explained to her. She should have the opportunity to discuss the prognosis with a neurosurgeon, and this may be best organized by referring her to a tertiary fetal medicine unit.

B   For women to make decisions about whether to continue with their pregnancy or not, they need an honest and realistic view of the likely outcome for their baby/child. It is always difficult to predict the outlook for the baby/child but lower lesions generally have a better prognosis. The main problems encountered are:

  * Problems with mobility – individuals with a neural tube defect tend to become wheelchair bound as they get older.
  * Continence and voiding – both bladder and bowel.
  * Low intelligence quotient (IQ).
  * Repeated surgery – shunts, bladder and bowel, orthopaedic.
  * Difficulty forming normal relationships and living independently.

C   Ms N may choose to continue with the pregnancy with support from health care professionals both before and after delivery. Parents who choose to continue with a pregnancy may benefit from contacting a parent support group such as ASBAH (Association for Spina Bifida and Hydrocephalus). Fetal surgery is now being offered in some countries to repair the myelomeningocoele defect during pregnancy. It involves extensive maternal surgery with an associated risk of spontaneous preterm birth, and there is limited outcome data to show benefit. Alternatively, she may opt for termination of pregnancy.

D   The risk of recurrence of a neural tube defect is 5% after one affected pregnancy (12% after two affected pregnancies and 20% after three affected pregnancies). Neural tube defects are more common in some geographical areas (e.g. Ireland, Scotland and North West England), if the mother has diabetes or epilepsy, if the mother is taking antiepileptic medication and in obese women.

Folic acid (400 µg) taken preconceptually and for the first trimester reduces the risk of neural tube defects.

E   By taking folic acid for at least 3 months preconceptually, the risk of recurrence can be reduced. Ms N should take a higher dose of preconceptual folic acid (5 mg instead of the usual 400 µg). She should also ensure that she eats healthily and that her weight is normal. Any medication she is taking should be reviewed.

CASE HISTORY 2

Ms G is an 18-year-old woman who had her first scan at 16 weeks' gestation. When the fetal abdomen was scanned, an irregular mass was seen to project from the anterior abdominal wall at the level of the umbilicus, to the right side of the umbilical cord insertion. **Figure 5.6** shows the herniated bowel (indicated by a white arrow) in the amniotic fluid. No other fetal abnormalities were noted.

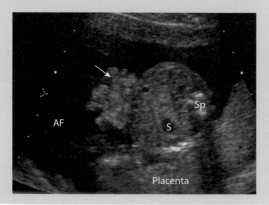

Figure 5.6 Ultrasound image of gastroschisis (arrow). AF, amniotic fluid; S, fetal stomach; Sp, fetal spine.

A   How should this patient be managed?

B   What should the consultant tell her about the outlook for her baby?

C   What plans would you make for delivery?

ANSWERS

A   A prenatal diagnosis of a gastroschisis has been made on ultrasound scan. Ultrasound scan will detect at least 90% of all gastroschisis defects. Ms G should be seen by the consultant and the ultrasound findings explained to her. She requires referral to a tertiary unit for ongoing management and planning of delivery. Involvement of a multidisciplinary team would be important.

B   The consultant should stress that the majority of babies born with gastroschisis will do well in the long term and lead normal lives. Gastroschisis is not usually associated with any other physical problems or with learning problems (Table 5.3). It should be explained that the fetus will need to be monitored regularly during the pregnancy as fetuses with gastroschisis are often small and may have oligohydramnios. In later pregnancy, the fetal bowel may dilate, which can be associated with bowel ischaemia and bowel atresia. This can make the postnatal surgery more difficult.

Following delivery, the baby would require an operation to repair the defect. Surgical repair ranges from reduction of bowel and suturing of defect under anaesthetic, to the need for a silo. This is a covering placed over the abdominal organs on the outside of the baby. Gradually, the organs are squeezed by hand through the silo into the opening and returned to the body. This method can take up to a week to return the abdominal organs to the body cavity. Severe cases may require bowel resection for atresias or volvulus. Survival rates of up to 97% are found for simple cases and the majority of babies are on full oral feeds by 4 weeks of age. For more complex severe cases there is a lower rate of survival with longer hospitalization.

Ms G should be given the opportunity to meet the paediatric surgeons during the pregnancy and visit the paediatric surgical unit. After delivery, she should be encouraged to express breast milk to feed to her baby.

C   Induction around 37 weeks' gestation enables delivery to be planned in a unit with appropriate paediatric surgical facilities, and may reduce the incidence of stillbirth late in pregnancy. There does not appear to be any benefit from delivery by caesarean section for babies with gastroschisis. If other organs such as the liver are also herniated, caesarean delivery may be indicated. If a woman has a normal delivery it makes it easier for her to visit her baby on the paediatric surgical unit in the first few days after birth.

Table 5.3 Key differences between abdominal wall defects

Exomphalos	Gastroschisis
Membrane covered herniation of abdominal contents – smooth outline	Not membrane covered Free floating bowel loops – irregular outline
Umbilical cord inserts into apex of sac	Herniation lateral (usually to the right) of the cord insertion
Very high incidence of associated abnormalities and genetic syndromes	Relatively low incidence of other abnormalities
High incidence of chromosomal abnormalities – karyotyping should be offered	No increase in incidence of chromosomal abnormalities
May contain stomach, liver, spleen	Usually only small bowel extra-abdominally
Associated with polyhydramnios	Associated with oligohydramnios

CASE HISTORY 3

Ms E is a 37-year-old woman who attended for her first scan at 18 weeks' gestation. On ultrasound scan, a smooth protrusion could be seen on the anterior abdominal wall of the fetus. It appeared to be covered by a membrane and the umbilical cord inserted into the apex of the protrusion. The sonographer described this as an exomphalos in her report. **Figure 5.7** shows an ultrasound image of an exomphalos with the sac containing the herniated bowel.

A How should this patient be managed?

B What options are available to Ms E?

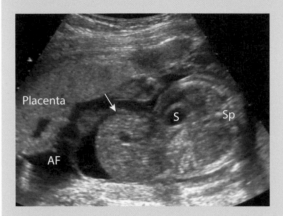

Figure 5.7 Ultrasound image of exomphalos, showing the sac containing the herniated bowel (white arrow). AF, amniotic fluid; S, fetal stomach; Sp, fetal spine.

ANSWERS

A A prenatal diagnosis of an exomphalos has been made on ultrasound scan. Ultrasound scan will detect at least 90% of all exomphalos defects, but this diagnosis cannot be made until after 12 weeks' gestation. Prior to 12 weeks, there is developmental physiological herniation of abdominal contents into the base of the umbilical cord. Ms E should be seen by the consultant and the ultrasound findings explained to her. As there is a high incidence of associated abnormalities (in 70–80% of fetuses), she should be referred to a tertiary unit for detailed ultrasound. The consultant should also explain that there is a high chance of chromosomal abnormality (approximately one-third of fetuses) and discuss the option of invasive testing (see *Table 5.3*).

B Ms E's options include:

- Do nothing.
- Termination of pregnancy.

- CVS now and continue if the chromosomes are normal. It is possible that other abnormalities may still be detected on ultrasound later in pregnancy. If the chromosomes are abnormal she would still have the option of a surgical termination of pregnancy up to 14 weeks' gestation in some hospitals.

- Wait until after 15 weeks' gestation, then have an amniocentesis with a lower risk of miscarriage. Even if the chromosomes are normal, it is still possible that other abnormalities may be detected on ultrasound later in pregnancy.

Ms E chose to have a CVS that showed that the fetus had trisomy 18. She then chose to terminate her pregnancy, as she knew that most fetuses with trisomy 18 were either stillborn or did not live beyond the first few months.

CASE HISTORY 4

Mrs D has a brother with Duchenne's muscular dystrophy (DMD). He has been under the care of the clinical geneticists, and Mrs D has been tested and found to be a carrier of the gene. She contacts her general practitioner (GP) when she is 7 weeks' pregnant as she wishes to have testing to see whether the fetus is affected by DMD.

A What are the chances of Mrs D having an affected fetus?

B How should Mrs D be managed?

ANSWERS

A   There is a 1:4 chance of an affected fetus. DMD is an X-linked recessive condition. There is a 1:2 chance that any baby will be a girl and a 1:2 chance that it will be a boy. If the fetus is male, there is a 1:2 chance that it has inherited a normal X chromosome from Mrs D (unaffected) and a 1:2 chance that it has inherited the X chromosome carrying the abnormal gene, in which case the boy would be affected. If the fetus is female there is a 1:2 chance that it will have inherited a normal X chromosome from Mrs D and therefore not be a carrier, and a 1:2 chance that it will have inherited the X chromosome carrying the abnormal gene and therefore be a carrier. A female fetus would not be affected as this is an X-linked recessive condition, and a female fetus would have inherited a normal X chromosome from the father.

B   The GP should arrange an urgent referral to the antenatal clinic and also contact the Clinical Genetics Department. Mrs D requires an initial ultrasound scan to confirm that the fetus is viable, to confirm the gestation and to confirm that it is a singleton pregnancy. Testing would be much more complex if this were a twin pregnancy.

Initially, a blood test can be performed on Mrs D to ascertain the sex of the fetus. All fetuses shed small quantities of DNA into the maternal circulation. This can be amplified by a PCR technique. By testing the maternal serum for cffDNA from the Y chromosome the sex of the fetus can be ascertained. If Y chromosome DNA is found in the maternal serum, it must have come from a male fetus. If no Y chromosome DNA is found then it is likely that it is a female fetus. However, there is also a small possibility that the test has not worked because there is insufficient cffDNA level in the maternal plasma. It is currently recommended that before 9 weeks of gestation, two samples should be collected, 1 week apart, to ensure that there is sufficient cffDNA to make a diagnosis.

Mrs D had a blood test at 8 weeks' gestation and a second blood test at 9 weeks that showed that she was carrying a female fetus. As this meant that she would not have an affected baby she did not need to have any further invasive testing. If the blood test had shown that she was carrying a male fetus, she would then have had a CVS to determine whether this was an affected or unaffected male. By having the blood test, she was able to avoid invasive testing.

EMQ

There are various invasive tests that can be used in prenatal diagnosis of genetic conditions. For each description, choose the SINGLE most appropriate answer from the list of options. Each option may be used once, more than once or not at all.

A Amniocentesis.

B CVS.

C Both amniocentesis and CVS.

D Neither amniocentesis nor CVS.

E Cordocentesis.

1 Which procedure is performed under continuous ultrasound guidance?

2 Which test can be performed at 9 weeks' gestation?

3 Which test is used to diagnose spina bifida?

4 Which test is used to diagnose single gene disorders in the fetus?

5 Which test is used to diagnose fetal anaemia?

6 Which test can be performed at 11 weeks' gestation?

ANSWERS

1C Both amniocentesis and CVS. Continuous ultrasound guidance must be used to perform both tests, to reduce the risk of complications such as miscarriage, fetal trauma and a failed sample collection.

2D Neither amniocentesis nor CVS. Early amniocentesis (before 15 weeks' gestation) is associated with a higher rate of miscarriage. Early CVS (before 11 weeks' gestation) is associated with limb defects and is not recommended. Non-invasive prenatal diagnosis using cffDNA may be performed at 9 weeks' gestation to test for fetal gender or RhD gene, but it is recommended that a repeat sample is collected 1 week later to confirm the diagnosis.

3D Neither amniocentesis nor CVS. Ultrasound is used to make the diagnosis of spina bifida. Invasive prenatal diagnostic tests are mainly used to diagnose aneuploidy, single gene disorders and some fetal infections. Fetal structural defects are not detected. Measuring the levels of AFP was used to screen for spina bifida in the past.

4C Both amniocentesis and CVS. Diagnosis of single gene disorders involves detection of a genetic mutation in fetal DNA, usually by PCR analysis. Fetal DNA can be extracted from the amniocytes that are present in the amniotic fluid. Since the placenta is derived from the blastocyst, the genetic makeup of the fetus is the same as that of the placenta. In chorion villus biopsy the trophoblast cells in the mesenchyme of the placental villi are collected and extracted DNA can be used for prenatal diagnosis.

5E Cordocentesis. Cordocentesis is collection of a sample of fetal blood from the umbilical cord under ultrasound guidance. Ultrasound can be used to screen for fetal anaemia using middle cerebral artery Doppler (see Chapter 4, Assessment of fetal wellbeing). Amniocentesis was used in the past to screen for fetal anaemia by measuring the change in optical density at a wavelength of 450 nm, which detects bilirubin, a breakdown product of fetal haemoglobin.

6B CVS. Amniocentesis before 14 weeks' gestation (early amniocentesis) has a higher fetal loss rate and increased incidence of fetal talipes and respiratory morbidity compared to chorion villus biopsy. Cordocentesis is usually performed after 20 weeks' gestation due to an increased risk of complications such as haemorrhage and miscarriage when it is performed earlier in gestation.

SBA QUESTION

There are two screening tests for Down's syndrome offered to pregnant women in England: first trimester combined screening and the quadruple test. These rely on the measurement of a number of factors in order for an estimation of the risk of that pregnancy being affected by Down's syndrome. Which of the following result in a low-chance result? Choose the single best answer.

A Beta-hCG levels above average for the gestation.
B AFP (alphafetoprotein) levels above average for the gestation.
C High maternal age.
D NT above average for the gestation.
E Previous history of Down's syndrome.
F PAPP-A levels below average for the gestation.

ANSWER

B Various maternal serum protein levels are altered in Down's syndrome:

- PAPP-A is produced by placental syncytiotrophoblasts; levels are reduced in pregnancies affected by Down's syndrome.
- Beta-hCG is produced by placental syncytiotrophoblasts; there are raised levels in pregnancies affected by Down's syndrome.
- AFP is produced by fetal yolk sac and liver; there are reduced levels in pregnancies affected by Down's syndrome.
- Unconjugated oestriol (uE3) is produced by placenta and fetal adrenals; levels are reduced in pregnancies affected by Down's syndrome.
- Inhibin-A is produced by placenta; there are raised levels in pregnancies affected by Down's syndrome.
- Fetuses with Down's syndrome tend to have a thicker NT for gestational age.

If a previous pregnancy was affected with Down's syndrome, the result will be classified as 'screen-positive' regardless of the level of the screening markers, so that further testing can be discussed with the woman.

Antenatal obstetric complications

LOUISE C KENNY

LEARNING OBJECTIVES

- To appreciate the causes and management of minor complications of pregnancy.
- To be able to provide a differential diagnosis for abdominal pain in pregnancy and a management plan.
- To understand the risk factors, presentation and management of venous thromboembolic disease in pregnancy.
- To understand the complications of drug abuse in pregnancy.
- To understand the causes, complications and management of oligohyramnios and polyhydramnios.
- To understand the causes and management of malpresentation in late pregnancy.
- To understand the causes, prevention and treatment of haemolytic disease of the fetus and newborn.

Introduction

There are a variety of maternal and fetal complications that can arise during pregnancy. Some of these 'minor' conditions arise because the physiological changes of pregnancy exacerbate many irritating symptoms that in the normal non-pregnant state would not require specific treatment. While these problems are not dangerous to the mother, they can be extremely troublesome and incapacitating. Some of the more major fetal and maternal complications are discussed in detail in other chapters. Here we discuss common complications, including malpresentation, rhesus disease and abnormalities of amniotic fluid production.

Minor problems of pregnancy

Musculoskeletal problems

Backache

Backache is extremely common in pregnancy and is caused by:

- Hormone induced laxity of spinal ligaments.
- A shifting in the centre of gravity as the uterus grows.
- Additional weight gain.

They cause an exaggerated lumbar lordosis. Pregnancy can exacerbate the symptoms of a prolapsed intervertebral disc, occasionally leading to complete immobility. Advice should include maintenance of correct posture, avoiding lifting heavy objects (including children), avoiding high-heels, regular physiotherapy and simple analgesia (paracetamol or paracetamol–codeine combinations).

Symphysis pubis dysfunction

This is an excruciatingly painful condition most common in the third trimester, although it can occur at any time during pregnancy. The symphysis pubis joint becomes 'loose', causing the two halves of the pelvis to rub on one another when walking or moving. The condition improves after delivery and the management revolves around simple analgesia. Under a physiotherapist's direction, a low stability belt may be worn.

Carpal tunnel syndrome

Compression neuropathies occur in pregnancy due to increased soft-tissue swelling. The most common of these is carpal tunnel syndrome. The median nerve, where it passes through the fibrous canal at the wrist before entering the hand, is most susceptible to compression. The symptoms include numbness, tingling and weakness of the thumb and forefinger, and often quite severe pain at night. Simple analgesia and splinting of the affected hand usually help, although there is no realistic prospect of cure until after delivery. Surgical decompression is very rarely performed in pregnancy.

Gastrointestinal symptoms

Constipation

Constipation is common in pregnancy and usually results from a combination of hormonal and mechanical factors that slow gut motility. Concomitantly administered iron tablets may exacerbate the condition. Women should be given clear explanations, reassurance and advice regarding the adoption of a high-fibre diet. Medications are best avoided but if necessary, mild (non-stimulant) laxatives such as lactulose may be suggested.

Hyperemesis gravidarum

Nausea and vomiting in pregnancy are extremely common; 70–80% of women experience these symptoms early in their pregnancy and approximately 35% of all pregnant patients are absent from work on at least one occasion through nausea and vomiting. Although the symptoms are often most pronounced in the first trimester, they are by no means confined to it. Similarly, despite common usage of the term 'morning sickness', in only a minority of cases are the symptoms solely confined to the morning. Nausea and vomiting in pregnancy tends to be mild and self-limited and is not associated with adverse pregnancy outcome.

Hyperemesis gravidarum, however, is a severe, intractable form of nausea and vomiting that affects 0.3–2.0% of pregnancies. It causes imbalances of fluid and electrolytes, disturbs nutritional intake and metabolism, causes physical and psychological debilitation and is associated with adverse pregnancy outcome, including an increased risk of preterm birth and low birthweight babies. The aetiology is unknown and various putative mechanisms have been proposed including an association with high levels of serum human chorionic gonadotrophin (hCG), oestrogen and thyroxine. The likely cause is multifactorial. Severe cases of hyperemesis gravidarum cause malnutrition and vitamin deficiencies including Wernicke's encephalopathy and intractable retching predisposes to oesophageal trauma and Mallory–Weiss tears. Treatment includes fluid replacement and thiamine supplementation. Antiemetics such as phenothiazines are safe and are commonly prescribed. Other proposed treatments including the administration of corticosteroids have not yet been adequately proven and remain empirical.

Gastroesophageal reflux

This is very common. Altered structure and function of the normal physiological barriers to reflux, namely the weight effect of the pregnant uterus and hormonally induced relaxation of the oesophageal sphincter, explain the extremely high incidence in the pregnant population. For the majority of patients, lifestyle modifications such as smoking cessation, frequent light meals and lying with the head propped up at night are helpful. When these prove insufficient to control symptoms medications can be added in a stepwise fashion, starting with simple antacids. Histamine-2 receptor antagonists and proton pump inhibitors have a good safety record in pregnancy and can be used.

Haemorrhoids

Several factors conspire to render haemorrhoids more common during pregnancy including the effects of circulating progesterone on the vasculature, pressure on the superior rectal veins by the gravid uterus and increased circulating volume. A conservative approach is usually advocated including local anaesthetic/anti-irritant creams and a high-fibre diet. Never overlook the 'warning' symptoms of tenesmus, mucus, blood mixed with stool and back passage discomfort that may suggest rectal carcinoma; a rectal digital examination should be carried out if these symptoms are suggested.

Obstetric cholestasis

Obstetric cholestasis (also referred to as intrahepatic cholestasis of pregnancy) affects 0.7% of pregnancies with some ethnic variation. It normally presents in the second half of pregnancy with pruritus and abnormal liver function tests (LFTs), neither of which has an alternative cause and both of which resolve after birth. The clinical importance of obstetric cholestasis lies in the potential fetal risks, which may include spontaneous preterm birth, iatrogenic preterm birth and fetal death. There can also be maternal morbidity in association with the intense pruritus and consequent sleep deprivation. It is normally treated with ursodeoxycholic acid (UDCA), which improves pruritus and liver function but has not been proven to improve fetal and neonatal outcomes. Women with obstetric cholestasis are therefore normally offered delivery after 37 weeks' gestation.

Varicose veins

Varicose veins may appear for the first time in pregnancy or pre-existing veins may become worse. They are thought to be due to the relaxant effect of progesterone on vascular smooth muscle and the dependent venous stasis caused by the weight of the pregnant uterus on the inferior vena cava (IVC).

Varicose veins of the legs may be symptomatically improved with support stockings, avoidance of standing for prolonged periods and simple analgesia. Thrombophlebitis may occur in a large varicose vein, more commonly after delivery. A large superficial varicose vein may bleed profusely if traumatized; the leg must be elevated and direct pressure applied. Vulval and vaginal varicosities are uncommon but symptomatically troublesome; trauma at the time of delivery (episiotomy, tear, instrumental delivery) may also cause considerable bleeding.

Oedema

This is common, occurring to some degree in approximately 80% of all pregnancies. There is generalized soft-tissue swelling and increased capillary permeability, which allows intravascular fluid to leak into the extravascular compartment. The fingers, toes and ankles are usually worst affected and the symptoms are aggravated by hot weather. Oedema is best dealt with by frequent periods of rest with leg elevation; occasionally, support stockings are indicated. Excessively swollen fingers may necessitate removal of rings and jewellery before they get stuck. It is important to remember that generalized (rather than lower limb) oedema may be a feature of pre-eclampsia, so remember to check the woman's blood pressure and urine for protein. More rarely, severe oedema may suggest underlying cardiac impairment or nephrotic syndrome.

Other common 'minor' disorders

- Itching.
- Urinary incontinence.
- Nose-bleeds.
- Thrush (vaginal candidiasis).
- Headache.
- Fainting.
- Breast soreness.
- Tiredness.
- Altered taste sensation.
- Insomnia.
- Leg cramps.
- Striae gravidarum and chloasma.

Problems due to abnormalities of the pelvic organs

Fibroids (leiomyomata)

Fibroids are compact masses of smooth muscle that lie in the cavity of the uterus (submucous), within the uterine muscle (intramural) or on the outside surface of the uterus (subserous). They may enlarge in pregnancy, and in so doing present problems later on in pregnancy or at delivery (**Figure 6.1**). A large fibroid at the cervix or in the lower uterine segment may prevent descent of the presenting part and obstruct vaginal delivery.

Red degeneration is one of the commonest complications of fibroids in pregnancy. As it grows, the fibroid may become ischaemic, which manifests clinically as acute pain, tenderness over the fibroid and frequent vomiting. If these symptoms are severe, it may precipitate uterine contractions, causing miscarriage or preterm labour. Red fibroid degeneration requires treatment in hospital, with potent analgesics (usually opiates and intravenous fluids). The symptoms usually settle within a few days. The differential diagnosis of red degeneration includes acute appendicitis, pyelonephritis/urinary tract infection, ovarian cyst accident and placental abruption.

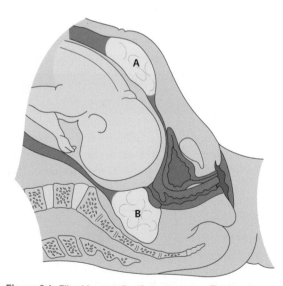

Figure 6.1 Fibroids complicating pregnancy. The tumour in the anterior wall of the uterus (**A**) has been drawn up and out of the pelvis as the lower segment formed, but the fibroid (**B**) arising from the cervix remains in the pelvis and will obstruct labour.

A subserous pedunculated fibroid may tort in the same way that a large ovarian cyst can. When this happens, acute abdominal pain and tenderness may make the two difficult to distinguish from one another. In this scenario, a pertinent history followed by ultrasound scan (transvaginal in the first trimester, transabdominal in the second and third) will aid the diagnosis.

Retroversion of the uterus

Fifteen percent of women have a retroverted uterus. In pregnancy, the uterus grows and a retroverted uterus will normally 'flip' out of the pelvis and begin to fill the abdominal cavity, as an anteverted uterus would. In a small proportion of cases, the uterus remains in retroversion and eventually fills up the entire pelvic cavity; as it does so, the base of the bladder and the urethra are stretched. Retention of urine may occur, classically at 12–14 weeks, and this is not only very painful but may also cause long-term bladder damage if the bladder becomes overdistended. In this situation, catheterization is essential until the position of the uterus has changed.

Congenital uterine anomalies

The shape of the uterus is embryologically determined by the fusion of the Müllerian ducts. Abnormalities of fusion may give rise to anything from a subseptate uterus through to a bicornuate uterus and even (very rarely) to a double uterus with two cervices. These findings are often discovered incidentally at the time of a pelvic operation, such as a laparoscopy, or an ultrasound scan.

The problems associated with bicornuate uterus are:

- Miscarriage.
- Preterm labour.
- Preterm premature rupture of membranes (PPROM).
- Abnormalities of lie and presentation.
- Higher caesarean section rate.

Ovarian cysts in pregnancy

Ovarian cysts are common in pregnant women; fortunately, the incidence of malignancy is uncommon in women of childbearing age. The most common types of pathological ovarian cyst are serous cysts and benign teratomas. Physiological cysts of the corpus luteum may grow to several centimetres but rarely require treatment. Asymptomatic cysts may be followed up by clinical and ultrasound examination, but large cysts (for example dermoids) may require surgery in pregnancy.

Surgery is usually postponed until the late second or early third trimester, when there is the potential that if the baby were delivered, it would be able to survive. The major problems are of large (>8 cm) ovarian cysts in pregnancy, which may undergo torsion, haemorrhage or rupture, causing acute abdominal pain. The resulting pain and inflammation may lead to a miscarriage or preterm labour. Symptomatic cysts, most commonly due to torsion, will require an emergency laparotomy and ovarian cystectomy or even oophorectomy if the cyst is torted. A full assessment must include a family history of ovarian or breast malignancy, tumour markers (although these are of limited value in pregnancy) and detailed ultrasound investigation of both ovaries. Surgery in late second and third trimester of pregnancy is normally performed through a midline or paramedian incision; a low transverse suprapubic incision would not allow access to the ovary, as it is drawn upwards in later pregnancy.

Cervical cancer

Cervical abnormalities are much more difficult to deal with in pregnancy, partly because the cervix itself is more difficult to visualize at colposcopy, and also because biopsy may cause considerable bleeding. Cervical carcinoma most commonly arises in poor attenders for cervical screening. The disease is commonly asymptomatic in early stages, but later stage presentation includes vaginal bleeding (especially postcoital). Examination may reveal a friable or ulcerated lesion with bleeding and purulent discharge. The prospect of cervical carcinoma in pregnancy leads to complex ethical and moral dilemmas concerning whether the pregnancy must be terminated (depending on the stage it has reached) to facilitate either surgical treatment (radical hysterectomy) or chemoradiotherapy. Cervical cancer is discussed in greater detail in Chapter 16, Premalignant and malignant disease of the lower genital tract, of *Gynaecology by Ten Teachers*, 20th edition.

Urinary tract infection

Urinary tract infections (UTIs) are common in pregnancy. Eight percent of women have asymptomatic bacteriuria; if this is untreated, it may progress to UTI or even pyelonephritis, with the attendant associations of low birthweight and preterm delivery.

The predisposing factors are:

- History of recurrent cystitis.
- Renal tract abnormalities: duplex system, scarred kidneys, ureteric damage and stones.
- Diabetes.
- Bladder emptying problems (e.g. multiple sclerosis).

The symptoms of UTI may be different in pregnancy; it occasionally presents as low back pain and general malaise with flu-like symptoms. The classic presentation of frequency, dysuria and haematuria is not often seen. On examination, tachycardia, pyrexia, dehydration and loin tenderness may be present. Investigations should include a full blood count and midstream specimen of urine (MSU) sent for urgent microscopy, culture and sensitivities. If there is a strong clinical suspicion of UTI, treatment with antibiotics should start straightaway. The woman should drink plenty of clear fluids and take a simple analgesic such as paracetamol.

The commonest organism for UTI is *Escherichia coli*; less commonly implicated are streptococci, *Proteus*, *Pseudomonas* and *Klebsiella* spp. Many laboratories define a UTI as the presence of >10^5 colony forming units (cfu)/ml. The commonly reported 'heavy mixed growth' is often associated with UTI symptoms and may be treated, or the MSU repeated after a week, depending on the clinical scenario. The first-line antibiotic for UTI is amoxycillin or oral cephalosporins.

Pyelonephritis is characterized by dehydration, a very high temperature (>38.5°C), systemic disturbance and occasionally shock. This requires urgent and aggressive treatment including intravenous fluids, opiate analgesia and intravenous antibiotics (such as cephalosporins or gentamicin). In addition, renal function should be determined, with at least baseline urea and electrolytes, and the baby must be monitored with cardiotocography (CTG). Recurrent UTIs in pregnancy require MSU specimens to be sent to the microbiology laboratory at each antenatal visit, and low-dose prophylactic oral antibiotics may be prescribed. Investigation should take place after delivery, unless frank haematuria or other symptoms suggest that an urgent diagnosis is essential. Investigations might include a renal ultrasound scan, renal dimercaptosuccinic acid (DMSA) function scan, creatinine clearance, intravenous urogram and cystoscopy.

Abdominal pain in pregnancy

Abdominal pain is one of the commonest minor disorders of pregnancy; the problem is in distinguishing pathological from 'physiological' pain. There are many possibilities to exclude and in addition, the anatomical and physiological changes of pregnancy may alter 'classical' presenting symptoms and signs, making clinical diagnosis challenging. The causes listed in *Table 6.1* are not exhaustive, but cover most possible diagnoses. The crucial point to make is that certain conditions are potentially so dangerous or debilitating (e.g. acute appendicitis), and may be masked by the altered anatomy and physiology of pregnancy, that obstetricians may have to perform X-rays and arrange invasive assessments to make a diagnosis. To avoid this, and risk not making an early diagnosis, means that women may not be treated appropriately for possibly very serious conditions.

Venous thromboembolism

Venous thromboembolism (VTE) is the most common cause of direct maternal death in the UK. In the most recent Confidential Enquiries into Maternal Deaths and Morbidity (2009–2012), there were 26 fatalities, giving a maternal mortality rate of 1.08 per 100,000, more than twice that of the next most common cause (genital tract sepsis).

Pregnancy is a hypercoagulable state because of an alteration in the thrombotic and fibrinolytic systems. There is an increase in clotting factors VIII, IX, X and fibrinogen levels, and a reduction in protein S and antithrombin (AT) III concentrations. The net result of these changes is thought to be an evolutionary response to reduce the likelihood of haemorrhage following delivery.

Table 6.1 Causes of abdominal pain in pregnancy

Obstetric conditions
Early pregnancy (<24 weeks)
Ligament stretching
Miscarriage
Ectopic pregnancy
Acute urinary retention due to retroverted gravid uterus
Later pregnancy (>24 weeks)
Labour
Placental abruption
HELLP syndrome
Uterine rupture
Chorioamnioitis
Pregnancy-unrelated conditions
Uterine/ovarian causes
Torsion or degeneration of fibroid
Ovarian cyst accident
Urinary tract disorders
Urinary tract infection (acute cystitis and acute pyelonephritis)
Renal colic
Gastrointestinal disorders
Medical gastric/duodenal ulcer
Acute appendicitis
Acute pancreatitis
Acute gastroenteritis
Intestinal obstruction or perforation
Medical causes
Sickle cell disease (abdominal crisis)
Diabetic ketoacidosis
Acute intermittent porphyria
Pneumonia (especially lower lobe)
Pulmonary embolus
Malaria

HELLP, haemolysis, elevated liver enzymes and low platelets.

These physiological changes predispose a woman to thromboembolism and this is further exacerbated by venous stasis in the lower limbs due to the weight of the gravid uterus placing pressure on the IVC in late pregnancy and immobility, particularly in the puerperium.

Pregnancy is associated with a 6–10-fold increase in the risk of VTE compared to the non-pregnant situation. Without thromboprophylaxis, the incidence of non-fatal pulmonary embolism (PE) and deep vein thrombosis (DVT) in pregnancy is about 0.1% in developed countries; this increases following delivery to around 1–2% and is further increased following emergency caesarean section.

Risk factors for thromboembolic disease

- Pre-existing:
  - maternal age (>35 years);
  - thrombophilia;
  - obesity (>80 kg);
  - previous thromboembolism;
  - severe varicose veins;
  - smoking;
  - malignancy.
- Specific to pregnancy:
  - multiple gestation;
  - pre-eclampsia;
  - grand multiparity;
  - caesarean section, especially if emergency;
  - damage to the pelvic veins;
  - sepsis;
  - prolonged bed rest.

Thrombophilia

Some women are predisposed to thrombosis through changes in the coagulation/fibrinolytic system that may be inherited or acquired. There is growing evidence that both heritable and acquired thrombophilias are associated with a range of adverse pregnancy outcomes, particularly recurrent fetal loss. The major hereditary forms of thrombophilia currently recognized include: deficiencies of the endogenous anticoagulants protein C, protein S and AT III; abnormalities of procoagulant factors, factor V Leiden (caused by a mutation in the factor V gene) and the prothrombin mutation G20210A. It seems probable that there are still some thrombophilias not yet discovered or described. Heritable thrombophilias are present in at least 15% of Western populations.

Acquired thrombophilia is most commonly associated with antiphospholipid syndrome (APS). APS is the combination of lupus anticoagulant with or without anticardiolipin antibodies, with a history of recurrent miscarriage and/or thrombosis. It may (or, more commonly, may not) be associated with other autoantibody disorders such as systemic lupus erythematosus (SLE).

If thrombophilic disorders are taken together, more than 50% of women with pregnancy-related VTE will have a thrombophilia. It is therefore vital that women with a history of thrombotic events are screened for thrombophilia. The presence of thrombophilia, with a history of thrombotic episode(s), means that prophylaxis should be considered for pregnancy.

Diagnosis of acute venous thromboembolism

Clinical diagnosis of VTE is unreliable. Therefore, women who are suspected of having a DVT or PE should be investigated promptly.

Deep vein thrombosis

The commonest symptoms are pain in the calf with varying degrees of redness or swelling. Women's legs are often swollen during pregnancy, therefore unilateral symptoms should ring alarm bells. The signs are few, except that often the calf is tender to gentle touch. It is mandatory to ask about symptoms of PE (see later), as a woman with PE might present initially with a DVT.

Compression ultrasound has a high sensitivity and specificity in diagnosing proximal thrombosis in the non-pregnant woman and should be the first investigation used in a suspected DVT. Calf veins are often poorly visualized; however, it is known that a thrombus confined purely to the calf veins with no extension is very unlikely to give rise to a PE.

Venography is invasive, requiring the injection of contrast medium and the use of X-rays. It does, however, allow excellent visualization of veins both below and above the knee.

Pulmonary embolus

It is crucial to recognize PE, as missing the diagnosis could have fatal implications. The most common presentation is of mild breathlessness or inspiratory chest pain in a woman who is not cyanosed but may be slightly tachycardic (>90 bpm) with a mild pyrexia (37.5°C). Rarely, massive PE may present with sudden cardiorespiratory collapse (see Chapter 14, Obstetric emergencies).

If PE is suspected, initial electrocardiogram (ECG), chest X-ray and arterial blood gases should be performed to exclude other respiratory diagnoses. However, these investigations are insufficient on their own to exclude or diagnose PE and it may be sensible to investigate the lower limbs for evidence of DVT by ultrasound, and if positive treat with a presumptive diagnosis of PE. If all the tests are normal but a high clinical suspicion of PE remains, a ventilation perfusion (V/Q) scan or computed tomography pulmonary angiogram (CTPA) should be performed. In both cases the radiation to the fetus is below the threshold considered potentially dangerous to the fetus.

D-dimer is now commonly used as a screening test for thromboembolic disease in non-pregnant women, in whom it has a high negative predictive value. Outwith pregnancy, a low level of D-dimer suggests the absence of a DVT or PE, and no further objective tests are necessary, while an increased level of D-dimer suggests that thrombosis may be present and an objective diagnostic test for DVT and/or PE should be performed. In pregnancy, however, D-dimer can be elevated due to the physiological changes in the coagulation system, limiting its clinical usefulness as a screening test in this situation.

Treatment of VTE

Warfarin is given orally and prolongs the prothrombin time (PT). Warfarin is rarely recommended for use in pregnancy (exceptions include women with mechanical heart valves) as it crosses the placenta and can cause limb and facial defects in the first trimester and fetal intracerebral haemorrhage in the second and third trimesters.

Low molecular weight heparins (LMWHs) are now the treatment of choice. They do not cross the placenta and have been shown to be at least as safe and effective as unfractionated heparin (UFH) in the treatment of VTE, with lower and fewer haemorrhagic complications in the initial treatment of non-pregnant subjects. In addition, LMWH is safe and easy to administer. Women are taught to inject themselves and can continue on this treatment for the duration of their pregnancy.

Following delivery, women can choose to convert to warfarin (with the need for stabilization of the doses initially and frequent checks of the international normalized ratio (INR) or remain on LMWH. Both warfarin and LMWH are safe in women who are breast feeding. Newer anticoagulants such as fondaparinux (a direct factor Xa inhibitor) and lepirudin (a direct thrombin inhibitor) are not licensed for use in pregnancy and experience with them is limited.

Graduated elastic stockings should be used for the initial treatment of DVT and should be worn for 2 years following a DVT to prevent post-thrombotic syndrome.

Prevention of VTE in pregnancy and postpartum

The Royal College of Obstetricians and Gynaecologists has recently released updated guidelines on the prevention of thrombosis and embolism in pregnancy and the puerperium (Green-top Guideline No. 37a, April 2015) and these are summarized in **Figure 6.2**.

KEY LEARNING POINTS

- Screening for thrombophilias should be carried out in those with a strong family or personal history of VTE.
- Rapid treatment of suspected VTE in pregnancy should be commenced while awaiting diagnosis.
- LMWHs are the treatment of choice.
- Graduated compression stockings should be fitted and worn for 2 years to reduce the incidence of post thrombotic syndrome.

Substance abuse in pregnancy

Approximately one-third of adults who access drug services are women of reproductive age. There are approximately 6,000 births to problem drug users in the UK

Antenatal assessment and management (to be assessed at booking and repeated if admitted)

HIGH RISK
Requires antenatal prophylaxis with LMWH
Refer to trust-nominated thrombosis in pregnancy expert/team

Any previous VTE except a single event related to major surgery

INTERMEDIATE RISK
Consider antenatal prophylaxis with LMWH

Hospital admission
Single previous VTE related to major surgery
High-risk thrombophilia + no VTE
Medical comorbidities (e.g. cancer, heart failure, active SLE, IBD or inflammatory polyarthropathy, nephrotic syndrome, type I DM with nephropathy, sickle cell disease, current IVDU)
Any surgical procedure (e.g. appendicectomy)
OHSS (first trimester only)

Four or more risk factors: prophylaxis from first trimester

Three risk factors: prophylaxis from 28 weeks

Obesity (BMI >30 kg/m²)
Age >35 years
Parity ≥3
Smoker
Gross varicose veins
Current pre-eclampsia
Immobility (e.g. paraplegia, PGP)
Family history of unprovoked or oestrogen provoked VTE in first-degree relative
Low-risk thrombophilia
Multiple pregnancy
IVF/ART

Fewer than three risk factors

LOWER RISK
Mobilization and avoidance of dehydration

Transient risk factors:
Dehydration/hyperemesis; current systemic infection; long-distance travel

APL, antiphospholipid antibodies (lupus anticoagulant, anticardiolipin antibodies, β₂-glycoprotein 1 antibodies); ART, assisted reproductive technology; BMI based on booking weight; DM, diabetes mellitus; FHx, family history; gross varicose veins, symptomatic, above knee or associated with phlebitis/oedema/skin changes; high-risk thrombophilia, antithrombin deficiency, protein C or S deficiency, compound or homozygous for low-risk thrombophilias; IBD, inflammatory bowel disease; immobility, ≥ 3 days; IVF, *in vitro* fertilisation; LMWH, low-molecular-weight heparin; long-distance travel, >4 hours; low-risk thrombophilia, heterozygous for factor V Leiden or prothrombin G20210A mutations; OHSS, ovarian hyperstimulation syndrome; PGP, pelvic girdle pain with reduced mobility; PPH, postpartum haemorrhage; thrombophilia, inherited or acquired; VTE, venous thromboembolism.

Postnatal assessment and management (to be assessed on delivery suite)

HIGH RISK
At least 6 weeks' postnatal prophylactic LMWH

Any previous VTE
Anyone requiring antenatal LMWH
High-risk thrombophilia
Low-risk thrombophilia + FHx

INTERMEDIATE RISK
At least 10 days' postnatal prophylactic LMWH

NB If persisting or >3 risk factors consider extending thromboprophylaxis with LMWH

Caesarean section in labour
BMI ≥40 kg/m²
Readmission or prolonged admission (≥3 days) in the puerperium
Any surgical procedure in the puerperium except immediate repair of the perineum
Medical comorbidities (e.g. cancer, heart failure, active SLE, IBD or inflammatory polyarthropathy; nephrotic syndrome, type I DM with nephropathy, sickle cell disease, current IVDU)

Two or more risk factors

Age >35 years
Obesity (BMI >30 kg/m²)
Parity ≥3
Smoker
Elective caesarean section
Family history of VTE
Low-risk thrombophilia
Gross varicose veins
Current systemic infection
Immobility (e.g. paraplegia, PGP, long-distance travel)
Current pre-eclampsia
Multiple pregnancy
Preterm delivery in this pregnancy (<37⁺⁰ weeks)
Stillbirth in this pregnancy
Midcavity rotational or operative delivery
Prolonged labour (>24 hours)
PPH >1 litre or blood transfusion

Fewer than two risk factors

LOWER RISK
Early mobilization and avoidance of dehydration

Antenatal and postnatal prophylactic dose of LMWH
Weight <50 kg = 20 mg enoxaparin/2,500 units dalteparin/3,500 units tinzaparin daily
Weight 50–90 kg = 40 mg enoxaparin/5,000 units dalteparin/4,500 units tinzaparin daily
Weight 91–130 kg = 60 mg enoxaparin/7,500 units dalteparin/7,000 units tinzaparin daily
Weight 131–170 kg = 80 mg enoxaparin/10,000 units dalteparin/9,000 units tinzaparin daily
Weight >170 kg = 0.6 mg/kg/day enoxaparin/ 75 u/kg/day dalteparin/ 75 u/kg/day tinzaparin

Figure 6.2 Obstetric thromboprophylaxis risk assessment and management. (Adapted from RCOG Green-top Guideline No. 37a, April 2015.)

each year (about 1% of all deliveries). Multidisciplinary care is often necessary to optimize outcomes because the financial, psychological, social and domestic problems associated with drug misuse are often greater than the physical and medical concerns.

Problems frequently encountered amongst drug addicts

- Social problems: housing, crime, other children in care or abused.
- Coexistent addictions: alcohol and smoking.
- Malnutrition: especially iron, vitamins B and C.
- Risk of viral infections (e.g. human immuno-deficiency virus [HIV] or hepatitis B).
- Specific fetal and neonatal risks.

Opioids, especially heroin, remain the most commonly used drugs in the UK, although many drug users take combinations of drugs that often include cocaine or crack cocaine. Amphetamines, benzodiazepines and cannabis are also common.

Most problem drug users smoke tobacco and are heavy users of alcohol and cannabis. Taking drugs in combination greatly increases the unpredictability of their effect on the user. Intravenous injection of drugs also puts drug users at greater risk of infection with blood-borne viruses (hepatitis B and C and HIV). Many drug users live in disadvantaged communities in conditions of poverty and social exclusion. Many have had poor parenting experiences, poor education and significant mental health problems. The aims of management are to stabilize the mother's drug-taking habits and ensure contact with social/care workers and psychiatric/drug liaison services as appropriate.

It is important not to try to reduce the opiate dose too rapidly in pregnancy. Sudden detoxification ('cold turkey') can be dangerous for the baby, especially in the third trimester when even mild maternal withdrawal is associated with fetal stress, fetal distress and stillbirth; the principle is to administer the lowest effective dose of methadone liquid in three divided doses every day.

Screening for infections such as hepatitis B and HIV is routinely offered in the UK. In many cases, multidisciplinary case conferences should be held to make arrangements and decisions for when the baby is delivered.

Alcohol

There is much debate about what a 'safe' dose of alcohol is during pregnancy. What is likely is that an intake of less than 100 g per week (approximately two drinks per day; for example, two medium glasses of wine or one pint of beer) is not associated with any adverse effects. Doses greater than this have been related to fetal growth restriction (FGR). Massive doses, in excess of 2 g/kg of body weight (17 drinks per day), have been associated with fetal alcohol syndrome. However, the syndrome is not seen consistently in infants born to women who are heavy consumers of alcohol, and occurs only in approximately 30–33% of children born to women who drink about 2 g/kg of body weight per day (equivalent to approximately 18 units of alcoholic drink per day). The differing susceptibility of fetuses to the syndrome is thought to be multifactorial and reflects the interplay of genetic factors, social deprivation, nutritional deficiencies, tobacco and other drug abuse, along with alcohol consumption.

If alcohol abuse is suspected, it may be necessary to involve social workers and arrange for formal psychiatric/addiction assessment. It is extremely difficult to 'test' for alcohol abuse, as even markers such as mean corpuscular volume and gamma-glutamyl transpeptidase (GGT) are not reliable in pregnancy. Malnutrition is very likely in heavy alcohol abuse and requires B vitamin supplements and iron. A common problem is that many women who abuse alcohol and other drugs not only do not take their medicines but also default antenatal appointments.

Smoking and pregnancy

Smoking acutely reduces placental perfusion. Overall perinatal mortality is increased, babies are smaller at delivery and there is a higher risk of placental abruption in smokers compared with non-smokers. It is estimated that a baby will weigh less than its target weight by a multiple of 15 g times the average number of cigarettes a woman smokes per day; smoking fewer than five cigarettes per day has a barely discernible obstetric effect and quitting by 15 weeks' gestation reduces the risk as much as quitting before pregnancy. Consequently, all women should be counselled regarding smoking cessation at their booking visit.

Oligohydramnios and polyhydramnios

Amniotic fluid is produced almost exclusively from fetal urine from the second trimester onwards. It serves a vital function in protecting the developing baby from pressure or trauma, allowing limb movement, hence normal postural development, and permitting the fetal lungs to expand and develop through breathing.

Oligohydramnios

Too little amniotic fluid (oligohydramnios) is commonly defined as amniotic fluid index (AFI) less than the 5th centile for gestation. The AFI is an ultrasound estimation of amniotic fluid derived by adding together the deepest vertical pool in four quadrants of the abdomen. The AFI (in cm) is therefore associated with some degree of error. In general, however, it is possible to differentiate subjectively on ultrasound between 'too much', 'too little' and 'normal looking'.

Oligohydramnios may be suspected antenatally following a history of clear fluid leaking from the vagina; this may represent PPROM (see Chapter 8, Preterm labour). Clinically, on abdominal palpation the fetal poles may be very obviously felt and 'hard', with a small for dates uterus.

Possible causes of oligohydramnios and anhydramnios

Too little production	Diagnosed by
Renal agenesis	Ultrasound: no renal tissue, no bladder
Multicystic kidneys	Ultrasound: enlarged kidneys with multiple cysts, no visible bladder
Urinary tract abnormality/ obstruction	Ultrasound: kidneys may be present, but urinary tract dilatation
FGR and placental insufficiency	Clinical: reduced SFH, reduced fetal movements, possibly abnormal CTG, Ultrasound: FGR, abnormal fetal Doppler wave forms

Too little production	Diagnosed by
Maternal drugs (e.g. NSAIDs)	Withholding NSAIDs may allow amniotic fluid to reaccumulate
Post-dates pregnancy	
Leakage	Diagnosed by
PPROM	Speculum examination: pool of amniotic fluid on posterior blade

NSAID, non-steroidal anti-inflammatory drug; SFH, symphysis–fundal height.

The fetal prognosis depends on the cause of oligohydramnios, but both pulmonary hypoplasia and limb deformities (contractures, talipes) are common to severe early-onset (<24 weeks' gestation) oligohydramnios. Renal agenesis and bilateral multicystic kidneys carry a lethal prognosis, as life after birth is impossible without functioning kidneys. In this situation, the fetal lungs would probably be hypoplastic; this may also be true of severe urinary tract obstruction. Oligohydramnios due to FGR/uteroplacental insufficiency is usually of a less severe degree and less commonly causes limb and lung problems.

Polyhydramnios

Polyhydramnios is the term given to an excess of amniotic fluid (i.e. AFI >95th centile for gestation on ultrasound estimation). It may present as severe abdominal swelling and discomfort. On examination, the abdomen will appear distended out of proportion to the woman's gestation (increased SFH). Furthermore, the abdomen may be tense and tender and the fetal poles will be hard to palpate. The condition may be caused by maternal, placental or fetal conditions.

Causes of polyhydramnios

Maternal
- Diabetes.
- Placental.
- Chorioangioma.
- Arteriovenous fistula.

Fetal

- Multiple gestation (in monochorionic twins it may be twin-to-twin transfusion syndrome).
- Idiopathic.
- Oesophageal atresia/tracheo-oesophageal fistula.
- Duodenal atresia.
- Neuromuscular fetal condition (preventing swallowing).
- Anencephaly.

The management of polyhydramnios is directed towards establishing the cause (and hence determining fetal prognosis), relieving the discomfort of the mother (if necessary by amniodrainage) and assessing the risk of preterm labour due to uterine overdistension.

Polyhydramnios due to maternal diabetes needs urgent investigation, as it often suggests high maternal blood glucose levels. In this context, polyhydramnios should correct itself when the mother's glycaemic control is optimized.

Twin-to-twin transfusion syndrome is a rare cause of acute polyhydramnios in the recipient sac of monochorionic twins. It is associated with oligohydramnios and a small baby in the other sac. The condition may be rapidly fatal for both twins; amniodrainage and removal by laser of the placental vascular connections are two therapeutic modalities employed in dealing with this condition. This is discussed further in Chapter 7, Multiple pregnancy.

Fetal malpresentation at term

Malpresentation is a presentation that is not cephalic. Breech presentation is the most commonly encountered malpresentation and occurs in 3–4% of term pregnancies, but is more common at earlier gestations. Similarly, oblique and transverse positions are not uncommon antenatally. They only become a problem if the baby (or first presenting baby in a multiple gestation) is not cephalic by 37 weeks' gestation.

Breech presentation

There are three types of breech: the commonest is extended (frank) breech (**Figure 6.3A**); less common is a flexed (complete) breech (**Figure 6.3B**); and least common is footling breech, in which a foot presents at the cervix (**Figure 6.3C**). Cord and foot prolapse are risks in this situation.

Predisposing factors for breech presentation

Maternal

- Fibroids.
- Congenital uterine abnormalities (e.g. bicornuate uterus).
- Uterine surgery.

Fetal/placental

- Multiple gestation.
- Prematurity.
- Placenta praevia.
- Abnormality (e.g. anencephaly or hydrocephalus).
- Fetal neuromuscular condition.
- Oligohydramnios.
- Polyhydramnios.

Antenatal management of breech presentation

If a breech presentation is clinically suspected at or after 36 weeks, this should be confirmed by ultrasound scan. The scan should document fetal biometry, amniotic fluid volume, the placental site and the position of the fetal legs. The scan should also look for any anomalies previously undetected.

The three management options available at this point should be discussed with the woman. These are external cephalic version (ECV), vaginal breech delivery and elective caesarean section. A previous large multicentre randomized controlled trial suggested that planned vaginal delivery of a breech presentation is associated with a 3% increased risk of death or serious morbidity to the baby. Although this trial did not evaluate long-term outcomes for child or mother, it has led to the recommendation that the best method of delivering a term breech singleton is by planned caesarean section. Despite this, either by choice or as a result of precipitous labour, a small proportion of women with breech presentations will deliver vaginally. It therefore remains important that clinicians and hospitals are prepared for vaginal breech delivery.

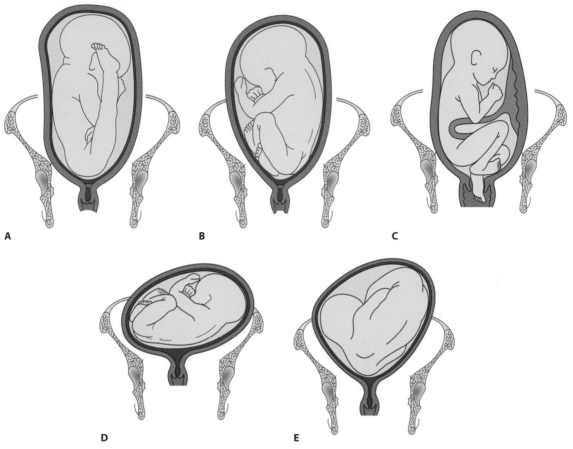

A   B   C

D   E

Figure 6.3 (**A**) Frank breech (also known as extended breech) presentation with extension of the legs; (**B**) breech presentation with flexion of the legs; (**C**) footling breech presentation; (**D**) transverse lie; (**E**) oblique lie.

External cephalic version

ECV is a relatively straightforward and safe technique and has been shown to reduce the number of caesarean sections due to breech presentations. Success rates vary according to the experience of the operator but in most units are around 50% (and are higher in multiparous women who tend to have lax abdominal musculature).

The procedure is performed at or after 37 completed weeks' gestation by an experienced obstetrician at or near delivery facilities. ECV should be performed with a tocolytic (e.g. nifedipine) as this has been shown to improve the success rate. The woman is laid flat with a left lateral tilt having ensured that she has emptied her bladder and is comfortable. With ultrasound guidance, the breech is elevated from the pelvis and one hand is used to

▶ **VIDEO 6.1**

External cephalic version (ECV): http://www.routledgetextbooks.com/textbooks/tenteachers/obstetricsv6.1.php

manipulate this upward in the direction of a forward role whilst the other hand applies gentle pressure to flex the fetal head and bring it down to the maternal pelvis (**Figure 6.4**).

The procedure can be mildly uncomfortable for the mother and should last no more than 10 minutes. If the procedure fails, or becomes difficult, it is abandoned. A fetal heart rate trace must be performed before and after the procedure and it is important to administer anti-D if the woman is rhesus negative.

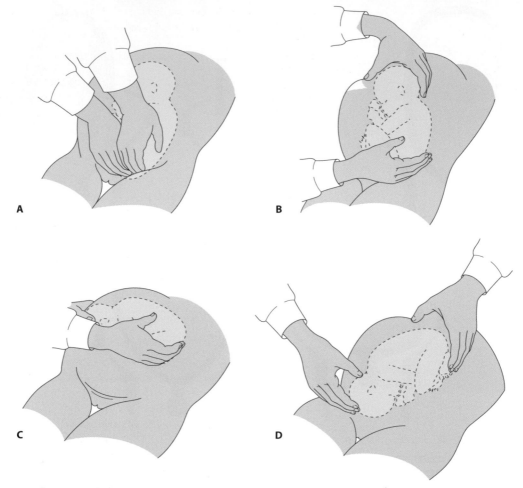

Figure 6.4 External cephalic version. (**A**) The breech is disengaged from the pelvic inlet; (**B**) version is usually performed in the direction that increases flexion of the fetus and makes it do a forward somersault; (**C**) on completion of version, the head is often not engaged for a time; (**D**) the fetal heart rate should be checked after the external version has been completed.

Contraindications to ECV

- Fetal abnormality (e.g. hydrocephalus).
- Placenta praevia.
- Oligohydramnios or polyhydramnios.
- History of antepartum haemorrhage.
- Previous caesarean or myomectomy scar on the uterus.
- Multiple gestation.
- Pre-eclampsia or hypertension.
- Plan to deliver by caesarean section anyway.

Risks of ECV

- Placental abruption.
- Premature rupture of the membranes.
- Cord accident.
- Transplacental haemorrhage (remember anti-D administration to rhesus-negative women).
- Fetal bradycardia.

Mode of delivery

If ECV fails, or is contraindicated, and caesarean section is nor indicated for other reasons, then women should be counselled regarding elective caesarean section and planned vaginal delivery. Although evidence suggests that it is probably safer for breech babies to be delivered by caesarean section, there is still a place for a vaginal breech delivery in certain circumstances. Maternal choice and the failure to detect breech presentation until very late in labour mean that obstetricians need to be expert in the skills of breech vaginal delivery and aware of the potential complications.

Pre-requisites for vaginal breech delivery

Feto-maternal

- The presentation should be either extended (hips flexed, knees extended) or flexed (hips flexed, knees flexed but feet not below the fetal buttocks).

- There should be no evidence of feto-pelvic disproportion with a pelvis clinically thought to be adequate and an estimated fetal weight of <3,500 g (ultrasound or clinical measurement).

- There should be no evidence of hyperextension of the fetal head, and fetal abnormalities that would preclude safe vaginal delivery (e.g. severe hydrocephalus) should be excluded.

Management of labour

- Fetal wellbeing and progress of labour should be carefully monitored.

- An epidural analgesia is not essential but may be advantageous; it can prevent pushing before full dilatation.

- Fetal blood sampling from the buttocks provides an accurate assessment of the acid–base status (when the fetal heart rate trace is suspect).

- There should be an operator experienced in delivering breech babies available in the hospital.

Although much emphasis is placed on adequate case selection prior to labour, a survey of outcome of the undiagnosed breech in labour managed by experienced medical staff showed that safe vaginal delivery can be achieved.

Technique

A vaginal breech delivery should be characterized by 'masterly inactivity' (hands-off). Problems are more likely to arise when the obstetrician tries to speed up the process by pulling on the baby, and this should be avoided.

Delivery of the buttocks

In most circumstances, full dilatation and descent of the breech will have occurred naturally. When the buttocks become visible and begin to distend the perineum, preparations for the delivery are made. The buttocks will lie in the anterior–posterior diameter. Once the anterior buttock is delivered and the anus is seen over the fourchette (and no sooner than this), an episiotomy can be cut.

Delivery of the legs and lower body

If the legs are flexed, they will deliver spontaneously. If extended, they may need to be delivered using Pinard's manoeuvre. This entails using a finger to flex the leg at the knee and then extend at the hip, first anteriorly then posteriorly. With contractions and maternal effort, the lower body will be delivered. Usually a loop of cord is drawn down to ensure that it is not too short.

Delivery of the shoulders

The baby will be lying with the shoulders in the transverse diameter of the pelvic midcavity. As the anterior shoulder rotates into the anterior–posterior diameter, the spine or the scapula will become visible. At this point, a finger gently placed above the shoulder will help to deliver the arm. As the posterior arm/shoulder reaches the pelvic floor, it too will rotate anteriorly (in the opposite direction). Once the spine becomes visible, delivery of the second arm will follow. This can be imagined as a 'rocking boat' with one side moving upwards and then the other. Loveset's manoeuvre essentially copies these natural movements (**Figure 6.5**). However, it is unnecessary and meddlesome to do routinely (one risks pulling the shoulders down but leaving the arms higher up, alongside the head).

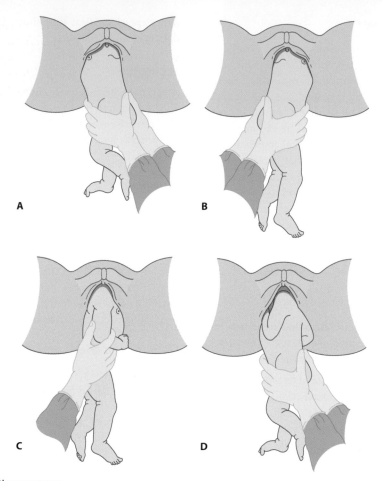

Figure 6.5 Loveset's manoeuvre.

Delivery of the head

The head is delivered using the Mauriceau–Smellie–Veit manoeuvre: the baby lies on the obstetrician's arm with downward traction being levelled on the head via a finger in the mouth and one on each maxilla (**Figure 6.6**). Delivery occurs with first downward and then upward movement (as with instrumental deliveries). If this manoeuvre proves difficult, forceps need to be applied. An assistant holds the baby's body upwards while the forceps are applied in the usual manner (**Figure 6.7**).

Complications

The greatest fear with a vaginal breech is that the baby will get 'stuck'. Interference in the natural process by the inappropriate use of oxytocic agents or by

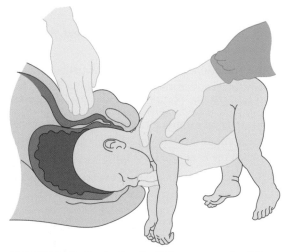

Figure 6.6 Mauriceau–Smellie–Veit manoeuvre for delivery of the head.

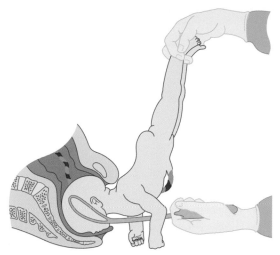

Figure 6.7 Delivery of the aftercoming head with forceps.

trying to pull the baby out (breech extraction) will paradoxically increase the risk of obstruction occurring. When delay occurs, particularly with delivery of the shoulders or head, the presence of an experienced obstetrician will reduce the risk of death or serious injury.

 KEY LEARNING POINTS

- Breech presentation: ECV should be offered at 36–37 weeks in selected women.
- Elective caesarean section is safer than vaginal delivery for a baby presenting by the breech at or close to term.
- Planned or unexpected vaginal breech deliveries should be attended by experienced clinicians.

Other fetal malpresentations

A transverse lie occurs when the fetal long axis lies perpendicular to that of the maternal long axis and classically results in a shoulder presentation (see **Figure 6.3D**). An oblique lie occurs when the long axis of the fetal body crosses the long axis of the maternal body at an angle close to 45° (see **Figure 6.3E**).

Any woman presenting at term with a transverse or oblique lie is at potential risk of cord prolapse following spontaneous rupture of the membranes, and prolapse of the hand, shoulder or foot once in labour. In most cases, the woman is multiparous with a lax

uterus and abdominal wall musculature, and gentle version of the baby's head in the clinic or on the ward will restore the presentation to cephalic. If this does not occur, or the lie is unstable (alternating between transverse, oblique and longitudinal), it is important to think of possible uterine or fetal causes of this.

The diagnosis of transverse or oblique lie might be suspected by abdominal inspection: the abdomen often appears asymmetrical. The SFH may be less than expected, and on palpation the fetal head or buttocks may be in the iliac fossa. Palpation over the pelvic brim will reveal an 'empty' pelvis.

It goes without saying that a woman in labour with the baby's lie anything other than longitudinal will not be able to deliver vaginally; this is one situation in which if caesarean section is not performed both the mother and baby are at considerable risk of morbidity and mortality. The only exception to this is for exceptionally preterm or small babies, where vaginal delivery may occur irrespective of lie or presentation.

A woman with an unstable lie at term should be admitted to the antenatal ward. The normal plan would be to deliver by caesarean section if the presentation is not cephalic in early labour or if spontaneous rupture of the membranes occurs. In a multiparous woman, an unstable lie will often correct itself in early labour (as long as the membranes are intact).

Post-term pregnancy

A pregnancy that has extended to or beyond 42 weeks' gestation is defined as a prolonged or post-term pregnancy. Accurate dating remains essential for the correct diagnosis and should ideally involve a first-trimester ultrasound estimation of crown–rump length.

Post-term pregnancy affects approximately 10% of all pregnancies and the aetiology is unknown. Post-term pregnancy is associated with increased risks to both the fetus and the mother, including an increased risk of stillbirth and perinatal death and an increased risk of prolonged labour and caesarean section.

Fetal surveillance and induction of labour are two strategies employed that may reduce the risk of adverse outcome. Unfortunately, there are no known tests that can accurately predict fetal outcome post-term; an ultrasound scan may give temporary reassurance if the amniotic fluid and fetal growth are normal. Similarly, a CTG should be performed at and after 42 weeks.

Immediate induction of labour or delivery postdates should take place if:

- There is reduced amniotic fluid on scan.
- Fetal growth is reduced.
- There are reduced fetal movements.
- The CTG is not perfect.
- The mother is hypertensive or suffers from a significant medical condition.

Induction of labour is discussed further in Chapter 12, Labour: normal and abnormal.

When counselling the parents regarding waiting for labour to start naturally after 42 weeks, it is important that the woman is aware that no test can guarantee the safety of her baby, and that perinatal mortality is increased (at least twofold) beyond 42 weeks. A labour induced post-term is more likely to require caesarean section; this may partly be due to the reluctance of the uterus to contract properly, and the possible compromise of the baby leading to abnormal CTG.

Vaginal bleeding in pregnancy

Bleeding in pregnancy is common but invariably causes anxiety in the pregnant woman. It should always be investigated to rule out significant and dangerous causes, but in many cases of minor bleeding, a cause is never found.

Vaginal bleeding less than 24 weeks' gestation is defined as a threatened miscarriage and the causes and management are described in more detail in Chapter 5, Implantation and early pregnancy, of *Gynaecology by Ten Teachers*, 20th edition. Vaginal bleeding from 24 weeks to delivery of the baby is defined as an antepartum haemorrhage (APH). The causes of APH are placental or local. The incidence of APH is 3%. It is estimated that 1% is attributable to placenta praevia, 1% is attributable to placental abruption and the remaining 1% is from other causes.

Causes of antepartum haemorrhage

Placental causes
- Placental abruption.
- Placenta praevia.
- Vasa praevia.

Local causes
- Cervicitis.
- Cervical ectropion.
- Cervical carcinoma.
- Vaginal trauma.
- Vaginal infection.

APH must always be taken seriously, and any woman presenting with a history of fresh vaginal bleeding must be investigated promptly and properly. The key questions are whether the bleeding is placental, and whether the bleeding is compromising the mother and/or fetus. A pale, tachycardic woman looking anxious with a painful, firm abdomen, underwear soaked in fresh blood and reduced fetal movements needs emergency assessment and management for a possible placental abruption. A woman having had a small postcoital bleed with no systemic signs or symptoms represents a different end of the spectrum.

History

- How much bleeding?
- Triggering factors (e.g. postcoital bleed).
- Associated with pain or contractions?
- Is the baby moving?
- Last cervical smear (date/normal or abnormal)?

Examination

- Pulse, blood pressure.
- Is the uterus soft or tender and firm?
- Fetal heart auscultation/CTG.
- Speculum vaginal examination, with particular importance placed on visualizing the cervix (having established that placenta is not a praevia, preferably using a portable ultrasound machine).

Investigations

- Depending on the degree of bleeding, full blood count, clotting and, if suspected praevia/abruption, cross-match 6 units of blood.
- Ultrasound (fetal size, presentation, amniotic fluid, placental position and morphology).

Management

If there is minimal bleeding and the cause is clearly local vaginal bleeding, symptomatic management may be given (e.g. antifungal preparations for candidiasis), as long as there is reasonable certainty that cervical carcinoma is excluded by smear history and direct visualization of the cervix. The management of significant APH is described in detail in Chapter 14, Obstetric emergencies.

Rhesus isoimmunization

Blood groups are defined in two ways. First, there is the ABO group, allowing four different permutations of blood group (O, A, B, AB). Second, there is the rhesus system, which consists of C, D and E antigens. The importance of these blood group systems is that a mismatch between the fetus and mother can mean that when fetal red cells pass across to the maternal circulation, as they do to a greater or lesser extent during pregnancy, sensitization of the maternal immune system to these fetal 'foreign' red blood cells may occur and subsequently give rise to haemolytic disease of the fetus and newborn (HDFN). The rhesus system is the one most commonly associated with severe haemolytic disease.

The aetiology of rhesus disease

The rhesus system comprises at least 40 antigens, the most clinically important of which are C, D and E. They are coded on two adjacent genes that sit within chromosome one. One gene codes for antigen polypeptides C/c and E/e while the other codes for the D polypeptide (rhesus antigen). The d (little d) antigen has not been identified so it is probable that women who are D negative lack the antigen altogether, as opposed to those with c (little c) or e (little e), where c is the allelic antigen of C and e is the allelic antigen of E. Antigen expression is usually dominant, whereas those who have a negative phenotype are either homozygous for the recessive allele or have a

deletion of that gene (**Figure 6.8**). In practice only anti-D and anti-c regularly cause HDFN and anti-D is much more common than anti-c.

Occurrence of HDFN as a result of rhesus isoimmunization involves three key stages (**Figure 6.9**). Firstly, a rhesus-negative mother must conceive a baby who has inherited the rhesus-positive phenotype from the father. Secondly, fetal cells must gain access to the maternal circulation in a sufficient volume to provoke a maternal antibody response. Finally, maternal antibodies must cross the placenta and cause immune destruction of red cells in the fetus.

Rhesus disease does not affect a first pregnancy as the primary response is usually weak and consists primarily of immunoglobulin (Ig) M antibodies that do not cross the placenta. However, in a subsequent pregnancy with a rhesus-positive baby, rhesus-positive red cells pass from the baby to the maternal circulation and cause maternal resensitization (**Figure 6.9**). On this occasion, the B-cells produce a much larger response, this time of IgG antibodies that can cross the placenta to the fetal circulation. If these antibodies are present in sufficient quantities, fetal haemolysis may occur, leading to such severe anaemia that the fetus may die unless a transfusion is performed.

> ▶ **VIDEO 6.2**
>
> Animation of the mechanism of rhesus sensitization and fetal red cell destruction: http://www.routledgetextbooks.com/textbooks/tenteachers/obstetricsv6.2.php

> **Potential sensitizing events for rhesus disease**
>
> - Miscarriage.
> - Termination of pregnancy.
> - Antepartum haemorrhage.
> - Invasive prenatal testing (chorion villus sampling, amniocentesis and cordocentesis).
> - Delivery.

Prevalence of rhesus disease

The prevalence of D-rhesus negativity is 15% in the UK Caucasian population, but lower in all other ethnic groups. Approximately 55% of UK Caucasian males are heterozygous for the D antigen; therefore, around two-thirds of rhesus-negative mothers would be expected

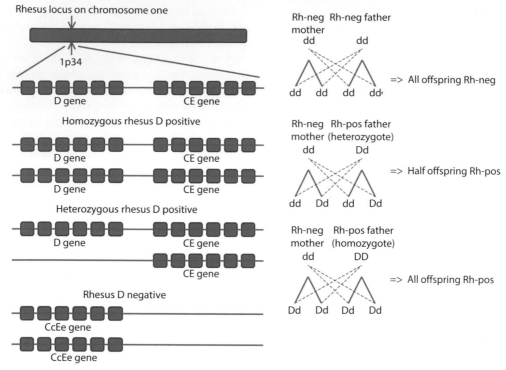

Figure 6.8 The parental genotype determinants of rhesus phenotype.

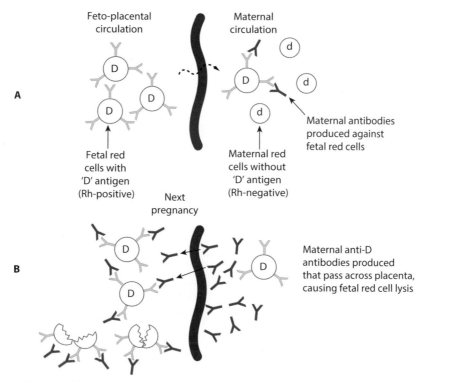

Figure 6.9 The mechanism of rhesus sensitization (**A**) and fetal red cell destruction (**B**).

to carry a rhesus-positive fetus. Rhesus disease is commonest in countries where anti-D prophylaxis is not widespread, such as the Middle East and Russia.

Preventing rhesus isoimmunization

The process of isoimmunization can be prevented by the intramuscular administration of anti-D immunoglobulins to a mother. Anti-D immunoglobulins 'mop up' any circulating rhesus-positive cells before an immune response is excited in the mother. It is normal practice to administer anti-D as soon as possible after any potential sensitizing events that may cause feto-maternal haemorrhage and preferably within 72 hours of exposure to fetal red cells. However, if, exceptionally, this deadline cannot be met, some protection may still be offered if anti-D Ig is given up to 10 days after the sensitizing event. The exact dose is determined by the gestation at which sensitization has occurred and the size of the feto-maternal haemorrhage. A Kleihauer test of maternal blood determines the proportion of fetal cells present in the maternal sample. It relies on the ability of fetal red blood cells to resist denaturation by alcohol or acid and it allows calculation of the size of the feto-maternal transfusion and the amount of extra anti-D Ig required.

The management of sensitizing events in the rhesus-negative pregnant woman

- In the first trimester of pregnancy, because the volume of fetal blood is so small, it is unlikely that sensitization would occur, and anti-D is only indicated following ectopic pregnancy, molar pregnancy, therapeutic termination of pregnancy and in cases of uterine bleeding where this is repeated, heavy or associated with abdominal pain. The dose that should be given is 250 IU.
- For potentially sensitizing events between 12 and 20 weeks' gestation, a minimum dose of 250 IU should be administered within 72 hours of the event and a Kleihauer test should be performed. Further anti-D can be given if indicated by the Kleihauer test.
- For potentially sensitizing events after 20 weeks' gestation, a Kleihauer test is required and pending the result, a minimum anti-D Ig dose of 500 IU should be administered within 72 hours of the event. Further anti-D can be given if indicated by the Kleihauer test.

A small number of rhesus-negative women become sensitized during pregnancy despite the administration of anti-D at delivery and without a clinically obvious sensitizing event. The likelihood is that a small feto-maternal haemorrhage occurs without any obvious clinical signs; therefore, prophylactic anti-D would reduce the risk of isoimmunization from this event. Current UK guidelines suggest that all rhesus-negative pregnant women who have not been previously sensitized should be offered routine antenatal prophylaxis with anti-D, either with a single dose regimen at around 28 weeks or a two-dose regimen given at 28 and 34 weeks' gestation.

Signs of fetal anaemia

Note: clinical and ultrasound features of fetal anaemia do not usually become evident unless fetal haemoglobin is more than 5 g/dl less than the mean for gestation. Usually, features are not obvious unless the fetal haemoglobin is less than 6 g/dl.

- Polyhydramnios.
- Enlarged fetal heart.
- Ascites and pericardial effusions.
- Hyperdynamic fetal circulation (can be detected by Doppler ultrasound by measuring increased velocities in the middle cerebral artery or aorta).
- Reduced fetal movements.
- Abnormal CTG with reduced variability, eventually a 'sinusoidal' trace.

The management of rhesus disease in a sensitized woman

Once a woman who is D-rhesus negative has been sensitized to the D-rhesus antigen, no amount of anti-D will ever turn the clock back. In a subsequent pregnancy, close surveillance is required. Rhesus disease gets worse with successive pregnancies, so it is important to note the severity of the disease in previous pregnancies. The management depends on the clinical scenario.

The father of the next baby is D-rhesus negative. In this situation there is no risk that the baby will be D-rhesus positive and therefore there is no chance of rhesus disease.

The father of the next baby is D-rhesus positive. He may be heterozygous and in this situation determining the paternal phenotype is useful in anticipating the likely fetal phenotype and, thus, the potential for development of HDFN. However, it is important to bear in mind that there are issues regarding paternal testing, and assuming paternity runs the risk of false prediction. Not withstanding this issue, paternal blood grouping is frequently used and often useful.

In a sensitized woman, if the father is D-rhesus positive or unknown, standard management involves monitoring antibody levels every 2–4 weeks from booking. Antibody levels or quantity can be described using the titre or by using IU (international units) as a standard quantification method. The titre simply refers to the number of times a sample has been diluted before the amount of antibody becomes undetectable; titre of 2, 4, 8, 16, 32, 64, 128, etc. Each time a sample is tested it should be checked in parallel with the previous sample to ensure the detection of significant changes in the antibody level. However, titrations of anti-D do not correlate well with the development of HDFN, and the standard quantification method (IU/ml) gives more clinically relevant levels (*Table 6.2*).

If antibody levels rise, the baby should be examined for signs of anaemia. In the past, the bilirubin concentration of amniotic fluid was determined optically to give an indirect measure of fetal haemolysis. This involved an invasive procedure with the attendant risks of miscarriage/preterm labour and further boosting of the alloimmune response. In the last decade, middle cerebral artery (MCA) Dopplers (peak velocity measurement) have been shown to correlate reliably with fetal anaemia. In practice, this means that the use of invasive tests to monitor disease progression once a critical antibody level has been reached have been replaced by non-invasive assessment using MCA Doppler. There are now substantial data to support the use of peak MCA velocity as a correlate of fetal anaemia. The sensitivity is reported at 100% with a false-positive rate of 12% (**Figure 6.10**).

A fetus with a raised peak MCA velocity has a high probability of anaemia. These cases are not common and the treatment should be in, or guided by, tertiary fetal medicine centres. Treatment options include delivery or fetal blood transfusion. Delivery of the fetus is an option if the fetus is sufficiently mature. However, delivery of an anaemic, rapidly haemolysing premature baby is a significant risk and should not be undertaken lightly. Delivery must take place in a unit where adequate neonatal support and expertise is available, and generally delivery should not be before 36–37 weeks' gestation unless there are specific reasons such as special difficulty with fetal transfusion.

Fetal blood transfusion is life saving in a severely anaemic fetus that is too premature for delivery to be contemplated. The aim is to restore haemoglobin levels, reversing or preventing hydrops or death. A side-effect is that transfusion will also suppress fetal erythropoiesis, which reduces the concentration of antigen-positive cells available for haemolysis. Blood can be transfused into a fetus in various ways depending on the gestation, the site of the cord insertion and the clinical situation. Routes of administration include:

- Into the umbilical vein at the point of the cord insertion (ideally through the placenta and not through the amniotic sac).

- Into the intrahepatic vein.

- Into the peritoneal cavity (not as effective but some blood is absorbed and this may be the only option, for example in early gestations).

- Into the fetal heart.

Once a decision has been made that the fetus is severely anaemic and requires a blood transfusion, the invasive procedure aims to first take a sample to confirm the anaemia and then infuse the blood during a single puncture.

Transfused blood is:

- RhD negative.

- Crossmatched with a maternal sample.

Table 6.2 Anti-D-rhesus titration

Anti-D level	Outcome
<4 IU/ml	HDFN unlikely
4–15 IU/ml	Moderate risk of HDFN
>15 IU/ml	High risk of hydrops fetalis

HDFN, haemolytic disease of the fetus and newborn.

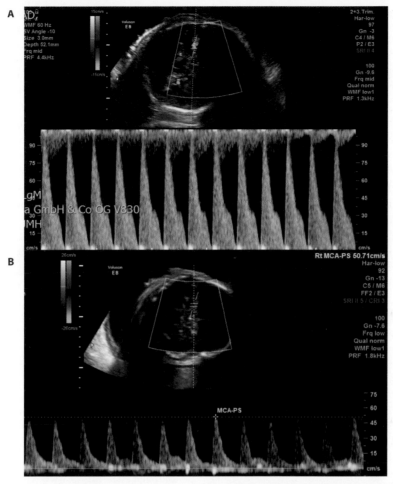

Figure 6.10 Middle cerebral artery Doppler waveform analysis (**A**) of a fetus with anaemia secondary to Rhesus disease demonstrating an increased peak systolic velocity, and the same fetus (**B**) 48 hours following an intrauterine transfusion.

- Densely packed (haemoglobin usually around 30 g/l) so that small volumes are used.
- White cell depleted and irradiated.
- Screened for infection including cytomegalovirus (CMV).

At delivery

If the baby is known to be anaemic or has had multiple transfusions, a neonatologist must be present at delivery should exchange transfusion be required. Blood must therefore always be ready for the delivery. All babies born to rhesus-negative women should have cord blood taken at delivery for a blood count, blood group and indirect Coombs test.

KEY LEARNING POINTS

- Rhesus disease gets worse with successive pregnancies.
- If the father of the fetus is rhesus negative, the fetus cannot be rhesus positive.
- If the father of the fetus is rhesus positive, he may be a heterozygote (50% likelihood that the baby is D-rhesus positive) or a homozygote (100% likelihood).
- Anti-D is given only as prophylaxis and is useless once sensitization has occurred.
- Prenatal diagnosis for karyotype, or attempts at determining fetal blood group by invasive testing (e.g. chorion villus sampling), may make the antibody levels higher in women who are already sensitized.

ABO incompatibility

ABO blood group isoimmunization may occur when the mother is blood group O and the baby is blood group A or B. Anti-A and anti-B antibodies are present in the maternal circulation naturally, usually secondary to sensitization against A or B substances in food or bacteria. This means that ABO incompatibility may occur in a first pregnancy. In this situation, anti-A or anti-B antibodies may pass to the fetal circulation, causing fetal haemolysis and anaemia. However, most anti-A and anti-B antibodies are mainly IgMs that do not cross the placenta. In addition, A and B antigens are not fully developed in the fetus. Therefore, ABO incompatibility generally causes mild haemolytic disease of the baby, but may sometimes explain unexpected jaundice in an otherwise healthy term infant.

New developments

When a fetus is at risk of HDFN in a sensitized rhesus-negative mother, the genotype of the fetus is very important. When the father is heterozygous for rhesus D, there is a 50% chance that the fetus will be rhesus positive. In this situation it is important to establish the fetal blood group to determine whether or not the baby is at risk. This can now be done non-invasively by examining cell-free fetal DNA (cffDNA) present in a maternal blood sample. Accuracies close to 100% are reported for rhesus genotyping.

A similar approach can be used to prevent unnecessary prophylaxis. Currently in the UK, all rhesus-negative pregnant women are offered anti-D. However, the disadvantage of this approach is that approximately 40% of D-negative women who are carrying a rhesus-negative child will be given routine prophylactic anti-D unnecessarily. This equates to approximately 40,000 women in the UK who are receiving prophylaxis unnecessarily each year. Fetal blood group genotyping using cffDNA from maternal blood samples taken between 16 and 20 weeks' gestation have made it possible to determine the fetal rhesus genotype type. Routine fetal rhesus typing for all rhesus-negative pregnant women has been introduced in Denmark and The Netherlands to allow selective use of anti-D, though this has not yet been recommended in the UK.

Further reading

Qureshi H, Massey E, Kirwan D, et al. (2014). BCSH guideline for the use of anti-D immunoglobulin for the prevention of haemolytic disease of the fetus and newborn. Transfusion Medicine 24:8–20.doi: 10.1111/tme.12091.

Royal College of Obstetricians and Gynaecologists Clinical Guideline No. 20a. External Cephalic Version and Reducing the Incidence of Breech Presentation. Published December 2006 and Reviewed 2010. https://www.rcog.org.uk/globalassets/documents/guidelines/gt20aexternalcephalicversion.pdf.

Royal College of Obstetricians and Gynaecologists Clinical Guideline No. 20b. The Management of Breech Presentation. Published 1999 and Revised in 2001 and 2006. https://www.rcog.org.uk/globalassets/documents/guidelines/gtg-no-20b-breech-presentation.pdf.

Royal College of Obstetricians and Gynaecologists Clinical Guideline No. 37a. Reducing the Risk of Venous Thromboembolism during Pregnancy and the Puerperium. Published April 2015. https://www.rcog.org.uk/globalassets/documents/guidelines/gtg-37a.pdf.

Self assessment

CASE HISTORY

The community midwife refers a 25-year-old woman in her second pregnancy to the antenatal clinic at 37 weeks' gestation. Clinical examination has shown the fetus to be in a breech position. An ultrasound scan confirms an extended breech presentation. You are asked to counsel this woman as to the possible options that are available for her management.

A What are the available options?

B What are the advantages and risks of each option?

ANSWERS

A There are three available management options that need to be discussed with this woman. These are:

- Elective caesarean section.
- External cephalic version (ECV).
- Vaginal breech delivery.

B Firstly, a brief history should be taken to determine whether there are any factors in the history that would be a contraindication to vaginal breech delivery or ECV.

The Term Breech Trial demonstrated that there was reduction in the perinatal mortality and morbidity with elective caesarean section over vaginal breech delivery. However, there are some factors that would increase and decrease the strength of the recommendation for a caesarean section, such as previous obstetric history and the presence of a large or small baby.

ECV is carried out at 36–37 weeks' gestation. The procedure has been shown to reduce the number of caesarean sections due to breech presentation. Contraindications to ECV are placenta praevia, oligohydramnios, previous caesarean section, multiple gestation and pre-eclampsia. The risks of the procedure, which need to be outlined, are placental abruption, premature rupture of the membranes, cord accident, transplacental haemorrhage and fetal bradycardia.

Vaginal breech delivery is still an acceptable option if the mother understands the increased risks to the fetus. There are a number of factors that increase the likelihood of a successful vaginal beech delivery: normal sized baby, flexed neck, multiparous, deeply engaged breech and positive mental attitude of the woman.

EMQ

A No intervention required.

B Lifelong anticoagulation.

C IV unfractionated heparin for 24 hours.

D LMWH for 6 weeks postnatally.

E Discussion with haematologist for specialist advice.

F LMWH for 10 days postnatally.

G Early mobilization and hydration.

H Antenatal prophylaxis with LMWH.

I None of the above.

For each description, choose the SINGLE most appropriate answer from the list of options. Each option may be used once, more than once or not at all.

1 A woman attends for booking at 6 weeks' gestation. She has had a previous metallic mitral valve replacement.

2 A 28-year-old woman who has had an emergency caesarean section in labour for fetal distress. She had a DVT in a previous pregnancy.

3 A healthy 30-year-old woman with a normal body mass index (BMI) who had a normal vaginal delivery of her fourth child 4 hours ago.

4 A healthy 36-year-old woman with a normal BMI who had a normal vaginal delivery of her fourth child 4 hours ago.

ANSWERS

1B   Thromboprophylaxis in pregnancy and the puerperium in the UK is usually based on the RCOG 2015 guidelines (**Figure 6.2**). The woman has a metallic mitral valve and should be on lifelong anti-coagulation. This is usually achieved with warfarin but may be switched to LMWH in pregnancy.

2D   The woman requires at least 6 weeks of postnatal prophylactic LMWH as she had a previous thrombotic event.

3G   The woman has single risk factor for VTE (parity >3) and therefore only needs sensible precautions.

4F   The woman has an additional risk factor being aged >35 and therefore needs postnatal LMWH for 10 days.

SBA QUESTION

On routine antenatal investigation, a 30-year-old woman is found to be rhesus negative. Which piece of advice regarding the management of her pregnancy is correct? Choose the single best answer.

A   Her fetus will also be rhesus negative.

B   If she experiences vaginal bleeding later in pregnancy, a Keilhauer test should be performed.

C   She should have a routine dose of anti-D at 23 weeks' gestation.

D   Once she has had two doses of anti-D, further administration will not be required.

E   If this pregnancy is not affected by rhesus disease, there should be no problem in subsequent pregnancies.

ANSWER

B   Approximately 15% of the Caucasian population are rhesus negative. The rhesus status of the fetus depends on the father's blood type. Exogenous anti-D immunoglobulin is administered in an attempt to prevent the manufacture of the endogenous antibody by the mother, as this would sensitize the immune system and put subsequent fetuses at risk, Routine doses of anti-D are normally given between 28 and 34 weeks' gestation, but should be considered after every sensitizing event. The Keilhauer test determines the portion of fetal cells within the maternal circulation and hence helps determine anti-D dosage.

Multiple pregnancy

FERGUS McCARTHY

LEARNING OBJECTIVES

- Understand classification of multiple pregnancies.
- Understand risk factors for multiple pregnancies and why prevalence is increasing.
- Understand the increased complications that occur in multiple pregnancies.
- Understand the antenatal care of women with multiple pregnancies.

Introduction

Rates of multiple pregnancies continue to increase and now constitute approximately 3% of live births. The high prevalence of multiple pregnancy is explained predominantly by increasing use of assisted fertility, with rates of multiple pregnancy being directly proportional to the number of embryos transferred. Regardless of chorionicity and amnionicity, complications in multiple pregnancies are higher than for singleton pregnancies and include preterm birth, fetal growth restriction (FGR), cerebral palsy and stillbirth. The maternal risks are also increased and include hypertensive and thromboembolic disease and antepartum and postpartum haemorrhage.

Epidemiology

The incidence of multiple pregnancy varies worldwide, with rates varying from approximately 6 per 1,000 births in Japan to rates of approximately 40 per 1,000 births in Nigeria. In the UK the rates of multiple pregnancy are approximately 16 per 1,000 births. The majority (97–99%) of these were twin pregnancies with the remainder being predominantly triplet pregnancies. Increasing maternal age is one of the key risk factors for multiple pregnancy, with multiple pregnancy occurring in approximately 1 in 10 women aged over 45 giving birth in the UK. Assisted conception is also responsible for the increasing incidence of multiple pregnancies, with approximately 1 in 5 successful *in vitro* fertilization (IVF)

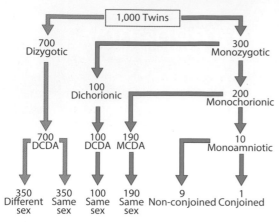

Figure 7.1 Incidence of monozygotic and dizygotic twin pregnancies. DCDA, dichorionic diamniotic; MCDA, monochorionic diamniotic.

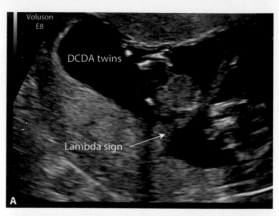

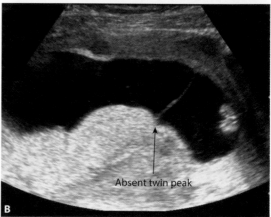

Figure 7.2 Ultrasound appearance of dichorionic (A) and monochorionic (B) twin pregnancies at 12 weeks' gestation. Note that there appears to be a single placental mass but in the dichorionic type there is an extension of placental tissue into the base of the inter-twin membrane, forming the lambda sign.

procedures resulting in multiple pregnancy. In the USA over one-third of twin pregnancies and approximately 80% of triplet (and higher order) pregnancies occur following treatment for infertility.

Figure 7.1 shows the relative contributions of the different types of twins to a hypothetical random selection of 1,000 twin pairs.

Aetiology

Multiple pregnancy may be classified according to:

- Number of fetuses: twins, triplets, quadruplets, etc.
- Number of fertilized eggs: zygosity.
- Number of placentae: chorionicity.
- Number of amniotic cavities: amnionicity.

Twin pregnancy may be dizygotic (70%) or monozygotic (30%). Dizygotic twins (non-identical) occur from ovulation and subsequent fertilization of two oocytes. This results in dichorionic diamniotic twins, where each fetus has its own placenta and amniotic cavity. Although they always have two functionally separate placentae (dichorionic), the placentae can become anatomically fused together and appear to the naked eye as a single placental mass. They always have separate amniotic cavities (diamniotic) and the two cavities are separated by a thick three-layer membrane (fused amnion in the middle with chorion on either side; **Figure 7.2A**). The fetuses can be either same-sex or different-sex pairings.

> ▶ VIDEO 7.1
>
> Ultrasound scan of dichorionic and monochorionic twin pregnancies:
> http://www.routledgetextbooks.com/textbooks/tenteachers/obstetricsv7.1.php

Monozygotic (identical) pregnancies result from fertilization of a single ovum with subsequent division of the zygote. If the zygote splits shortly after fertilization, the twins will each have a separate placenta and thus will be dichorionic diamniotic. Monochorionic diamniotic (20%) pregnancies occur when division of the zygote occurs between days four and eight postfertilization. The vast majority of monochorionic twins have two amniotic cavities (diamniotic) but the dividing membrane is thin, as it consists of a single layer of amnion alone (**Figure 7.2B**).

Monochorionic monoamniotic (1%) pregnancy occurs when division occurs between days 8 and 12 postfertilization and finally conjoined twins occur when division of the zygote happens after day 13.

Care of women with a multiple pregnancy

According to the National Institute for Health and Care Excellence (NICE) guidelines, treatment and care should take into account a woman's needs and preferences.

Due to an increased risk of pregnancy complications, women with multiple pregnancies that involve a shared amnion should be offered individualized care in a tertiary level fetal medicine.

- Women with multiple pregnancies should be cared for by a multidisciplinary team consisting of a core team of named specialist obstetricians, specialist midwives and ultrasonographers.
- Regular ultrasound assessment is used to date the pregnancy, perform first trimester screening and to monitor growth. Abdominal palpation or symphysis–fundal height (SFH) measurements should not be used to predict FGR.
- There is no benefit in using untargeted administration of corticosteroids.
- Gestation and mode of delivery depends on the type of multiple pregnancy.
- Women with multiple pregnancies should receive the same advice about diet, lifestyle and nutritional supplements as in routine antenatal care.
- Women with multiple pregnancies are at higher risk of anaemia compared with singleton pregnancies and a full blood count should be checked at 20 and 28 weeks' gestation and supplementation with iron, folic acid or vitamin B12 initiated.

Complications of multiple pregnancy

All the physiological changes of pregnancy, including increased cardiac output, volume expansion, relative haemodilution, diaphragmatic splinting, weight gain and lordosis, are exaggerated in multiple gestations. This results in much greater stresses being placed on maternal reserves. The 'minor' symptoms of pregnancy may be exaggerated, such as nausea and vomiting and heartburn. However, for women with pre-existing health problems, such as cardiac disease, a multiple pregnancy may substantially increase their risk of morbidity.

One of the commonest and most serious complications of dichorionic diamniotic pregnancies is preterm delivery, either spontaneous or iatrogenic due to the occurrence of other adverse pregnancy complications such as pre-eclampsia or FGR (**Figure 7.3**). Overall, approximately 60% of twin pregnancies result in spontaneous birth before 37 weeks' gestation. In a dichorionic pregnancy, the chance of late miscarriage is 2%. In 15% of cases, delivery will be very preterm. For monochorionic twins, the chance of preterm delivery is increased even further, with 12% born before viability and 25% delivering between 24 and 32 weeks. With two or more babies resulting from each delivery, multiple gestations account for 20–25% of Neonatal Intensive Care Unit (NICU) admissions. In addition to the other complications of twin pregnancy described above, monochorionic diamniotic pregnancies are also at risk of twin-to-twin transfusion syndrome (TTTS) and, more rarely, twin anaemia–polycythaemia sequence (TAPS).

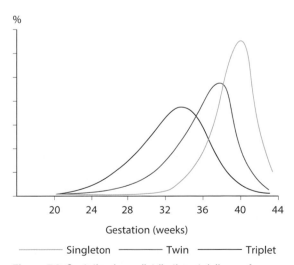

Figure 7.3 Gestational age distribution at delivery of singleton, twin and triplet pregnancies.

Perinatal mortality

Overall perinatal mortality for monochorionic twins is estimated at 30 per 1,000 (compared with 3.8 per 1,000 among dichorionic twins). The overall infant mortality rate for twins is approximately 5.5 times higher than for singletons, mainly as a result of extreme prematurity. The survival at any given gestation is similar for singletons and multiple pregnancies. The stillbirth rate is 12 per 1,000 twin births and 31 per 1,000 triplet births. This compares with about five in 1,000 singleton pregnancies. With the increasing use of early pregnancy scanning, it has been recognized that up to 25% of twins may suffer an early demise and subsequently 'vanish' well before they would have previously been detected. After the first trimester, the intrauterine death of one fetus in a twin pregnancy may be associated with a poor outcome for the remaining co-twin. Maternal complications such as disseminated intravascular coagulation have been reported, but the incidence of this appears to be very low. In dichorionic twins, the second or third trimester intrauterine death of one fetus may be associated with the onset of labour, although in some cases the pregnancy may continue uneventfully and even result in delivery at term. Careful fetal and maternal monitoring is required. By contrast, fetal death of one twin in monochorionic twins may result in immediate complications in the survivor. These include death or brain damage with subsequent neurodevelopmental handicap. Acute hypotensive episodes, secondary to placental vascular anastomoses between the two fetuses, result in haemodynamic volume shifts from the live to the dead fetus. The acute release of vasoactive substances into the survivor's circulation may also play a role. Death or handicap of the co-twin occurs in up to 30% of cases.

Fetal growth restriction

Compared to singletons, the risk of FGR is higher in each individual twin alone and substantially raised in the pregnancy as a whole. This increased incidence of growth restriction creates several management difficulties as the interpretation of and performing detailed Doppler studies, including ductus venosus (DV) and middle cerebral artery Dopplers, become increasingly difficult as gestation progresses. When a fetus is growth restricted, the main aims of antenatal care become prediction of the severity of impaired fetal oxygenation and selecting the appropriate time for delivery. In singletons, this is a balance between the relative risks of intrauterine death versus the risk of neonatal death or handicap from elective preterm delivery. The situation is much more complicated in twin pregnancies. The potential benefit of expectant management or elective delivery for the small fetus must also be weighed against the risk of the same policy for the normally grown co-twin. In a dichorionic pregnancy, each fetus runs twice the risk of a low birthweight and there is a 25% chance that at least one of the fetuses will be small for gestational age. The chance of suboptimal fetal growth for monochorionic twins is almost double that for dichorionic twins. In dichorionic twin pregnancies where one fetus has growth restriction, elective preterm delivery may lead to iatrogenic complications of prematurity in the previously healthy co-twin. In general, delivery should be avoided before 28–30 weeks' gestation, even if there is evidence of imminent intrauterine death of the smaller twin; however, this may not be applicable in the management of monochorionic twins.

The death of one of a monochorionic twin pair may result in either death or handicap of the co-twin because of acute hypotension secondary to placental vascular anastomoses between the two circulations. As the damage potentially happens at the moment of death of the first twin, the timing of delivery may be a very difficult decision. Below 30 weeks' gestation, the aim is to prolong the pregnancy as far as possible without risking the death of the growth-restricted twin.

Complications unique to monochorionic twin pregnancies

Twin-to-twin transfusion syndrome

Unique to monochorionic pregnancy is a complication involving the development of abnormal unbalanced vascular anastomoses leading to the development of TTTS. Although vascular connections are found in nearly all monochorionic twins, approximately 10% of monochorionic diamniotic pregnancies and 5% of monoamniotic pregnancies will subsequently develop TTTS. Four types of vascular connections have been identified in monochorionic pregnancies: arteriovenous (AV), venoarterial (VA), arterioarterial (AA) and venovenous (VV).

If the connections are unbalanced with more AV connections occurring in one direction than the other, alterations in the hydrostatic and osmotic forces occur, resulting in the manifestations seen in TTTS. An equal number of bidirectional anastomoses results in balanced connections and TTTS does not occur under these circumstances. AA anastomoses are protective against the development of TTTS.

TTTS is diagnosed based on the following ultrasound criteria:

- Single placental mass.
- Concordant gender.
- Oligohydramnios with maximum vertical pool (MVP) less than 2 cm in one sac and polyhydramnios in the other sac (MVP >8 cm).
- Discordant bladder appearances.
- Haemodynamic and cardiac compromise.

TTTS may be graded in severity according to the widely accepted Quintero staging:

- Stage I: Oligohydramnios and polyhydramnios sequence and the bladder of the donor twin is visible. Dopplers in both twins are normal.
- Stage II: Oligohydramnios and polyhydramnios sequence, but the bladder of the donor is not visualized. Dopplers in both twins are normal.
- Stage III: Oligohydramnios and polyhydramnios sequence, non-visualized bladder and abnormal Dopplers. There is absent/reversed end-diastolic velocity in the umbilical artery, reversed flow in a-wave of the DV or pulsatile flow in the umbilical vein in either fetus.
- Stage IV: One or both fetuses show signs of hydrops.
- Stage V: One or both fetuses have died.

TAPS is a rarer chronic form of TTTS in which a large inter-twin haemoglobin difference occurs but the oligohydramnios polyhydramnios sequence that is observed with TTTS is not seen. It is thought to occur from residual small (<1 mm) unidirectional AV anastomoses without accompanying AA anastomoses. The small residual anastomoses lead to the gradual development of anaemia in one twin and polycythaemia in the other twin. As the vessels are small, this allows haemodynamic compensation, which is thought to be why the characteristic oligohydramnios polyhydramnios pattern does not occur.

Severe polycythaemia can occur, leading to fetal and placental thrombosis and hydrops fetalis in the anaemic twin. Rarely, mirror syndrome, the combination of fetal hydrops and maternal pre-eclampsia, has been reported.

Serial ultrasound is recommended to assess growth in multiple pregnancies. The optimal scanning schedule has not yet been identified. Generally, in monochorionic pregnancies the aim of ultrasound assessment is to detect early signs of TTTS, enabling early intervention and optimizing outcomes. As a result, generally monochorionic pregnancies will be assessed using ultrasound fortnightly from 16 weeks' gestation to at least 24 weeks' gestation. Although the risk of TTTS reduces after this gestation, it is still possible. However, the occurrence of discordant growth is more likely as pregnancy progresses. As a result, continued surveillance with growth assessments remains essential.

Treatment of TTTS

When TTTS is suspected or diagnosed patients should be referred for a tertiary referral. When TTTS is confirmed, management options include: expectant management; amnioreduction; septostomy; selective feticide, fetoscopic laser ablation of vascular anastomoses. Fetoscopic laser ablation is now generally considered the definitive treatment for severe (defined as Quintero stage II or above) TTTS between 16 and 26 weeks' gestation. Above 26 weeks, delivery may be considered. These recommendations are based on the results of a meta-analysis that demonstrated that fetuses undergoing laser ablation rather than amnioreduction were twice as likely to survive and had an 80% reduction in neurological morbidity (overall survival odds ratio [OR] 2.04, 95% CI 1.52–2.76; neonatal death: OR 0.24, 95% CI 0.15–0.40; and neurological morbidity OR 0.20, 95% CI 0.12–0.33).

The procedure is performed either under local anaesthetic with intravenous sedation, with regional anaesthesia or occasionally under general anaesthesia. Under ultrasound guidance a 2–3 mm diameter fetoscope is introduced into the amniotic cavity of the recipient twin. The location of the dividing twin membrane between the two amniotic cavities at the placental interface and the placental insertions of the umbilical cords are visualized. AV anastomoses are ablated using laser energy.

Following the laser therapy, the fetoscope is removed and an amnioreduction is performed until the amniotic fluid volume appears normal by ultrasound assessment.

Monochorionic monoamniotic twin pregnancy

Monoamniotic twin pregnancies result from division of a single fertilized oocyte. The incidence of monoamniotic twins is approximately 1 in 10,000 pregnancies. It is the least common pattern of placentation but is associated with high morbidity and mortality due to the high rate of perinatal mortality that occurs secondary to cord entanglement resulting in fetal loss or neurological morbidity. Monochorionic monoamniotic (MCMA) twins have increased risk of congenital anomalies including neural tube defects and abdominal wall and urinary tract malformations. Discordant birthweight affects approximately 20% of surviving monoamniotic twin pairs without congenital anomalies. As a result, close surveillance with ultrasound is essential. Monochorionic monoamniotic pregnancies are monitored closely with antenatal fetal surveillance and delivery by caesarean section generally at 32–34 weeks' gestation. The ideal method for surveillance is unclear. Generally, patients are hospitalized from 28 weeks' gestation and fetal heart auscultation performed several times daily using cardiotocography in an effort to detect signs of cord compression. Perinatal mortality occurs in approximately 20% of fetuses and infants.

Antenatal care

The NICE guidelines recommend that women with uncomplicated dichorionic twin pregnancies be offered at least eight antenatal appointments with a health care professional from the core team (at least nine antenatal appointments for uncomplicated monochorionic diamniotic twin pregnancies). Routine antenatal care for all women involves screening for hypertension and gestational diabetes. These conditions occur more frequently in twin pregnancies and there is also a higher risk of other problems (such as antepartum haemorrhage and thromboembolic disease); however, the management is the same as for a singleton. Due to the increased fetoplacental demand for iron and folic acid, many

would recommend routine (as opposed to selective) supplementation in multiple pregnancies. Minor symptoms of pregnancy are more common, but management is again unchanged compared to singletons.

Screening in multiple pregnancy

Women with multiple pregnancy should be offered a first trimester scan when the crown–rump length (CRL) measures 45–84 mm, which equates to approximately 11 weeks 0 days to 13 weeks 6 days. The purpose of this is threefold:

- To accurately estimate gestational age.
- To determine chorionicity.
- To screen for Down's syndrome.

Gestational age is assessed by measuring the CRL. Chorionicity is determined by assessing the number of placental masses and assessing for the lambda or T-sign and membrane thickness (**Figures 7.2A, B**). At this stage the fetuses are mapped and it is documented clearly which fetus is where, to ensure consistency with future scans throughout pregnancy, for example, triplet two maternal upper right side. With dichorionic pregnancies calculate the risk of Down's syndrome for each baby. With monochorionic pregnancies the risk of Down's syndrome is calculated for the pregnancy as a whole. Assessment of the a-wave in the DV at 11–13 weeks' gestation may help identify monochorionic pregnancies at risk of severe TTTS as reversed a-wave is associated with an increased risk of developing severe TTTS, as well as other complications including aneuploidy. However, due to high false positives, this is not widely advocated or must be interpreted with caution. Both amniocentesis and chorion villous sampling (CVS) can be performed in twin pregnancies, but in dichorionic pregnancies, it is essential that both fetuses are sampled.

Anomaly scan

Fetuses of multiple pregnancies have higher rates of congenital anomalies compared to singleton fetuses. Monozygotic twins are two to three times more likely to have structural defects than dizygotic twins or singleton fetuses. These include anencephaly and holoprosencephaly. In general, only one fetus is affected by the congenital malformations should they occur. In 5–20% of cases the defect is present in both twins. Multiple gestations with an abnormality in one fetus can be managed expectantly or by selective fetocide of the affected twin. In cases where the abnormality is non-lethal but may well result in handicap, the parents may need to decide whether the potential burden of a handicapped child outweighs the risk of loss of the normal twin from fetocide-related complications, which occur after 5–10% of procedures. In cases where the abnormality is lethal, it may be best to avoid such risk to the normal fetus, unless the condition itself threatens the survival of the normal twin. Anencephaly is a good example of a lethal abnormality that can threaten the survival of the normal twin. At least 50% of pregnancies affected by anencephaly are complicated by polyhydramnios, which can lead to the spontaneous preterm delivery of both babies.

Fetocide in monochorionic pregnancies carries increased risk and requires a different technique such as cord occlusion. As there are potential vascular anastomoses between the two fetal circulations, intracardiac injections cannot be employed. Methods have evolved that employ cord occlusion techniques. These require significant instrumentation of the uterus and are therefore associated with a higher complication rate.

In twins, as in singletons, the risk for chromosomal abnormalities increases with maternal age. The rate of spontaneous dizygotic twinning also increases with maternal age. Many women undergoing assisted conception techniques (that increase the chance of dizygotic twinning) are also older than the mean maternal age. Chromosomal defects may be more likely in a multiple pregnancy for various reasons, and couples should be counselled accordingly.

Growth assessments

Multiple pregnancies are at high risk of FGR. As a result, fetal weight should be calculated from 20 weeks' gestation at a maximum of 4 week intervals. A growth discrepancy of 25% or greater should be considered clinically significant, a tertiary referral opinion sought and additional monitoring or delivery depending on gestation planned.

Other indications for a tertiary level fetal medicine opinion include discordant fetal growth, fetal anomaly, discordant fetal death or TTTS.

Delivery

A delivery plan should be discussed and made with the patient, ideally throughout pregnancy, with a clear delivery plan discussed and documented early in the third trimester. This is essential as multiple pregnancies have a high prevalence of preterm delivery. The discussion with the patient should include desired mode for delivery, gestation for induction of labour if no spontaneous onset of labour, process for delivery of twin one and twin two including internal podalic version, risk of caesarean section, complications following delivery including postpartum haemorrhage and desire to breast feed or not.

Intrapartum management

General management of a patient with twin pregnancy in labour involves:

- Antenatal education and a preagreed birth plan.
- Continuous fetal heart monitoring.
- Two neonatal resuscitation trolleys, two obstetricians and two paediatricians are available and that the special care baby unit and anaesthetist are informed well in advance of the delivery.
- Analgesia, ideally in the form of an early epidural, to allow for internal podalic version (if needed) for twin 2.
- A standard oxytocin solution for augmentation should be prepared, run through an intravenous giving-set and clearly labelled 'for augmentation', for use for delivery of the second twin.
- Oxytocin infusion in anticipation of postpartum haemorrhage.
- Portable ultrasound.

With uncomplicated dichorionic diamniotic pregnancies vaginal delivery is advocated provided the presenting twin is cephalic. The risk of requiring emergency caesarean section for delivery of the second twin following vaginal delivery of the first twin is approximately 4%.

If the second twin is non-vertex, which occurs in about 40% of twins, a vaginal delivery can be safely considered. If the second twin is a breech, the membranes can be ruptured once the breech is fixed in the birth canal. A breech extraction may be performed if fetal distress occurs or if a footling breech is encountered, but this requires considerable expertise. Complications are less likely if the membranes are not ruptured until the feet are held by the operator. Where the fetus is transverse, external cephalic version can be successful in more than 70% of cases. The fetal heart rate should be closely monitored, and ultrasound can be helpful to demonstrate the final position of the baby. If external cephalic version is unsuccessful, and assuming that the operator is experienced, an internal podalic version can be undertaken (**Figure 7.4**).

Internal podalic version is performed by identifying a fetal foot through intact membranes. The foot is grasped and pulled gently and continuously into the birth canal. The membranes are ruptured as late as possible. This procedure is easiest when the transverse lie is with the back superior or posterior. If the back is inferior or if the limbs are not immediately palpable, ultrasound may help to show the operator

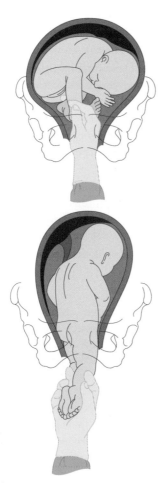

Figure 7.4 Internal podalic version.

where they would be found. This will minimize the unwanted experience of bringing down a fetal hand in the mistaken belief that it is a foot.

Generally, with dichorionic twin pregnancies delivery from 37 weeks' gestation is advocated.

Women with uncomplicated monochorionic twin pregnancies should be offered elective delivery from 36 weeks' gestation and this should be performed after a course of antenatal corticosteroids has been given. However, this approach carries a 1.5% risk of late *in utero* death for monochorionic twins. Continuing uncomplicated twin pregnancies beyond 38 weeks' gestation increases the risk of intrauterine fetal death. The indications for instrumental delivery of the second twin are as for singletons.

Higher order multiples

The incidence of spontaneous triplet pregnancy is 1 in 6,000–8,000 births. However, as a result of assisted fertility, in the UK in 2012, 221 sets of triplets were delivered. Triplets are associated with a high morbidity and mortality. According to UK data, they have an average gestation of 34 weeks at delivery, average birthweight of 1.8 kg and cerebral palsy rate of 26.7 per 1,000 live births. When performing first trimester screening in monochorionic triplet pregnancies, calculate the risk of Down's syndrome for each baby in dichorionic and trichorionic triplet pregnancies. NICE recommends that women with uncomplicated monochorionic triamniotic and dichorionic triamniotic triplet pregnancies be offered at least 11 antenatal appointments with a health care professional from the core team. It is not recommended to prolong pregnancy beyond 36 weeks' gestation.

Multiple pregnancy support groups

Twin pregnancies are associated with a number of financial, personal and social costs for families that continue long beyond the neonatal period. A significant contribution to these costs comes from the increased incidence of handicap, largely secondary to preterm delivery. Several specialized support groups for multiple pregnancy exist. In the UK, these include the Twins and Multiple Birth Association (TAMBA) and the Multiple Birth Foundation. All parents expecting twins should be given contact details for such resources locally.

KEY LEARNING POINTS

- Multiple pregnancy rates continue to increase worldwide.
- Multiple pregnancies are associated with increased incidence of almost every pregnancy complication, with the exception of macrosomia and postdates pregnancy.
- Preterm birth, growth restriction and stillbirth are key causes of the raised fetal morbidity and mortality associated with multiple pregnancies.
- Maternal morbidity and mortality is also increased in multiple pregnancies.
- Early ultrasound assessment is key in the management of multiple pregnancy as it can correctly classify the type of pregnancy according to chorionicity and amnionicity, allowing risk to be stratified.

Further reading

Multiple pregnancy. The management of twin and triplet pregnancies in the antenatal period. Issued: September 2011 NICE Clinical Guideline 129. guidance.nice.org.uk/cg129. https://www.nice.org.uk/guidance/cg129/resources/guidance-multiple-pregnancy-pdf

Management of monochorionic twin pregnancy. Green top guideline No. 51. December 2008. https://www.rcog.org.uk/globalassets/documents/guidelines/t51managementmonochorionictwin-pregnancy2008a.pdf.

Self assessment

CASE HISTORY

Ms B is 38 weeks' gestation in her second pregnancy. This is a dichorionic diamniotic pregnancy that has been uncomplicated to date. Ms B presents contracting every 5 minutes. Twin 1 (the presenting twin) is cephalic and twin 2 is cephalic. Her first pregnancy was a term delivery, delivered 11 months previously as a spontaneous vaginal delivery. On examination Ms B is 6 cm dilated and both fetal heart recordings are reassuring. An epidural has just been inserted and is providing good analgesia.

A What would you do next?

Ms B waters rupture and she proceeds to have a spontaneous vaginal delivery. On delivering twin 1, the abdomen is palpated and ultrasound confirms that twin 2 is cephalic. The fetal heart rate remains reassuring.

B How would you proceed?

After 25 minutes of reassuring heart monitoring Ms B is contracting once every 10 minutes. Fetal heart monitoring remains reassuring.

C How would you proceed?

The membranes surrounding twin 2 rupture. Vaginal examination reveals that Ms B remains fully dilated. However, twin 2 is now transverse with its back upwards. The fetal heart tracing shows prolonged fetal decelerations.

D How would you proceed?

ANSWER

A There is no indication to intervene in this situation. Ms B has laboured spontaneously and is progressing quickly. Fetal heart rate is reassuring. Allow labour to progress naturally. Continue fetal monitoring.

B Again, there is no indication to intervene. Ms B has successfully delivered twin 1. Waiting allows the head of twin 2 to descend, which will increase the likelihood of a spontaneous vaginal delivery.

C There are now two options. First would be to perform an amniotomy to rupture the membranes of twin 2, which will likely increase the frequency of contractions, allowing twin 2 to be delivered. The second option would be to start oxytocin infusion to try to increase the frequency of contractions and allow delivery of twin 2 to proceed. As the membranes are intact one must be cautious with the use of oxytocin, therefore the ideal option is to perform a vaginal examination and, when a contraction occurs (which will push the fetal head into the pelvis), perform artificial rupture of the membranes. Oxytocin may be used at this stage to augment contractions.

D This is now an obstetric emergency. Ensure senior obstetric help is present. There are two options on how to manage this situation. The first is to perform internal podalic version as described above by performing vaginal examination; follow the fetal spine towards the legs and on palpating a foot apply gentle traction to the foot to encourage delivery of the fetus by breech extraction. The second option is to transfer the mother to the operating theatre and perform a category 1 caesarean section. As Ms B is multiparous, internal podalic version and breech extraction would be the quickest way to deliver twin B and ensure a quick recovery for Ms B. External cephalic version would be a third option, but in the presence of a non-reassuring fetal heart rate this would be contraindicated.

EMQ

A External cephalic version.
B Emergency caesarean section.
C Internal podalic version.
D Allow spontaneous delivery.
E Start oxytocin infusion.
F Elective caesarean section at 32–34 weeks.
G Administer corticosteroid injection.
H Refer for tertiary referral opinion.
I Recommend septostomy.
J Refer for laser ablation therapy.
K Delivery by caesarean section at 37 weeks.

For each description, choose the SINGLE most appropriate answer from the list of options. Each option may be used once, more than once or not at all.

1 You review a woman who is 18 weeks pregnant with MCDA twins. The ultrasound has reported the deepest volume pool (DVP) of twin 1 of <2 cm with the second twin having a DVP of 10 cm. The bladder of twin 1 is also not possible to visualize.

2 You review a woman who is 20 weeks pregnant with MCMA twins at her booking appointment. She asks your opinion regarding timing and mode of delivery. She had hoped for a vaginal delivery. How would you advise her?

3 You are called to the labour ward for the delivery of 37-week DCDA twins. Twin 1 has delivered cephalic. Twin 2 is cephalic but high in the pelvis with the membranes intact. When you arrive there are decelerations on the CTG.

4 You are on duty in the emergency department and a woman presents contracting every 15 minutes. Examination reveals a long closed cervix with a reassuring fetal heart trace.

ANSWER

1H From the description this pregnancy is likely affected by TTTS stage 1 (oligohydramnios and polyhydramnios sequence, and the bladder of the donor twin is visible). These findings first of all need confirmation. Therefore, referral for tertiary referral opinion would be appropriate as there is a high possibility that intervention in the form of laser ablation may be necessary.

2F The risk of cord entanglement and death with MCMA twins is very high. As a result, delivery by caesarean section is recommended and this would be performed normally at 32–34 weeks, after a course of corticosteroids.

3C There are three possible options here: amniotomy and cephalic delivery, internal podalic version and amniotomy and finally emergency caesarean section. Amniotomy and cephalic delivery may take a prolonged amount of time and as the head is high in the pelvis it is unpredictable.

4G As this is a twin pregnancy the risk of preterm delivery is increased. Although the cervix is closed, if the patient is contracting every 15 minutes she may deliver prematurely. As a result it would be reasonable to administer antenatal corticosteroids.

SBA QUESTIONS

Choose the single best answer.

1 Which of the following pregnancy complications does NOT increase in incidence in multiple pregnancy?
   A   Pre-eclampsia.
   B   Obstetric cholestasis.
   C   Preterm delivery.
   D   Macrosomia.
   E   FGR.

ANSWER

D Macrosomia. Multiple pregnancy is associated with an increased risk of most pregnancy complications including pre-eclampsia, which is in part caused by the increased placental volume present in multiple pregnancies. The risk of FGR is also increased. This occurs secondary to placental insufficiency. Preterm delivery is significantly more common in twin pregnancies, as is obstetric cholestasis. The presence of a macrosomic fetus is less likely in a multiple pregnancy than in a singleton pregnancy.

2 Which of the following is NOT a Quintero stage for TTTS?
   A   Oligohydramnios and polyhydramnios sequence and the bladder of the donor twin is visible. Dopplers in both twins are normal.
   B   Growth restriction in both twins, raised middle cerebral artery Dopplers and reduced fetal movements in both twins.
   C   Oligohydramnios and polyhydramnios sequence, non-visualized bladder and abnormal Dopplers. There is absent/reversed end-diastolic velocity in the umbilical artery, reversed flow in a-wave of the DV or pulsatile flow in the umbilical vein in either fetus.
   D   One or both fetuses have died.
   E   One or both fetuses show signs of hydrops.

ANSWER

B A describes stage Quintero stage I, C describes stage III, D describes stage V and E describes stage IV. Stage II is not listed and is defined as oligohydramnios and polyhydramnios sequence, but the bladder of the donor is not visualized. Dopplers in both twins are normal. B does fit the characteristic description any stage of Quintero's staging for TTTS.

MARK R JOHNSON

LEARNING OBJECTIVES

- To understand the extent of the problem, its causes and consequences.
- To be aware of the limitations of our current understanding.

- To appreciate the problems and potential complications associated with our current management of preterm labour.
- To grasp the potential for improvements in our management of preterm labour.

Introduction

Preterm labour (PTL) is the onset of labour before 37 weeks' gestation. This chapter will describe the current understanding of preterm delivery (PTD) due to PTL and preterm premature rupture of the membranes (PPROM). It will give a background to the occurrence of PTL and a global perspective of the problem, while considering the limitations of our current approaches in prediction and management and the potential of future innovations.

Why does preterm labour occur?

Compared to other species, human pregnancy is complicated by PTL more frequently. A possible explanation lies in human evolution, specifically involving bipedalism and encephalization. Bipedalism, where humans assumed an upright posture, is associated with a narrower pelvis. Encephalization, where the human brain increased in volume, is associated with a larger head circumference (**Figure 8.1**). Each has the potential to increase the chance of obstructed labour and the death of

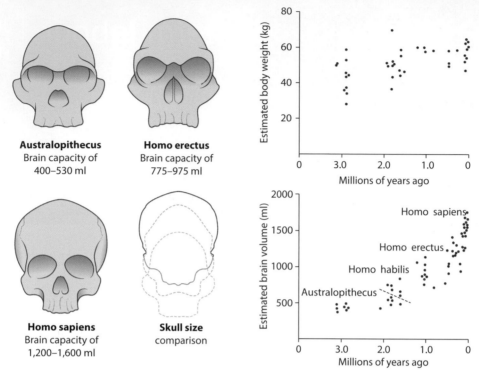

Australopithecus
Brain capacity of
400–530 ml

Homo erectus
Brain capacity of
775–975 ml

Homo sapiens
Brain capacity of
1,200–1,600 ml

Skull size
comparison

Figure 8.1 Evolution of the human skull.

both mother and baby. Consequently, evolution would favour the emergence of earlier delivery and the ability to survive an earlier delivery, potentially explaining why PTL is more common in humans.

Epidemiology

Worldwide, 15 million babies are born preterm every year and of these 1.1 million will die. Of the survivors, many will be left with lifelong disability. The vast majority of these births occur in countries with emerging economies (**Figure 8.2**) where PTL is up to three times more common and the prognosis of those born preterm far worse. In high-income countries, a baby born at 24 weeks has a 50% chance of surviving. In low-income countries, a similar survival rate is not achieved until 34 weeks. PTD can be categorized into spontaneous PTL, PPROM and delivery for maternal or fetal indications. Approximately 25% of PTDs are for maternal or fetal indications, 50% follow spontaneous PTL and 25% follow PPROM. Iatrogenic or medically-indicated deliveries are typically for diagnoses such as pre-eclampsia, fetal growth

restriction (FGR) and maternal cardiac or renal conditions. The risk of PTD is greater in teenagers and women with advanced maternal age, and there is a higher incidence of preterm deliveries in first pregnancies. Socioeconomic factors, marital status, environmental stress, cigarette smoking, illegal substance (i.e. cocaine) abuse, alcohol and poor nutrition have all been linked to an increased risk of preterm birth. Intervention studies have shown that smoking cessation programmes can reduce the risk of preterm birth.

The incidence of PTDs is greater in African or Afro-Caribbean women, but it is difficult to differentiate between social deprivation and genetic variation. Specific genetic polymorphisms have been recently linked with increased risk of PTL (albeit rarely), suggesting that genetic as well as environmental factors can explain increased rates of preterm birth in specific ethnic groups.

The rate of preterm birth overall has risen progressively from the 1960s, when rates were in the region of 6%, to the early years of the new millennium, when the rates peaked at around 10%. More recently, rates have stabilized and even declined in some countries (**Figure 8.3**).

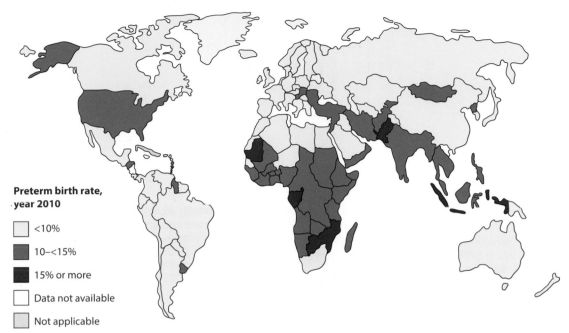

Figure 8.2 Global incidence of preterm birth. (Source: Born Too Soon Executive Summary Group; Kenney MV, Howson CP, McDougall L, Lawn JE (2012). Executive summary for *Born Too Soon: The Global Action Report on Pre-term Birth*. March of Dimes, PMNCH, Save the Children, World Health Organization.)

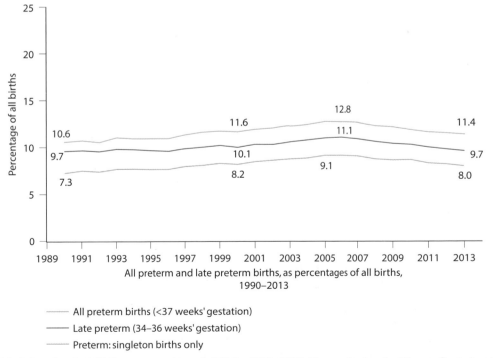

Figure 8.3 Rates of preterm birth as a percentage of all births 1990–2013. (Source: Centers for Disease Control and Prevention.)

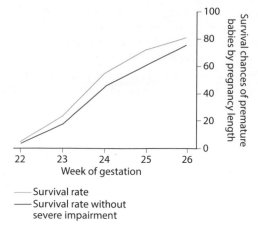

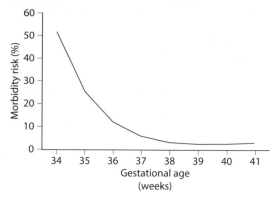

Figure 8.4 Survival chances of preterm infants by gestational age at birth. (Source: Rysavy MA, Li L, Bell EF, *et al.* [2015]. Between-hospital variation in treatment and outcomes in extremely preterm infants. *N Engl J Med* **372**(19):1801–11.)

Figure 8.5 Morbidity according to gestational age at birth. Gestational age was significantly correlated with morbidity risk. (Source: Shapiro-Mendoza CK, Tomashek KM, Kotelchuk M, *et al.* [2008]. Effect of late-preterm birth and maternal medical conditions on newborn morbidity risk. *Pediatrics* **121**:e223–32.)

Neonatal outcomes have improved too, with better survival and reduced morbidity, but rates of neonatal mortality and morbidity remain considerable (**Figures 8.4, 8.5**). Neonatal care will continue to advance, but to improve these figures substantially we have to work to prevent preterm birth.

Improvements in other areas of paediatric care mean that PTL is now not only the most important cause of perinatal morbidity and mortality worldwide, but also of infant mortality less than 5 years of age. The World Health Organization (WHO) stated in 2010 "The largest barrier to the development of diagnostic, treatment and prevention strategies for preterm birth and stillbirth is our inability to comprehend the biological processes of pregnancy and childbirth". This statement is as true now is was then; substantial work needs to be performed to achieve an improvement in pregnancy outcomes worldwide.

Endocrinology and biochemistry of labour

The mechanisms that control the length of human pregnancy and signal the onset of labour have been the subject of extensive research, but are not yet determined. During pregnancy the uterus undergoes marked biochemical and physiological changes while expanding to accommodate the growing fetus

and remaining uiescent. At the same time the cervix remains rigid and closed to retain the developing fetus within the uterus. Throughout pregnancy, 'pro-pregnancy' factors such as progesterone, relaxin, human chorionic gonadotrophin (hCG) and prorelaxation prostaglandins (PGs), such as prostacyclin, inhibit myometrial contractility.

The onset of labour involves the synchronization of myometrial activity through greater expression of gap junctions that connect myometrial cells. Labour onset is diagnosed by the occurrence of painful uterine contractions with changes in the structure of the cervix, leading to cervical dilatation and effacement. It is a gradual process that begins several weeks before delivery with changes in the lower pole of the uterus, which cause cervical ripening and effacement. The changes in the cervix occur through breakdown of collagen, changes in proteoglycan concentrations, infiltration of leucocytes and macrophages and an increase in water content. Increased myometrial activity results from the activation of a 'cassette of contraction-associated proteins' (CAPs), which convert the myometrium from a quiescent to a contractile state. CAPs include gap junction proteins, oxytocin and prostanoid receptors, enzymes for PG synthesis and cell signalling proteins. The latter mediate the uterine response to receptor activation. It is likely that CAPs also activate fetal membrane PG and cytokine production, as well as cervical remodelling and ripening. Contractions are a relatively late event in this process, preceded by cervical remodelling and fetal membrane activation.

Progesterone maintains uterine quiescence

Progesterone is considered to play a major role in the maintenance of pregnancy. In most pregnant mammals, the onset of parturition is associated with a decrease in circulating progesterone through a variety of mechanisms including corpus luteum lysis in rodents and a reduction in placental progesterone synthesis in the sheep. However, in humans the levels of circulating progesterone remain elevated throughout pregnancy, but the administration of the progesterone receptor antagonist RU486 can induce labour. This suggests that although progesterone is involved in pregnancy maintenance, the onset of human labour either involves a functional withdrawal of progesterone action or occurs independent of any loss in progesterone activity. Current theories favour the former, invoking a change in progesterone receptor (PR) isoform expression, an increase in the antagonist PRA isoform and decline in the agonist PRB isoform, or a repression in PRB activity through activation of the inflammatory transcription factor nuclear factor kappa B (NFκB).

Labour as an inflammatory process

Consistent with the theory that progesterone action is repressed by inflammation, several studies have shown that human labour is associated with a global increase in a number of proinflammatory factors including PGs, cytokines and chemokines. Elevated levels of interleukin-1β (IL-1β), IL-6 and tumor necrosis factor-α (TNFα) have been shown in amnion, myometrium and choriodecidua. The influx of inflammatory cells such as neutrophils, macrophages and T-lymphocytes into the labouring uterine tissues may result in the increased levels of proinflammatory cytokines. In addition, inflammation has been strongly implicated in infection-driven preterm labour.

The roles of oxytocin and prostaglandins

The oxytocin/oxytocin receptor (OTR) system within the pregnant uterus serves two distinct physiological functions, stimulation of contractions and production of PGs. There is no increase in the production of oxytocin associated with the onset or progression of labour; however, the sensitivity of the myometrium to oxytocin at term increases dramatically and this is mediated via increased expression of OTR. Activation of OTR triggers the release of intracellular Ca^{2+}, leading to a calmodulin-mediated activation of myosin light chain kinase, which phosphorylates myosin, promoting the interaction with actin and the onset of contractions.

PGs are derived from arachidonic acid (AA), which is found in cell membrane phospholipids. They play a key role in the onset and progression of human labour, promoting cervical ripening and myometrial contractility. Their importance is shown by the widespread use of different formulations of PGE to induce labour and the success of PG inhibitors in the inhibition of PTL. However, in the case of the latter, their use is limited by their adverse fetal effects (premature closure of the ductus arteriosus and renal impairment). The PG family is large with procontractile ($PGF_{2\alpha}$) and prorelaxatory (PGI_2) members. PGE_2 can have both effects depending on whether it acts via its procontractile receptors (EP1 and 3) or its prorelaxatory receptors (EP2 and 4). Consequently, although the PG synthetic enzyme PGHS-2 is the rate-limiting step in PG synthesis and increases with the onset of labour, it is the down-stream synthetic enzymes, such as PGES (PGE_2) and PGFS ($PGF_{2\alpha}$), and the expression of specific receptor isoforms that determine the effect of increased PGHS-2 activity. Further, the amnion is the dominant site of PG synthesis, while the prime site of PG action is the myometrium. The chorion lies between these tissues and expresses the enzyme responsible for PG metabolism, 15-hydroxyprostaglandin dehydrogenase (PGDH). The expression of this enzyme falls with onset of labour, facilitating the transfer of PGs from amnion to myometrium.

Causes of preterm labour

PTL is not a single condition; it has multiple causes (**Figure 8.6**). Many risk factors have obvious biophysical correlates; multiple pregnancy is associated with prematurity through its effect on myometrial stretch. However, in many other cases this is not clear and more work needs to be performed to understand the mechanisms involved.

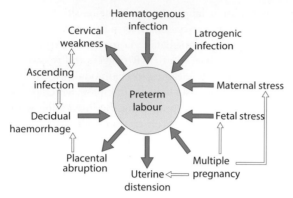

Figure 8.6 Causes of preterm birth.

Cervical weakness

Cervical weakness is classically associated with painless premature cervical dilatation and is suggested by a history of painless second trimester pregnancy loss. There is almost certainly an overlap between cervical weakness and other factors such as ascending infection, as during pregnancy, the cervix not only acts as a physical obstacle, keeping the pregnancy in the uterus, but also as a barrier to ascending infection through the synthesis of a thick mucus plug in the cervical canal that has bactericidal properties. Several studies have demonstrated a strong relationship between cervical length and the risk for PTD, and a previous history of cervical surgery is a common risk factor for cervical weakness.

Infection

Infection of the fetal membranes, chorioamnionitis, is a major cause of preterm birth particularly in deliveries before <32 weeks' gestation. It is associated with a threefold increased risk of PTD with intact membranes, and a fourfold increased risk with ruptured membranes. In most cases, infection ascends from the vagina, although the route of infection may be transplacental or introduced during invasive procedures. Cervical weakness, resulting in early shortening, as described earlier, can predispose to ascending bacterial infection. However, it is possible for vaginal pathogens to ascend through a normal cervix. Overall, 33% of all pregnancies delivered after PPROM are complicated by infection. This rate rises the earlier the PPROM occurs, with positive amniotic fluid cultures found in 83% of babies delivered

weighing <1 kg, which approximates to a gestation of less than 28 weeks. Abnormal vaginal flora, for example bacterial vaginosis (BV), affects 16% of pregnant women and is associated with PPROM and PTL, with a greater risk the earlier in gestation it is identified (relative risk [RR]: 5–7.5 if identified <16 weeks' gestation). The relationship with PTD is not direct, since antibiotic treatment of BV does not consistently reduce the risk of PTD. Current recommendations are to screen high-risk women for BV and treat those found to be positive.

Chorioamnionitis not only drives PTL, but it is also associated with fetal brain damage, since intrauterine infection drives a fetal inflammatory response, involving a proinflammatory cytokinaemia and, morphologically, a vasculitis of the umbilical cord and/or the vessels of the chorionic plate. The release of inflammatory cytokines during maternal infection is harmful to the developing brain of the unborn infant, causing periventricular white matter damage also known as periventricular leukomalacia (PVL; **Figure 8.7**). Indeed, increased amniotic fluid IL-6 levels are associated with intraventricular haemorrhage (IVH) and PVL and high levels of cytokines have been found in brains of infants who die with evidence of PVL (**Figure 8.8**).

Multiple pregnancy and uterine distension

Overall, 56% of multiple births deliver before 37 weeks and 10–15% before 32 weeks. Consequently, although multiple pregnancies only make up 2% of the pregnant population, they contribute disproportionately to PTDs and, consequently, Neonatal Intensive Care Unit (NICU) admissions. The risk of PTD rises with fetal number, with triplets delivering on average at 32 weeks and quadruplets delivering at 28 weeks. Multiple pregnancies have an increased risk of preeclampsia, FGR and other medical complications of pregnancy, explaining the observation in one study that of the 54% of the twins delivered preterm, 23% were for medical reasons and 76% were after PTL or PPROM. Twins have a six- to sevenfold increased risk of cerebral palsy and this rises to 100-fold if one twin dies antenatally (see Chapter 7, Multiple pregnancy).

Polyhydramnios, the presence of too much amniotic fluid, also increases the risk of PTL and PPROM, although the effect is not as great as with twins, with

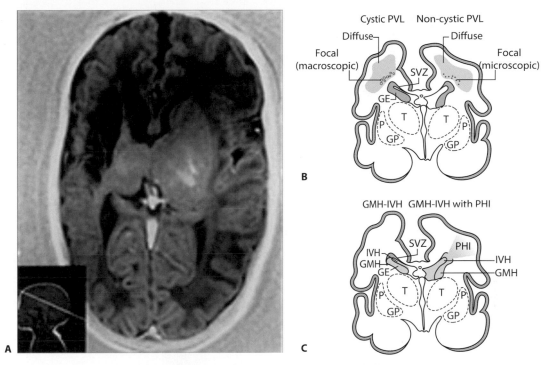

Figure 8.7 (**A**) Magnetic resonance imaging (MRI) in a preterm infant with a gestational age at birth of 32 weeks. Routine ultrasound performed at 2 weeks of age shows cystic changes in the distribution of the right middle cerebral artery. MRI, inversion recovery, axial slice, performed at 40 weeks postmenstrual age, shows an area of cavitation and *ex-vacuo* dilatation of the right ventricle. Also note the absence of myelination of the posterior limb of the right internal capsule. The infant developed a moderate hemiplegia and has a Developmental Quotient of 91 at 24 months of age. (**B**, **C**) Cystic and non-cystic periventricular leukomalacia (PVL) and germinal matrix haemorrhage–intraventricular haemorrhage (GMH-IVH) and GMH-IVH with periventricular haemorrhagic infarction (PHI). Coronal sections from the brain of a 28-week-old premature infant. GE: ganglionic eminence; GP: globus pallidus; P: putamen; SVZ: subventricular zone; T: thalamus.(From Volpe JJ [2009]. Brain injury in premature infants: a complex amalgam of destructive and developmental disturbances. *Lancet Neurol* **8**:110–24.)

PTD occurring in between 7 and 25% of fetuses depending on the degree. Severe polyhydramnios can be managed with amnio-drainage, but this may itself precipitate PTL and/or PPROM. Alternatively, indomethacin, a non-steroidal anti-inflammatory drug (NSAID), may be used as it reduces fetal urine production, but flow through the ductus arteriosus has to be closely monitored as the inhibition of PGE production by indomethacin may result in premature closure.

Uterine müllerian anomalies

Congenital müllerian anomalies are often unrecognized but are estimated to occur in up to 4% of women of reproductive age. They occur as a consequence of abnormal embryologic fusion and canalization of the müllerian ducts and result in an abnormally formed uterine cavity, which can range from an arcuate uterus, which results in minimal

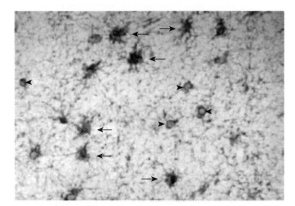

Figure 8.8 An example of white matter injury due to periventricular leukomalacia. Two cell types are shown staining positive for TNF-alpha, the larger more densely stained cells with prominent cytoplasmic processes (astrocytes, arrows) and smaller, less densely stained cells with fewer cytoplasmic processes (microglial cells, arrowheads).

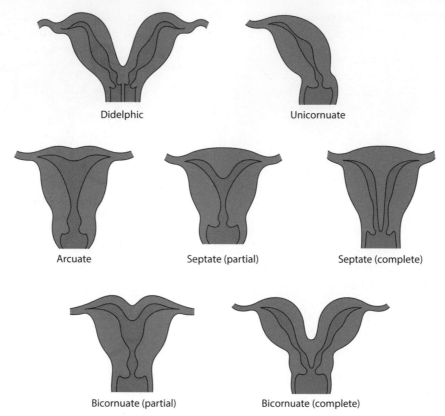

Figure 8.9 Schematic diagram of different types of congenital uterine anomalies. Uterine müllerian anomalies are associated with an increased risk of preterm delivery.

fundal cavity indentation, to complete failure of fusion resulting in uterine didelphys (**Figure 8.9**). They are associated with adverse pregnancy outcome in up to 25% of women, including first and second trimester miscarriage, PPROM, preterm birth, FGR, breech presentation and caesarean section.

Haemorrhage

Antepartum haemorrhage and placental abruption may lead to spontaneous PTL. The presence of a sub-chorionic haematoma in early pregnancy increases the risk of later PPROM, either through an effect of thrombin on membrane strength or through the occurrence of infection in the haematoma. Acute bleeding leads to the release thrombin that directly stimulates myometrial contractions. Placental abruption complicates 1% of all pregnancies and the maternal or fetal effects depend primarily on its severity and the gestational age when it occurs. Risk factors include pre-eclampsia and hypertension,

previous abruption, trauma, smoking, cocaine use, multiple pregnancy, polyhydramnios, thrombophilias, advanced maternal age and PPROM. When an abruption involves 50% or more of the placenta it is frequently associated with fetal death.

Stress

There is growing evidence that either maternal or fetal stress may be associated with PTL. Major life events have an association with prematurity, as does the fetal stress of FGR. A link between maternal stress and PTL is suggested by its increased prevalence among unmarried and poor mothers, as well as in stressful sociodemographic conditions (such as loss of employment, housing or partner). Prematurity is also more common among women reporting increased stress or anxiety. The biochemical pathway through which maternal and fetal stress promotes PTL is uncertain, but may involve a premature increase in circulating corticotrophin-releasing hormone (CRH).

Management of preterm labour

Up to 70% of women who present with threatened PTL to the labour ward will not deliver during the current admission, and up to 50% will not deliver until term. Deciding who is and who is not in PTL has been helped by testing the cervicovaginal fluid levels of fetal fibronectin (fFN), a glycoprotein found in cervicovaginal fluid, amniotic fluid, placental tissue and in the interface between the chorion and decidua. It acts like 'glue' at the maternal–fetal interface and its presence in cervicovaginal fluid between 22 and 36 weeks' gestation has been shown to be a predictor of PTD. Negative fFN testing has a very high negative predictive value, enabling most women with threatened PTL and a negative fFN test to be sent home. Those with a positive fFN test can be admitted for tocolysis and steroids for fetal lung maturation.

Tocolytics are used to delay delivery long enough for corticosteroid administration to improve neonatal lung function and, if necessary, for *in utero* transfer to a NICU. The current guidelines from the Royal College of Obstetricians and Gynecologists suggest that if tocolytics are administered for the medical treatment of PTL, the first choice should be a calcium channel blocker (nifedipine) or an OTR antagonist (atosiban). However, a recent review and network meta-analysis on trials of tocolysis found that PG inhibitors and calcium channel blockers are most likely the best therapy for PTD on the basis of delaying delivery by 48 hours, neonatal mortality, neonatal respiratory distress syndrome (RDS) and maternal side-effects. The different types of tocolytics are discussed briefly below.

Beta-sympathomimetics

Beta-agonists (ritodrine, salbutamol and terbutaline) are predominantly β2 adreno-receptor agonists), which mediate myometrial relaxation by stimulating cyclic adenyl monophospate (AMP) production. They are effective in delaying delivery, but do not improve neonatal outcome or ultimate PTD rates. Further, they have significant maternal side-effects, which means that they are rarely used in the context of threatened PTL in the UK, although globally they are still widely used. The most serious side-effect is pulmonary oedema, with an estimated incidence of 1:350–1:400 treated patients. Maternal deaths from acute cardiopulmonary compromise are described, with greater risks if beta-agonists are given in large fluid volumes, in multiple pregnancies and in women with cardiac disease.

Magnesium sulphate

Magnesium decreases the frequency of depolarization of smooth muscle by modulating calcium uptake, binding and distribution in smooth muscle cells and results in inhibition of uterine contractions. However, although magnesium sulphate is widely used as a tocolytic in the USA, there has only been one randomized trial comparing its effect to placebo and that failed to demonstrate a beneficial effect on the duration of pregnancy. Similarly, the 2014 Cochrane review on magnesium sulphate tocolysis found no effect favouring magnesium sulphate over controls. However, the American College of Obstetricians and Gynecologists (ACOG) supports the use of magnesium sulphate for neuroprotection stating that "magnesium sulphate reduces the risk of cerebral palsy in surviving infants".

Non-steroidal anti-inflammatory drugs

The first NSAID to be widely used in the management of PTL was indomethacin. It is a reversible, non-specific competitive cyclooxygenase (COX) inhibitor. In a series of studies, indomethacin has been shown to effectively delay delivery for 48 hours, 7–10 days and beyond 37 weeks, so reducing the incidence of low birthweight (<2,500 g). However, although PG inhibitors are effective in delaying PTD, they do have several adverse fetal effects. As mentioned above, PG synthesis is responsible for the maintenance of a patent ductus arteriosus and inhibition can lead to its premature closure. This can occur as early as the late second trimester, with the incidence increasing dramatically from 32 weeks. This may lead to persistent pulmonary hypertension in the fetal circulation of the neonate. The effect is completely reversible with early identification and discontinuation of treatment. In addition, indomethacin use has been associated with an increased risk of necrotizing enterocolitis and neonatal renal dysfunction. The latter probably occurs because inhibition of fetal PG synthesis reduces renal perfusion and fetal urine output, resulting in reversible (after discontinuation of the drug) oligohydramnios.

Calcium channel blockers

The effects of calcium channel blockers in relaxing the contractions of the human myometrium have been known for several years. They exert their effect by binding to L-type channels, reducing intracellular levels of calcium and blocking the transmembrane influx of calcium ions into muscle cells. Comparing nifedipine with other tocolytics (including beta-sympathomimetics, NSAIDs, magnesium sulphate and OTR antagonist [OTR-A]), no significant reductions were shown in the primary outcome measures of birth within 48 hours of treatment or in perinatal mortality. However, adverse drug reactions, discontinuation due to side-effects, neonatal RDS, necrotizing enterocolitis, intraventricular haemorrhage and neonatal jaundice were least for OTR-A, intermediate for nifedipine and greatest for beta-sympathomimetics.

Oxytocin receptor antagonists

OTRs play an important role in the onset and progression of labour as described above. The OTR-A atosiban is a competitive antagonist of oxytocin and vasopressin, binding to both the OTRs and the vasopressin V1a receptors within the myometrium. Administration of atosiban results in a dose-dependent inhibition of uterine contractility and oxytocin-mediated PG release. In pregnant women, atosiban is 46–48% plasma protein bound and only a small amount appears to cross the placenta into the fetal circulation. It has a similar efficacy as beta-sympathomimetics, but is much better tolerated. Compared to placebo, more atosiban-treated patients remained undelivered at 24 hours, 48 hours and 7 days.

Corticosteroid therapy

The administration of corticosteroids has the greatest influence on preterm neonatal outcome. Although the use of recombinant surfactant in neonates has also had a major impact on the incidence and consequences of RDS, antenatal corticosteroids are still associated with significant reduction in neonatal mortality principally through reduced rates of RDS and IVH. A 2006 *Cochrane Database Review* confirmed significant reductions in the risks of mortality, RDS and IVH in preterm infants of 31, 44 and 46%, respectively, after a single course of steroids. Their mechanism of action is complex; they affect not only fetal lung maturation, but also fetal growth, organ system maturation, fetal brain development, immune function and the fetal hypothalamic–pituitary–adrenocortical axis. Currently, betamethasone or dexamethasone are recommended; both are able to cross the placenta in their active form and have comparable properties, but some dexamethasone preparations contain a sulphite preservative that has been linked with neurotoxicity and should be avoided.

Enthusiasm for their use has been tempered by recent concerns, based on animal and some human data, that repeated antenatal doses could lead to a decrease in birthweight, brain size and abnormal neuronal development. However, the long-term outcomes related to their use have been largely positive and overall, antenatal corticosteroid treatment has been associated with less developmental delay in childhood and a trend towards fewer children having cerebral palsy when compared with no corticosteroid treatment. While 30 years follow-up showed no clinical differences in adults who were exposed *in utero* to betamethasone, there are no comparable data for dexamethasone.

Antibiotics

Despite a clear link between bacterial infection and preterm birth, the results of antibiotic treatment as an attempt to prevent PTL have been disappointing. The ORACLE trials focused on the use of antibiotics in PPROM (over 4,000 women) and spontaneous PTL with intact membranes (over 6,000 women). These trials demonstrated that, in singleton pregnancies with PPROM, erythromycin improved neonatal outcomes, but that antibiotic treatment in women with intact membranes had no benefit. As a result of these trials, 10 days of erythromycin has been adopted as the treatment of choice for PPROM in many obstetric units in the UK. However, concerns have been raised over widespread use of broad-spectrum antibiotics for all patients with PPROM.

Management of PPROM

PPROM occurs in approximately 2% of all pregnancies and accounts for up to one-third of preterm deliveries. Fifty percent of women deliver within 1 week and 75% within 2 weeks of PPROM. The earlier in pregnancy that PPROM occurs the shorter the interval to delivery.

Although postnatal survival following PPROM is directly related to birthweight and gestational age at delivery, in pregnancies complicated by PPROM prior to 23 weeks, pulmonary hypoplasia may develop leading to an increased risk of neonatal death, even if delivery occurs at later gestational ages. Pulmonary hypoplasia following PPROM occurs in approximately 50% of women with PPROM at 19 weeks, falling to about 10% at 25 weeks. The presence of amniotic fluid greater than 2 cm on ultrasound is associated with a lower incidence of pulmonary hypoplasia.

PPROM is diagnosed through clinical history and the demonstration of a pool of liquor in the vagina on speculum examination. Management balances the risk of prematurity (if delivery is encouraged) versus the risk of maternal and fetal infection (if delivery is delayed). In general, conservative management is followed in PPROM before 34 weeks' gestation unless there is evidence of chorioamnionitis and immediate induction of labour is advised in women after 37 weeks' gestation.

Conservative management includes intensive clinical surveillance for signs of chorioamnionitis including regular recording of maternal temperature, heart rate, cardiotocography and maternal biochemistry, with a rising white cell count or a rising C-reactive protein indicating development of chorioamnionitis. Lower genital tract swabs are routinely taken, but cultures do not correlate well with the risk of chorioamnionitis. In the majority of cases of PPROM there is time for administration of corticosteroids and *in utero* transfer before the onset of PTL. Tocolysis is contraindicated due to the increased risk of maternal and fetal infection in patients with PPROM.

Prediction of preterm delivery

Since the current management of PTL has little impact on neonatal outcome, research has focused on detecting those women who are at high risk of PTL and intervening to reduce their risk. Risk scoring systems rely heavily on previous obstetric history and are therefore not useful in women having their first baby.

Past obstetric history

Having had a previous PTD increases the risk of PTL in a subsequent pregnancy four times in comparison to a woman who had a previous delivery at term (*Table 8.1*).

Ultrasound measurement of cervical length

Cervical length measured by transvaginal ultrasound has been shown to be more accurate than transabdominal ultrasound or digital examination. There is a direct relationship between cervical length and the risk of PTD (**Figure 8.10**). Cervical length surveillance with serial measurement of cervical length throughout the second and early third

Table 8.1 Risk of preterm delivery in subsequent pregnancies

First delivery	Second delivery	Relative risk of preterm labour
Term		1
Preterm		4
Term	Term	0.5
Preterm	Term	1.3
Term	Preterm	2.5
Preterm	Preterm	6.5

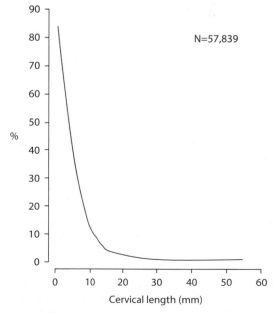

Figure 8.10 Cervical length and the risk of preterm (<34 weeks) delivery.

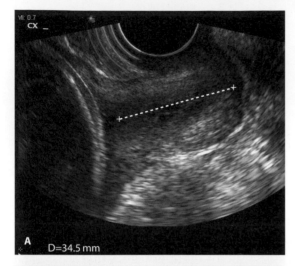

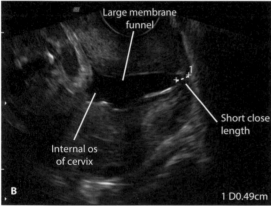

Figure 8.11 (**A**) Normal cervix; (**B**) cervical length and funnelling on ultrasound.

Prevention of preterm delivery

In those found to be at high risk of PTD, two interventions are currently available, progesterone and cervical cerclage.

Progesterone

Progesterone has been known to be important in maintaining pregnancy for more than 80 years and is thought to promote uterine quiescence and inhibit the production of proinflammatory cytokines and PGs within the uterus. In women with a previous preterm birth, there is some evidence that intramuscular hydroxyprogesterone caproate is effective in reducing the risk of recurrence. Hydroxyprogesterone caproate is licenced in the USA for preterm birth prevention in women with a previous preterm birth. In women with a short cervix, some studies have suggested that vaginal progesterone may prevent preterm birth. The largest study to date (OPPTIMUM) failed to find any benefit of vaginal progesterone in any patient group. Crucially, there is no evidence from any study that progesterone can reduce the longer-term adverse effects of preterm birth, that of neurodevelopmental disability and respiratory morbidity.

Cervical cerclage

Tranvaginal cervical cerclage may be placed in three different circumstances: following multiple midtrimester losses or preterm deliveries (history indicated cerclage); when the cervix shortens (usually <25 mm) in women with a history of cervical surgery or previous preterm birth (ultrasound indicated cerclage); or when the cervix is dilating in the absence of contractions (rescue cerclage).

trimester is now used to monitor women at high risk of PTD (**Figure 8.11**). The combination of cervical length and obstetric history can predict 80.6% of extremely early spontaneous PTD (10% screen-positive rate). However, currently universal cervical length screening has not been approved as it has not been shown to be cost effective.

Table 8.2 Types of cerclage

McDonald transvaginal cerclage	Transvaginal purse-string suture inserted at the cervicovaginal junction without bladder mobilization
Shirodkar (high transvaginal) cerclage	Transvaginal purse-string suture inserted following bladder mobilization, to allow insertion above the level of cardinal ligaments
Transabdominal cerclage	Suture inserted at the cervicoisthmic junction via laparotomy or laparoscopy. Transabdominal cerclages can either be inserted preconceptionally or in the first trimester of pregnancy

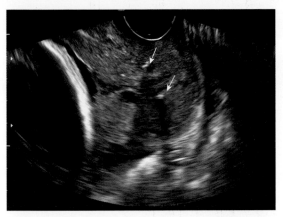

Figure 8.12 Cervical cerclage seen on ultrasound (arrows).

The exact mechanism by which cerclage helps to prevent or delay PTL is not entirely understood. It is likely, however, that cerclage provides structural support to a weakened cervix, and enhances the cervical immunological barrier by improving retention of the mucous plug and preventing ascending infection by maintaining cervical length. Similar to progesterone, cervical cerclage does not appear to reduce the risk of PTD in multiple pregnancies. The different types of cerclage are described in *Table 8.2* and an ultrasound image of a cervical cerclage *in situ* is shown in **Figure 8.12**.

A transabdominal cerclage is usually inserted following a failed vaginal cerclage or extensive cervical surgery. There are no randomized studies comparing the effectiveness of transabdominal cerclage with that of expectant management or transvaginal cerclage. Any potential benefits of transabdominal cerclage must be weighed against its increased operative risks. Patients must undergo two laparotomies during pregnancy, one for suture insertion and the other for caesarean section. Transabdominal cerclage should be therefore performed only by experienced operators and only for clear and defined indications.

Conclusion

Currently, the management of PTL is inadequate. Interventions in women who present in PTL do not improve neonatal outcomes. We are able to reduce the risk of PTD in those who are recognized to be high risk, but since 85% of PTD (due to PTL and PPROM) occurs in low-risk women who we do not screen, our impact on the overall rate of PTD is limited. We could effectively screen the low-risk population using transvaginal ultrasound to identify those at risk of PTD and give progesterone to reduce their risk, but this approach is yet to be proven to be cost effective. In order to manage PTD due to PTL and PPROM more effectively, we need to fully understand the mechanisms responsible. Only then will we be able to design targeted therapies that will make a significant impact on the risk of PTD.

 KEY LEARNING POINTS

- Preterm labour has multiple causes.
- Worldwide, preterm delivery is the most important cause of infant (<5 years) mortality.
- Tocolysis does not improve neonatal outcomes.
- Antenatal steroids reduce the risk of RDS.
- Screening with transvaginal ultrasound can detect women at high risk of preterm delivery.
- Progesterone reduces the risk of preterm birth in women with a short cervix.
- Cervical cerclage reduces the risk of preterm birth in high-risk women.

New developments

Recent data suggest that the arabin pessary may reduce the risk of PTD in women with a singleton or multiple pregnancy. Further studies are ongoing. An abnormal vaginal microbiome has been linked to an increased risk of PTD.

Further reading

Cervical Cerclage (Green-top Guideline No. 60). https://www.rcog.org.uk/en/guidelines-research-services/guidelines/gtg60/
NICE Guideline on Preterm labour and birth. https://www.nice.org.uk/guidance/ng25.
Smith R (2007). Parturition. *N Engl J Med* **356**(3):271–83.
WHO: The worldwide incidence of preterm birth: a systematic review of maternal mortality and morbidity. http://www.who.int/bulletin/volumes/88/1/08-062554/en/

Self assessment

CASE HISTORY

Mrs A, a 39-year-old Caucasian woman, works as a secretary in a bank. She has no known medical problems but is a smoker. This is her 5th pregnancy. At the age of 18, she had a termination of pregnancy at 10 weeks' gestation. She had two spontaneous first trimester miscarriages, aged 36 and 37. Both required dilation and curettage (D&C) for retained products of conception. Just over 1 year ago, she had a late miscarriage at 22 weeks. She has been trying to conceive since the last miscarriage.

She is now 8 weeks pregnant, fit and well, and is taking iron supplements. When seen in the antenatal booking clinic, concerns were raised about her risks of an early delivery.

A What risk factors does Mrs A have for PTL?

B What care should Mrs A receive?

C Discuss specific elements of her antenatal care that may be beneficial.

ANSWER

A Her greatest risk factor is the 22 week loss in her last pregnancy. Although a single operative cervical dilatation is unlikely to lead to any significant degree of cervical weakness, there is some evidence that three or more such procedures pose a risk for early delivery. Finally, smoking is associated with increased risks of antepartum haemorrhage and spontaneous membrane rupture, either of which can lead to early birth.

B In view of her high risk of PTD, she should receive consultant-led care in a hospital. It may be a good idea for her to meet a neonatologist and to be shown around the neonatal unit, particularly if any antenatal investigations further elevate her risk.

C A careful history should be taken regarding the events surrounding her last delivery. Presentation in advanced labour or with bulging membranes despite little or no pain may suggest a degree of cervical weakness. Although cerclage could be contemplated for such a history, the use of ultrasound assessment of cervical length may allow her to avoid surgery. Even if cerclage is not contemplated, cervical length measurements can guide interventions such as maternal steroids. Cervicovaginal fFN may allow even greater predictive accuracy. Screening for BV between 12 and 18 weeks may allow a specific intervention (i.e. targeted antibiotics) that reduces risk and improves outcome.

EMQ

Risk factors for preterm labour:

A Smoking.
B Uterine abnormality.
C Appendicitis.
D Parity >5.
E Previous preterm delivery.
F Intrauterine bleeding.
G Cervical fibroids.
H Poor socioeconomic background.
I Interpregnancy interval <1 year.
J Afro-Caribbean origin.
K Multiple pregnancy.
L Previous cervical cone biopsy.

For each description, choose the SINGLE most appropriate answer from the list of options. Each option may be used once, more than once or not at all.

1 Risk of PTL is primarily due to uterine overdistension.
2 Linked to recurrent episodes of threatened miscarriage early in pregnancy.
3 May require surgery during pregnancy with associated risk of PTL.
4 Modifiable risk factor for which help and advice can be given in antenatal clinic.

ANSWER

1K   2F   3C   4A

The main risk of PTL in multiple pregnancy is the increased intrauterine volume, which leads to overdistension. Intrauterine bleeding, such as a subchorionic haemorrhage, is irritant to the uterus and may contribute to episodes of abdominal pain and bleeding. Surgery such as appendicectomy is relatively safe in pregnancy, but does increase the risk of PTL. Smoking is the only modifiable risk factor in the list. Help and encouragement to stop smoking should be offered.

SBA QUESTION

Which statement is most accurate regarding cervical cerclage? Choose the single best answer.

A In a high-risk patient should be performed as soon as practical after confirmation of intra-uterine pregnancy.
B It is a suitable procedure in any woman with a prior history of delivery between 20 and 26 weeks.
C Should be performed using an absorbable suture material.
D May be placed using a transvaginal approach.
E Requires a second anaesthetic procedure for removal when delivery is imminent.

ANSWER

D Cervical clerclage should be considered in a small group of carefully selected patients. Studies suggest benefit in women with a prior history of three or more late miscarriages or PTD. It is best performed after 12–14 weeks to avoid the problems of early pregnancy loss. The most common suture material is a Mercilene tape, which is non-absorbable. Transvaginal or transabdominal approaches are possible. A cervical suture placed vaginally can usually be removed without recourse to regional anaesthesia.

Hypertensive disorders of pregnancy

LOUISE C KENNY

LEARNING OBJECTIVES

- To understand the classification of hypertension in pregnancy.
- To appreciate and be able to differentiate the different risks associated with various types of hypertensive disorders in pregnancy.
- To understand the pathophysiology of pre-eclampsia.

- To be aware of the clinical presentation of pre-eclampsia and understand the principles of management.
- To understand the long-term risks to both mother and baby from pre-eclampsia.

Introduction

Hypertension is common in pregnancy. Approximately 1 in 10 women will have one or more episodes of raised blood pressure prior to delivery. The majority have a benign condition called gestational hypertension, which is not associated with adverse outcomes. However, about one-third of these women (3% overall) will develop pre-eclampsia. Pre-eclampsia is a leading cause of maternal death. The World Health Organization (WHO) estimates that globally between 50,000 and 75,000 women die of this condition each year. Furthermore, pre-eclampsia is frequently accompanied by fetal growth restriction (FGR), which is responsible for considerable perinatal morbidity and mortality. An increasing number of women enter pregnancy with chronic hypertension and this is associated with increased risks for both mother and baby, including an increased risk of pre-eclampsia and FGR. In this chapter, the various types of hypertension and their respective management are discussed.

Classification of hypertension in pregnancy

There is now a widely agreed classification system for hypertension in pregnancy. Simply put, pregnant women who develop or present with hypertension in pregnancy have one of three conditions:

- Non-proteinuric pregnancy-induced hypertension.
- Pre-eclampsia.
- Chronic hypertension.

133

Non-proteinuric pregnancy-induced hypertension (otherwise known as gestational hypertension) is hypertension that arises for the first time in the second half of pregnancy and in the absence of proteinuria. It is not associated with adverse pregnancy outcome and mild and moderate increases in blood pressure in this setting do not require treatment. However, up to one-third of women who present with gestational hypertension will progress to pre-eclampsia.

Women who have confirmed hypertension in the first half of pregnancy most likely have chronic hypertension. The majority will have essential hypertension but this is a diagnosis of exclusion and secondary causes should be excluded. Chronic hypertension, of whatever type, can predispose to the later development of superimposed pre-eclampsia. Even in the absence of superimposed pre-eclampsia, chronic hypertension is associated with increased maternal and fetal morbidity and pregnancies complicated by chronic hypertension should therefore be regarded as high risk. The physiological fall in blood pressure that occurs in the first trimester secondary to peripheral vasodilatation can mask chronic hypertension. For example, a booking blood pressure of 138/88 mmHg, while still technically within normal limits, raises the suspicion of an underlying hypertensive tendency.

Degrees of hypertension

- Mild: diastolic blood pressure 90–99 mmHg, systolic blood pressure 140–149 mmHg.
- Moderate: diastolic blood pressure 100–109 mmHg, systolic blood pressure 150–159 mmHg.
- Severe: diastolic blood pressure ≥110 mmHg, systolic blood pressure ≥160 mmHg

Pre-eclampsia

Incidence

Pre-eclampsia complicates approximately 2–3% of pregnancies, but the incidence varies depending on the exact definition used and the population studied. In the most recent UK Confidential Enquiry (2010–2012)

there were nine deaths due to pre-eclampsia, which represents a significant fall from 19 deaths in 2006–2008. However, globally, around 70,000 women die annually of pre-eclampsia, making it a leading cause of maternal death in low-resource settings.

Pre-eclampsia is defined as hypertension of at least 140/90 mmHg recorded on at least two separate occasions and at least 4 hours apart and in the presence of at least 300 mg protein in a 24-hour collection of urine, arising *de novo* after the 20th week of pregnancy in a previously normotensive woman and resolving completely by the sixth postpartum week.

Risk factors

Pre-eclampsia is more common in first-time mothers. It is thought that the normal fetal–maternal transfusion that occurs during pregnancy and particularly during delivery exposes the mother to products of the fetal (and hence paternal) genome, protecting her in subsequent pregnancies.

Risk factors for pre-eclampsia

- First pregnancy.
- Multiparous with a previous history of pre-eclampsia.
- Pre-eclampsia in any previous pregnancy.
- 10 years or more since last baby.
- Age 40 years or more.
- Body mass index (BMI) of 35 or more.
- Family history of pre-eclampsia (in mother or sister).
- Booking diastolic blood pressure of 80 mmHg or more.
- Booking proteinuria (of ≥1+ on more than one occasion or quantified at ≥0.3 g/24 h).
- Multiple pregnancy.
- Certain underlying medical conditions:
  - pre-existing hypertension;
  - pre-existing renal disease;
  - pre-existing diabetes;
  - antiphospholipid antibodies.

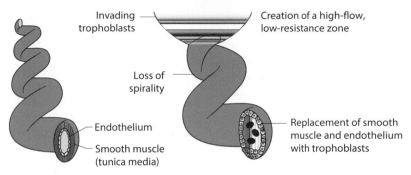

Figure 9.1 Physiological change of spiral arteries by invading trophoblasts.

In line with this, the protective effect of first pregnancy seems to be lost if a woman has a child with a new partner. There also appears to be a maternal genetic predisposition to pre-eclampsia as there is a three- to fourfold increase in the incidence of pre-eclampsia in the first-degree relatives of affected women. Finally, there are a number of general medical conditions and pregnancy-specific factors that predispose to the development of pre-eclampsia.

Pathophysiology

Pre-eclampsia only occurs in pregnancy, but has been described in pregnancies lacking a fetus (molar pregnancies) and in the absence of a uterus (abdominal pregnancies), suggesting that it is the presence of trophoblast tissue that provides the stimulus for the disorder. General thinking suggests that the development of pre-eclampsia is a two-stage process, which originates in early pregnancy (**Figure 9.1**). In the first stage, trophoblast invasion is patchy and the spiral arteries retain their muscular walls. This is thought to prevent the development of a high-flow, low-impedance uteroplacental circulation and leads to uteroplacental ischaemia (**Figure 9.2**). The reason why trophoblasts invade less effectively in these pregnancies is not known but may reflect an abnormal adaptation of the maternal immune system.

In the second stage, uteroplacental ischaemia results in oxidative and inflammatory stress, with the involvement of secondary mediators leading to endothelial dysfunction, vasospasm and activation of the coagulation system (**Figure 9.1**). As the target cell of the disease process, the vascular endothelial cell, is so ubiquitous, pre-eclampsia is a truly multisystem disorder, affecting multiple organ systems, often concurrently.

Cardiovascular system

Normal pregnancy is characterized by marked peripheral vasodilatation resulting in a fall in total peripheral resistance despite an increase in plasma volume and cardiac rate. Pre-eclampsia is characterized by marked peripheral vasoconstriction, resulting in hypertension. The intravascular high pressure and loss of endothelial cell integrity results in greater vascular permeability and contributes to the formation of generalized oedema.

Renal system

In the kidney, a highly characteristic lesion called glomeruloendotheliosis is seen. This is relatively specific for pre-eclampsia (it is not seen with other

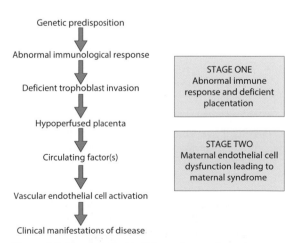

Figure 9.2 The proposed aetiology of pre-eclampsia.

hypertensive disorders) and is associated with impaired glomerular filtration and selective loss of intermediate weight proteins, such as albumin and transferrin, leading to proteinuria. This is turn causes a reduction in plasma oncotic pressure and exacerbates the development of oedema.

Haematological system

In the event of endothelial damage, platelets adhere to the damaged area. Furthermore, diffuse vascular damage is associated with the laying down of fibrin. Pre-eclampsia is association with increased fibrin deposition and a reduction in the platelet count may accompany and occasionally predate the onset of disease.

The liver

In the liver, subendothelial fibrin deposition is associated with elevation of liver enzymes. This can be associated with haemolysis and a low platelet count due to platelet consumption (and subsequent widespread activation of the coagulation system). The presence of these finding is called HELLP syndrome (haemolysis, elevation of liver enzymes and low platelets). HELLP syndrome is a particularly severe form of pre-eclampsia, occurring in just 2–4% of women with the disease. It is associated with a high fetal loss rate (of up to 60%) (see Box).

Neurological system

The development of convulsions in a woman with pre-eclampsia is defined as eclampsia. Vasospasm and cerebral oedema have both been implicated in the pathogenesis of eclampsia. Retinal haemorrhages, exudates and papilloedema are characteristic of hypertensive encephalopathy and are rare in pre-eclampsia, suggesting that hypertension alone is not responsible for the cerebral pathology.

Clinical presentation

The classic symptoms of pre-eclampsia include a frontal headache, visual disturbance and epigastric pain. However, the majority of women with pre-eclampsia are asymptomatic or merely complain of general vague 'flu-like' symptoms.

Clinical examination should include a complete obstetric and neurological examination (see Chapter 1, Obstetric history and examination). Hypertension is usually the first sign but occasionally is absent or transient until the late stages of the disease. Dependent oedema of the feet is very common in healthy pregnant women. However, rapidly progressive oedema of the face and hands may suggest pre-eclampsia. Epigastric tenderness is a worrying sign and suggests liver involvement. Neurological examination may reveal hyperreflexia and clonus in severe cases. Urine testing for protein should be considered part of the clinical examination (*Table 9.1*).

HELLP syndrome

- HELLP syndrome is an acronym for haemolysis, elevation of liver enzymes and low platelets.
- Women with HELLP syndrome typically present with epigastric pain, nausea and vomiting.
- Hypertension may be mild or even absent.
- HELLP syndrome is associated with a range of serious complications including acute renal failure, placental abruption and stillbirth.
- The management of HELLP syndrome involves stabilizing the mother, correcting any coagulation deficits and assessing the fetus for delivery.

Table 9.1 Testing for proteinuria

Dipstick urinalysis	Instant result but quantitatively inaccurate
Trace	Seldom significant
1+	Possible significant proteinuria, warrants quantifying
≥2+	Probable significant proteinuria, warrants quantifying
Protein:creatinine ratio	Fast (within 1 hour)
	Results semiquantitave
>30 mg/mol	Probable significant proteinuria
24-hour collection	Slow
300 mg/24 h	Confirmed significant proteinuria

Management and treatment

There is no cure for pre-eclampsia other than to end the pregnancy by delivering the baby (and placenta). This can be a significant problem if pre-eclampsia occurs early in pregnancy, particularly at gestations below 34 weeks. Therefore, management strategies are aimed at minimizing risk to the mother in order to permit continued fetal growth. In severe cases this is often not possible.

The principles of management of pre-eclampsia are:

- Early recognition of the symptomless syndrome.
- Awareness of the serious nature of the condition in its severest form.
- Adherence to agreed guidelines for admission to hospital, investigation and the use of antihypertensive and anticonvulsant therapy.
- Well-timed delivery to pre-empt serious maternal or fetal complications.
- Postnatal follow-up and counselling for future pregnancies.

A diagnosis of pre-eclampsia usually requires admission (*Table 9.2*). Patients with mild hypertension, minimal protein and normal haematological and biochemical parameters may be monitored as outpatients, but will require frequent attendance for fetal and maternal assessment. Women with moderate or severe hypertension, significant proteinuria or abnormal haematological or biochemical parameters require admission and inpatient management.

Investigations

To monitor maternal complications:

- Full blood count (with particular emphasis on falling platelet count and rising haematocrit).
- If platelet values are normal, additional clotting studies are not indicated.
- Serum renal profile (including serum uric acid levels).
- Serum liver profile.
- Frequent repeat proteinuria quantification is probably unhelpful once a diagnosis of pre-eclampsia has been made.

Table 9.2 The management of pregnancy complicated by pre-eclampsia

Degree of hypertension	Mild hypertension (140/90—149/99 mmHg)	Moderate hypertension (150/100—159/109 mmHg)	Severe hypertension (160/110 mmHg or higher)
Admit to hospital	Yes	Yes	Yes
Treat	No	With oral labetalol† as first-line treatment to keep: • diastolic blood pressure between 80 and 100 mmHg • systolic blood pressure less than 150 mmHg	With oral labetalol† as first-line treatment to keep: • diastolic blood pressure between 80 and 100 mmHg • systolic blood pressure less than 150 mmHg
Measure blood pressure	At least four times a day	At least four times a day	More than four times a day, depending on clinical circumstances
Test for proteinuria	Do not repeat quantification of proteinuria	Do not repeat quantification of proteinuria	Do not repeat quantification of proteinuria
Blood tests	Monitor using the following tests twice a week: kidney function, electrolytes, full blood count, transaminases, bilirubin	Monitor using the following tests three times a week: kidney function, electrolytes, full blood count, transaminases, bilirubin	Monitor using the following tests three times a week: kidney function, electrolytes, full blood count, transaminases, bilirubin

† Only offer women with pre-eclampsia antihypertensive treatment other than labetalol after considering side-effect profiles for the woman, fetus and newborn baby. Alternatives include methyldopa and nifedipine.
(Adapted from the National Institute for Health and Care Excellence (NICE) guideline, Hypertension Pregnancy.)

To monitor fetal complications:

- Ultrasound assessment of:
  - fetal size;
  - amniotic fluid volume;
  - maternal and fetal Dopplers.
- Antenatal cardiotocography, used in conjunction with ultrasound surveillance, provides a useful but by no means infallible indication of fetal well-being. A loss of baseline variability or decelerations may indicate fetal hypoxia.

Treatment of hypertension

The commonest cause of death in women who die of pre-eclampsia in the UK is cerebral bleeding secondary to uncontrolled systolic blood pressure. Therefore, the aim of antihypertensive therapy is to lower the blood pressure and reduce the risk of maternal cerebrovascular accident without reducing uterine blood flow and compromising the fetus. There are a variety of antihypertensives used in the management of pre-eclampsia. Methyldopa is a centrally acting antihypertensive agent. It has a long-established safety record in pregnancy. However, it can only be given orally, it takes upwards of 24 hours to take effect and has a range of unpleasant side-effects including sedation and depression. These properties limit its usefulness. Labetalol is an alpha-blocking and beta-blocking agent. It has a good safety record in pregnancy and can be given orally and intravenously. It is the first drug of choice in most national guidelines including the current National Institute for Health and Care Excellence (NICE) guideline, Hypertension in Pregnancy. Nifedipine is a calcium-channel blocker with a rapid onset of action. It can, however, cause severe headache that may mimic worsening disease. In severe cases of fulminating disease, an intravenous infusion of hydralazine or labetalol can be titrated rapidly against changes in the blood pressure.

Treatment and prevention of eclampsia

Eclampsia is defined as the presence of tonic–clonic convulsions in a woman with pre-eclampsia and in the absence of any other identifiable cause. The drug of choice for the treatment of eclampsia is magnesium sulphate. This is given intravenously and has been shown to reduce the incidence of further convulsions in women with eclampsia. Magnesium sulphate should also be used in women with severe pre-eclampsia to prevent the onset of convulsions. The management of eclampsia is described in further detail in Chapter 14, Obstetric emergencies.

Screening and prevention

The accurate prediction of women at risk of developing pre-eclampsia will facilitate targeting of increased antenatal surveillance while allowing women at low risk to participate in community-based antenatal care. In addition, a predictive test would in turn facilitate the development of novel therapeutic preventive interventions.

Unfortunately there is currently no screening test for pre-eclampsia. Despite intensive research in this area, no single blood biomarker has emerged that either alone or in combination with other biomarkers or clinical data possesses sufficient sensitivity and specificity to be clinically useful.

The ability of Doppler ultrasound uterine artery waveform analysis to identify women at risk of pre-eclampsia (and other adverse pregnancy outcomes) has been investigated with varying success. In pregnancies with incomplete trophoblast remodelling of the spiral arteries, a characteristic 'notch' can often be seen in the waveform pattern that frequently also demonstrates high resistance (see Chapter 4, Assessment of fetal wellbeing, and **Figure 4.20**). This screening test may have a role in women who have already been identified as being at risk of the disease because of their medical or past obstetric history. However, it is not of value in screening low-risk women.

Established preventive interventions include low-dose aspirin (typically 75 mg daily), which modestly reduces the risk of pre-eclampsia in high-risk women; calcium supplementation may also reduce risk, but only in women with low dietary intake.

Additional points in management

Iatrogenic premature delivery of the fetus is often required in severe pre-eclampsia. If her condition allows, the mother should be transferred to a centre with adequate facilities to care for her baby, and prior to 34 weeks' gestation steroids should be given intramuscularly to the mother to reduce the chance of neonatal respiratory distress syndrome. Delivery before term is often by caesarean section. Such patients are at particularly high risk for thromboembolism and should be given prophylactic subcutaneous heparin and issued with antithromboembolic stockings. In the case of spontaneous or induced labour and if clotting studies are normal, epidural anaesthesia is indicated as it helps control blood pressure. Ergometrine is avoided in the management of the third stage as it can significantly increase blood pressure.

Postnatally, blood pressure and proteinuria will resolve. However, in a minority of cases one or both persist beyond 6 weeks and this suggests the presence of underlying chronic hypertension or renal disease. Additionally, a careful search should be made postnatally for underlying medical disorders in women who present with severe pre-eclampsia before 34 weeks' gestation.

KEY LEARNING POINTS

- Pre-eclampsia is a multisystem disorder that likely originates in the placenta and is a significant cause of maternal and perinatal morbidity and mortality.
- There is no cure other than delivery; the aim of management is to stabilize the maternal blood pressure and prevent seizures and cerebral bleeding.

Chronic hypertension

Essential hypertension is the underlying cause of chronic hypertension in 90% of cases. However, before a diagnosis is made, other causes need to be excluded. Appropriate investigations include serum creatinine, electrolytes, urine analysis (blood, protein and glucose), protein quantification and renal ultrasound. Autoantibody screen and cardiac investigations including electrocardiography (ECG) and echocardiography should be considered where there is clinical suspicion (history, examination or investigation results) of a secondary cause. Renal causes account for over 80% of cases of secondary hypertension (see Chapter 10, Medical complications of pregnancy).

Causes

- Idiopathic.
- Essential hypertension.
- Vascular disorders.
- Renal artery stenosis.
- Coarctation of the aorta.
- Renal disease.
- Polycystic disease.
- Diabetic nephropathy.
- Chronic glomerulonephritis.
- Nephrotic and nephritic syndrome.
- Collagen vascular disease.
- Systemic sclerosis.
- Systemic lupus erythematosus.
- Rheumatoid disease.
- Endocrine disease.
- Phaeochromocytoma.
- Conn's syndrome.
- Cushing's syndrome.
- Diabetes mellitus.

The maternal risks of pre-existing hypertension include pre-eclampsia, abruption, heart failure and intracerebral haemorrhage. Pre-eclampsia develops in around one-third of women with pre-existing hypertension and is more likely to affect those with severe hypertension and/or renal disease.

Management

In mild cases (<150/100 mmHg) there is no immediate indication to treat; however, the pregnancy should be monitored carefully to detect changes in blood pressure or features of pre-eclampsia (usually indicated by new proteinuria), as well as FGR by serial ultrasound scans. Antihypertensive medication taken before pregnancy can often be discontinued in the first half of pregnancy as there is a physiological reduction in blood pressure. Angiotensin-converting enzyme (ACE) inhibitors, angiotensin-receptor blockers and atenolol should be discontinued because of concerns of teratogenicity and negative effects on fetal growth.

If the blood pressure is consistently >150/100 mmHg, antihypertensive medication should be offered to reduce the risk of severe hypertension and the attendant risks of intracerebral haemorrhage, although treatment does not prevent placental abruption or superimposed pre-eclampsia, nor does it influence perinatal outcome. Preferred antihypertensive agents include labetolol, nifedipine and methyldopa (centrally acting agent). The aim of antihypertensive medication is to maintain the blood pressure below 160 mmHg systolic and 80–100 mmHg diastolic.

The obstetric management of pre-existing hypertension involves close monitoring for the development of superimposed pre-eclampsia and FGR. In women requiring antihypertensive medication, delivery is usually offered around 39 weeks, but may need to be earlier if complications have developed.

Following delivery, the maternal blood pressure often decreases, but careful surveillance is required as it tends to increase again on the third or fourth postpartum day. Breastfeeding is encouraged and medication should be changed to those drugs that are considered safe.

Risk factors for developing superimposed pre-eclampsia

- Renal disease.
- Maternal age >40 years.
- Pre-existing diabetes.
- Multiple pregnancy.
- Connective tissue disease (e.g. antiphospholipid syndrome).
- Coarctation of the aorta.
- Blood pressure ≥160/100 mmHg in early pregnancy.
- Prepregnancy BMI >35.
- Previous pre-eclampsia.
- Antiphospholipid syndrome.

KEY LEARNING POINTS

- Chronic hypertension is associated with a range of adverse maternal and perinatal outcomes and it should be regarded as a high-risk pregnancy.
- Chronic hypertension may present for the first time in pregnancy and it may initially be masked by the profound vasodilatation and decrease in peripheral vascular resistance seen in the first trimester of pregnancy.

Fetal growth restriction

Definition and incidence

FGR is defined as a failure of a fetus to achieve its genetic growth potential. This usually results in a fetus that is small for gestational age (SGA). SGA means that the weight of the fetus is less than the 10th centile for its gestation. Other cut-off points (e.g. the third centile) can be used. The terms SGA and FGR are not synonymous. It is important to remember that most SGA fetuses are constitutionally small and are not compromised. FGR indicates that there is a pathological process operating to restrict the growth rate of the fetus. Consequently, some FGR fetuses may not actually be SGA, but nevertheless will have failed to fulfil their growth potential.

There are a wide variety of reasons why a baby may be born small including congenital anomalies, fetal infections and chromosomal abnormalities (these are discussed in more detail in Chapter 5, Prenatal diagnosis). However, most babies that are born small are either constitutionally small (i.e. healthy, but born to small parents and fulfilling their genetic growth potential) or are small secondary to abnormal placenta function and have FGR.

FGR is a major cause of neonatal and infant morbidity and mortality. There is a significant cost associated with providing adequate facilities to look after these babies. In addition, there is an increasing body of evidence that certain adult diseases (such as diabetes and hypertension) are more common in adults who were born with FGR.

Aetiology

The common causes of FGR are listed in *Table 9.3*. They are grouped into two main categories: factors that directly affect the intrinsic growth potential of the fetus and external influences that reduce the support for fetal growth. Chromosome abnormalities, genetic syndromes and fetal infections can alter intrinsic fetal growth potential. External influences that affect fetal growth can be subdivided into maternal systemic factors and placental insufficiency.

Maternal undernutrition is globally the major cause of FGR. Low maternal oxygen saturation, which can occur with cyanotic heart disease or at

Table 9.3 Causes of fetal growth restriction

Reduced fetal growth potential	Aneuploidies, e.g. trisomy 18 Single gene defects (e.g. Seckel's syndrome) Structural abnormalities (e.g. renal agenesis) Intrauterine infections (e.g. cytomegalovirus, toxoplasmosis)
Reduced fetal growth support	
Maternal factors	Undernutrition (e.g. poverty, eating disorders) Maternal hypoxia (e.g. living at altitude, cyanotic heart disease) Drugs (e.g. alcohol, cigarettes, cocaine)
Placental factors	Reduced uteroplacental perfusion (e.g. inadequate trophoblast invasion, sickle cell disease, multiple gestation) Reduced fetoplacental perfusion (e.g. single umbilical artery, twin-to-twin transfusion syndrome)

high altitude, will reduce fetal pO_2 levels and fetal metabolism. Smoking, by increasing the amount of carboxyhaemoglobin in the maternal circulation, effectively reduces the amount of oxygen available to the fetus, thus causing FGR. A wide variety of drugs other than tobacco can affect fetal growth including alcohol and cocaine, probably through multiple mechanisms affecting fetal enzyme systems, placental blood flow and maternal substrate levels.

In developed countries, the most common cause of FGR is poor placental function secondary to inadequate trophoblast invasion of the spiral arteries. This results in reduced perfusion of the intracotyledon space, which in turn leads to abnormal development of the terminal villi and impaired transfer of oxygen and nutrients to the fetus. The placental pathology of this is similar to that seen in pre-eclampsia and accounts for why pre-eclampsia and FGR commonly present together. Less frequently, reduced perfusion can occur from other conditions such as maternal sickle cell disease and the antiphospholipid syndrome (see Chapter 10, Medical complications of pregnancy). Multiple pregnancy usually results in a sharing of the uterine vascularity, which causes a relative reduction in the blood flow to each placenta. On the fetal side of the placental circulation, abnormalities of the umbilical cord, such as a single umbilical artery, are associated with FGR as are the intraplacental vascular connections found in monochorionic twinning.

Pathophysiology

FGR is frequently classified as symmetrical or asymmetrical. Symmetrically small fetuses are normally associated with factors that directly impair fetal growth such as chromosomal disorders and fetal infections. Asymmetrical growth restriction is classically associated with uteroplacental insufficiency that leads to reduced oxygen transfer to the fetus and impaired excretion of carbon dioxide by the placenta. A fall in pO_2 and a rise in pCO_2 in the fetal blood induces a chemoreceptor response in the fetal carotid bodies, with resulting vasodilatation in the fetal brain, myocardium and adrenal glands, and vasoconstriction in the kidneys, splanchnic vessels, limbs and subcutaneous tissues. The liver circulation is also severely reduced. Normally, 50% of the well-oxygenated blood in the umbilical vein passes to the right atrium through the ductus venosus, eventually to reach the fetal brain, with the remainder going to the portal circulation in the liver. When there is fetal hypoxia, more of the well-oxygenated blood from the umbilical vein is diverted through the ductus venosus, which means that the liver receives less. The result of all these circulatory changes is an asymmetrical fetus with relative brain sparing and reduced abdominal girth and skin thickness. The vasoconstriction in the fetal kidneys results in impaired urine production and oligohydramnios. The fetal hypoxaemia also leads to severe metabolic changes in the fetus reflecting intrauterine starvation. Antenatal fetal blood sampling has shown reduced levels of nutrients such as glucose and amino acids (especially essential amino acids) and of hormones such as thyroxine and insulin. There are increased levels of corticosteroids and catecholamines, which reflect the increased perfusion of the adrenal gland. Haematological changes also reflect the chronic hypoxia, with increased levels of erythropoietin and nucleated red blood cells.

Chronic fetal hypoxia in FGR may eventually lead to fetal acidaemia, both respiratory and metabolic, which if prolonged can lead to intrauterine death if the fetus is not removed from its hostile environment. FGR fetuses are especially at risk from profound asphyxia in labour due to further compromise of the uteroplacental circulation by uterine contractions.

Management

The assessment of fetal well-being is described in detail in Chapter 4, Assessment of fetal wellbeing.

In brief, the detection of an SGA infant contains two elements: first the accurate assessment of gestational age and second, the recognition of fetal smallness.

Early measurement of the fetal crown–rump length before 13 weeks plus 6 days gestation or head circumference between 13 weeks plus 6 days and 20 weeks' gestation remains the method of choice for confirming gestational age. Thereafter the most precise way of assessing fetal growth is by ultrasound biometry (biparietal diameter, head circumference, abdominal circumference and femur length) serially at set time intervals (usually of 4 weeks and no less than 2 weeks). As resources in most units do not permit comprehensive serial ultrasound in all pregnancies, serial ultrasound biometry is usually performed in 'at risk' pregnancies (see box below).

Pregnancies at risk of FGR

- Multiple pregnancies (see Chapter 7, Multiple pregnancy).
- History of FGR in previous pregnancy.
- Current heavy smokers.
- Current drug users.
- Women with underlying medical disorders:
    - hypertension;
    - diabetes;
    - cyanotic heart disease;
    - antiphospholipid syndrome.
- Pregnancies where the symphysis–fundal height is less than expected.

When a diagnosis of SGA has been made, the next step is to clarify whether the baby is normal and simply constitutionally small or whether it is FGR. A comprehensive ultrasound examination of the fetal anatomy should be made looking for fetal abnormalities that may explain the size. Even if the anatomy appears normal, the presence of symmetrical growth restriction in the presence of a normal amniotic fluid volume raises the suspicion of a fetal genetic defect and the parents should be counselled accordingly. Amniocentesis and rapid fetal karyotyping should be offered. Features suspicious of uteroplacental insufficiency are an asymmetrically growth restricted fetus with a relatively small abdominal circumference, oligohydramnios and a high umbilical artery resistance (see Chapter 4, Assessment of fetal wellbeing, **Figures 4.14–4.16**).

At present there are no widely accepted treatments available for FGR related to uteroplacental insufficiency. Obvious contributing factors such as smoking, alcohol and drug abuse should be stopped and the health of the women should be optimized. Low-dose aspirin may have a role in the prevention of FGR in high-risk pregnancies but is not effective in the treatment of established cases.

When growth restriction is severe and the fetus is too immature to be delivered safely, bed rest in hospital is usually advised in an effort to maximize placental blood flow, although the evidence supporting this practice is limited. The aim of these interventions is to gain as much maturity as possible before delivering the fetus, thereby reducing the morbidity associated with prematurity. However, timing the delivery in such a way that maximizes gestation without risking the baby dying *in utero* demands intensive fetal surveillance. The most widely accepted methods of monitoring the fetus are discussed in detail in Chapter 4, Assessment of fetal wellbeing, and summarized briefly in the following box.

Prognosis

The prognosis of FGR is highly dependent upon the cause, severity and the gestation at delivery. When FGR is related to a congenital infection or chromosomal abnormality, subsequent development of the child will be determined by the precise abnormality.

Surveillance of the FGR fetus

- Serial biometry and amniotic fluid volume measurement performed at no less than 2-weekly intervals.
- In the FGR fetus dynamic tests of fetal well-being include:
  - umbilical artery Doppler wave form analysis: absence or reversed flow of blood in the umbilical artery during fetal diastole requires delivery in the near future;
  - in extremely preterm or previable infants with absent or reversed end-diastolic flow in the umbilical artery, other fetal arterial and venous Doppler studies can be performed, although their use has not yet been proven by large prospective trials;
  - fetal cardiotocography.

Of babies with FGR secondary to uteroplacental insufficiency, some will suffer morbidity or mortality as a result of prematurity. For the survivors, the long-term prognosis is good with low incidences of mental and physical disability and most infants demonstrate 'catch-up growth' after delivery when feeding is established.

A link between FGR and the adult onset of hypertension and diabetes has been established. It remains to be seen whether other associations will be found in the future.

KEY LEARNING POINTS

- SGA refers to those fetuses whose estimated weight is less than 10th centile for their gestational age. Most SGA fetuses are healthy.
- FGR refers to any fetus failing to achieve its growth potential. Not all SGA fetuses are FGR and some FGR fetuses are not SGA.
- FGR carries an increased risk of intrapartum asphyxia, stillbirth and possible long-term risk of hypertension and other cardiovascular diseases.
- There is no effective treatment and the management involves appropriate monitoring and timely delivery.

New developments

There is intense interest in the development of screening and better diagnostic tests for pre-eclampsia. Placental growth factor (PlGF) belongs to the vascular endothelial growth factor (VEGF) family and represents a key regulator of angiogenic events in pathological conditions. PlGF is low in pregnancy-complicated pre-eclampsia and early data suggest that a low PlGF has a high sensitivity for predicting adverse outcomes in women presenting with suspected pre-eclampsia. The results of a larger trial are awaited.

There is also an urgent need to develop treatments for FGR. Sildenafil citrate potentiates the effect of nitrous oxide (NO) and thus may cause vasodilatation of vessels responsive to NO. The incomplete remodelling of maternal spiral arteries in FGR results in vessels with intact or partially intact muscular layers, which remain responsive to regional vascular control. Sildenafil has the potential to increase uteroplacental circulation and perfusion, resulting in improved gaseous and nutrient exchange and improved fetal growth and wellbeing. There are a series of coordinated trials of sildenafil citrate in progress for the treatment of severe early-onset FGR.

Further reading

National Institute for Health and care Excellence (NICE) Hypertension in pregnancy: diagnosis and management. Clinical guideline. Published: 25 August 2010. Available at www.nice.org.uk/guidance/cg107.

Royal College of Obstetricians and Gyneacologists (RCOG) Green-top Guideline No. 31. The Investigation and Management of the Small-for-Gestational-Age Fetus, 2nd Edition, February 2013 Revised January 2014. Available at https://www.rcog.org.uk/globalassets/documents/guidelines/gtg_31.pdf.

Self assessment

CASE HISTORY

Mrs B was a 34-year-old Caucasian primigravid teacher. She was seen in the hospital antenatal clinic for the first time at 11 weeks' gestation. She was noted to be a non-smoker. There was no relevant past history, but family history revealed that her mother has had hypertension since her late forties. Mrs B was 1.56 m tall and weighed 83 kg. Her booking blood pressure was 110/74 mmHg and urinalysis was normal.

The antenatal period was uneventful until 37 weeks. At 37 weeks' gestation, a community midwife noted that Mrs B's blood pressure had risen to 150/100 mmHg and that there was 1+ of protein in the urine. Mrs B was referred to the hospital as an emergency admission.

On arrival at the hospital, Mrs B's blood pressure was 160/110 mmHg and there was 3+ of protein in the urine. She was complaining of some upper abdominal pain and there was hyperreflexia. The fetal heart rate was normal.

What are the risks in this case?

ANSWER

Mrs B was hypertensive and had marked proteinuria, having previously been normotensive. The diagnosis is pre-eclampsia. The level of the blood pressure denotes severe disease. The pregnancy is at term.

Mrs B is at risk of developing a worsening condition. A further rise in her blood pressure will put her at risk of intracranial haemorrhage. She may have an eclamptic fit, develop a coagulopathy and HELLP syndrome, and possibly renal failure. There is a further risk of placental abruption and severe haemorrhage. The fetus is at risk secondary to the mother's condition.

Plan of action

- The patient does not require resuscitation.
- The fetus does not require emergency delivery.
- Call for help.
- Establish an intravenous line with a wide-bore cannula.
- Take blood for clotting studies, full blood count and blood biochemistry and save serum.
- Prevent an eclamptic fit from occurring: give magnesium sulphate intravenously 4 g bolus over 20 minutes. Continue with 1 g/h.
- At these doses, monitoring blood levels is not necessary unless the urine output falls to less than 20 ml/h (magnesium sulphate is excreted via the kidneys).
- Lower the blood pressure. The aim is to achieve a diastolic blood pressure of 90–100 mmHg and the systolic blood pressure should be treated if above 160 mmHg. Check the blood pressure every 5 minutes. Oral labetalol or nifedipine can be used to treat blood pressure. If unsuccessful, intravenous hydralazine or labetalol, as a bolus followed by an infusion, will be needed.
- Measure input and output of fluids.
- Put a Foley catheter into the bladder.
- Restrict input from all sources to 80 ml/h (or 1 ml/kg/h).
- If the clotting becomes deranged (platelets $<50 \times 10^9/l$), contact a consultant haematologist for advice.

Management of the case

In this case, the blood pressure fell to 145/96 mmHg on treatment with labetalol. Treatment with magnesium sulphate was started and the urine output averaged 35 ml/h. Clotting studies, full blood count and biochemistry remained normal. The cardiotocograph showed a normal fetal heart pattern.

Once stabilization had been achieved, delivery was planned. Because the clotting studies were normal, an epidural was put in place. Vaginal examination showed that the cervix was favourable, with the fetus presenting by the head. Therefore, induction of labour was commenced, and after a rapid labour a 3.2 kg boy was delivered, with normal Apgar scores. The estimated blood loss was 600 ml.

After delivery, Mrs B was nursed in the delivery suite for 36 hours. The magnesium sulphate infusion was continued for 24 hours after delivery. Oral labetalol was commenced and the infusion was discontinued. There was initial concern with regard to the urine output, which remained at 25 ml/h for the first 6 hours after delivery. The position was watched, but no active steps were taken to redress the issue and, between 6 and 12 hours after delivery, the patient began to have a marked diuresis. Seven days after delivery, Mrs B's blood pressure had returned to normal without medication.

Conclusion

This case demonstrates appropriate management of moderate to severe pre-eclampsia at term. Major problems were prevented by swift action. Mrs B is at risk of pre-eclampsia in her next pregnancy, although it is likely to be less severe. She is also at risk of developing hypertension later in life.

EMQ

Features of abnormal placentation:

A HELLP syndrome.

B Pre-eclampsia.

C Eclampsia.

D Disseminated intravascular coagulation.

E Glomeruloendotheliosis.

F Gestational hypertension.

G Chronic hypertension.

H Placental abruption.

I None of the above.

For each description, choose the SINGLE most appropriate answer from the list of options. Each option may be used once, more than once or not at all.

1 A 40-year-old woman in her first pregnancy presents in labour. Her blood pressure is 145/90 mmHg. Shortly after beginning regular contractions she has a tonic–clonic seizure.

2 A 32-year-old woman presents with epigastric pain at 38/40 in her second pregnancy, her first having been complicated by pre-eclampsia. Her blood pressure is 130/86 mmHg, her alanine aminotransferase (ALT) is 170 IU/L and her platelet count is 40×10^9/l.

3 A 24-year-old woman in her first pregnancy presents at 32/40 with sudden onset severe abdominal pain and vaginal bleeding. Her blood pressure is 160/95 mmHg.

4 A 36-year-old woman in her first pregnancy is noted to have a blood pressure of 140/86 mmHg at 32/40. There is no protein in her urine and she is asymptomatic.

ANSWERS

1C A seizure in labour in a non-epileptic with a raised blood pressure is highly likely to represent eclampsia.

2A A mildly elevated blood pressure with a high ALT, a low platelet count and epigastric pain make HELLP syndrome the most likely diagnosis.

3H Sudden onset of severe abdominal pain and bleeding in late pregnancy should always raise the suspicion of placental abruption. This is more common in the context of pre-eclampsia, and this may be the cause of her elevated blood pressure.

4F This patient has a mildly elevated blood pressure but no protein in the urine, which suggests the diagnosis of gestational hypertension.

SBA QUESTION

Which of the following is not useful in the treatment or prevention of pre-eclampsia?

Choose the single best answer.

A Hydralazine.
B Aspirin.
C Labetalol.
D Methyldopa.
E Rantidine.

ANSWER

E Hydralazine, labetalol and methyldopa are all used to treat hypertension. Aspirin can reduce the risk of pre-eclampsia in high-risk women. Ranitidine is a histamine-2 blocker used to reduce gastric acid. It is not helpful in the management or prevention of pre-eclampsia.

Medical complications of pregnancy

JENNY E MYERS, DAVID WILLIAMS AND LOUISE C KENNY

LEARNING OBJECTIVES

- Understand the importance of medical conditions in pregnancy in relation to maternal and infant health.
- Appreciate the importance of preconceptual counselling and its impact on improving pregnancy outcomes.
- Understand the impact of common medical conditions such as hypertension, kidney disease, cardiac disease and diabetes on pregnancy.
- Appreciate the contribution of maternal medical disease to maternal mortality.

Overview

Pregnancy in women with pre-existing medical diseases is becoming increasingly common as the treatment of many chronic conditions improves. Women with underlying medical conditions are at increased risk of developing complications in pregnancy and pre-existing medical conditions may, in some circumstances, be associated with significant maternal and fetal morbidity and, more rarely, mortality. In this chapter, the risks and management of the more common pre-existing medical disorders that are seen in pregnancy are discussed.

Introduction

Women with pre-existing medical problems can often pose complex management issues in pregnancy. Ideally, such women should be seen for preconceptual care with a multidisciplinary approach. Unfortunately, while such counselling is available and does occur, many women present with unplanned pregnancies. It is therefore vital to be aware of the most common medical disorders that occur in women of reproductive age and to have an appreciation of the associated risks and the appropriate management.

Renal disease

Women with chronic kidney disease (CKD) are less able to make the renal adaptations necessary for a healthy pregnancy and pregnancy in women with renal disease therefore requires increased maternal and fetal surveillance.

Prepregnancy counselling

Prepregnancy counselling is recommended in all women with chronic kidney disease and they should be made aware of the risks to the fetus and to their long-term renal function before conception.

Prepregnancy counselling discussion should include:

- Safe contraception until pregnancy advised.
- Fertility issues if indicated.
- Genetic counselling if inherited disorder.
- Risks to mother and fetus during pregnancy.
- Avoid known teratogens and contraindicated drugs.
- Treatment of blood pressure and adjustment of antihypertensives.
- Low-dose aspirin.
- Need for anticoagulation once pregnant in women with significant proteinuria:
  - need for compliance with strict surveillance;
  - likelihood of prolonged admission or early delivery;
  - possibility of accelerated decline in maternal renal function;
  - need for postpartum follow-up.

Chronic kidney disease

CKD is classified into five stages based on the level of renal function (*Table 10.1*). Stages 1 and 2 affect around 3% of women of childbearing age (20–39), and while stages 3–5 affect 1 in 150 women in this age group, pregnancy in these women is less common. Some women are found to have CKD for the first time in their pregnancy, and pregnancy can unmask previously unrecognized renal disease.

Effect of pregnancy on CKD

Women with CKD stages 1–2 have mild renal dysfunction and usually have an uneventful pregnancy and good renal outcome. Pregnancy with a serum creatinine <110 µmol/l, minimal proteinuria (<1 g/24 hours) and absent or well-controlled hypertension pre-pregnancy has been shown to have little or no adverse effect on long-term maternal renal function. Women with moderate to severe disease (stages 3–5) are at highest risk of complications during pregnancy and of an accelerated decline in their renal function. In summary, therefore, women with the most impaired renal function have the worst pregnancy outcome. Clinical complications including hypertension, proteinuria and recurrent urinary infections independently and additively enhance the risk of a poor pregnancy outcome.

The diagnosis of pre-eclampsia is often difficult due to the presence of pre-existing hypertension and/or proteinuria. If pre-eclampsia develops, maternal renal function often deteriorates further, but any other additional complications, such as postpartum haemorrhage or use of non-steroidal anti-inflammatory drugs (NSAIDs), can critically threaten maternal renal function.

Table 10.1 Stages of chronic kidney disease

Stage	Description	Estimated GFR (ml/min/1.73m²)
1	Kidney damage with normal/raised GFR	>90
2	Kidney damage with mildly low GFR	60–89
3	Moderately low GFR	30–59
4	Severely low GFR	15–29
5	Kidney failure	<15 or dialysis

GFR, glomerular filtration rate.

Effect of CKD on pregnancy outcome

Pregnancies in mothers with CKD have increased risks of preterm delivery, delivery by caesarean section and fetal growth restriction (FGR) dependent on the degree of renal impairment. The risk of adverse pregnancy outcome correlates with the degree of renal dysfunction (*Table 10.2*).

Monitoring of patients with CKD during pregnancy

- Blood pressure.
- Renal function:
  - creatinine.
- Urine:
  - infection;
  - proteinuria.
- Full blood count:
  - haemoglobin;
  - ferritin.
- Renal ultrasound.
- Fetal ultrasound:
  - anatomy;
  - uterine artery Doppler 20–24 weeks;
  - growth.

Table 10.2 Estimated effects of renal function on pregnancy outcome and maternal renal function

	Mean prepregnancy serum creatinine value (mg/dl)		
	<125	125–180	>180
Fetal growth restriction (%)	25	40	65
Preterm delivery (%)	30	60	>90
Pre-eclampsia (%)	22	40	60
Loss of >25% renal function postpartum (%)	0	20	50
End-stage renal failure after 1 year (%)	0	2	35

Data adapted from Williams and Davidson (2008). *BMJ* **326**:211–15.

Dialysis

The incidence of pregnancy on dialysis (stage 5 CKD) is increasing. Dialysis must be adjusted to allow for the physiological changes of pregnancy (plasma volume, fluid retention, electrolytes), and haemodialysis is usually more effective then peritoneal dialysis in achieving this. Complications include preterm delivery, polyhydramnios (30–60%), pre-eclampsia (40–80%) and caesarean delivery (50%).

Pregnancy in women with renal transplants

Women with end-stage kidney disease have hypothalamic–gonadal dysfunction and infertility, so conception is rare. Female fertility returns rapidly after renal transplantation and it is estimated that 2–10% of female recipients conceive. Of pregnancies progressing beyond the third trimester, the vast majority (>90%) result in a successful pregnancy outcome. Most transplantation centres advise that conception is safe after the second post-transplantation year, provide the graft is functioning well.

All pregnancies in transplant recipients are high risk and should be managed by a multidisciplinary team. Lower doses of immunosuppressive therapy, longer time since transplantation and better graft function with absence of chronic rejection are all associated with better maternal outcomes. There is an increased risk of complications in women with renal transplants, often related to residual underlying disease; complications include preterm delivery, pre-eclampsia and urinary tract infection. The risk

Monitoring of renal transplant patients during pregnancy

- Renal function:
  - proteinuria;
  - creatinine.
- Blood pressure.
- Drug levels.
- Fetal growth.
- If renal function declines, exclude:
  - obstruction;
  - infection;
  - rejection.

of acute rejection in pregnancy is estimated at 2%, and allograft dysfunction may also be difficult to detect during pregnancy. Vaginal delivery is considered safe, although there is a small risk of damage to the transplant during a caesarean section, which is slightly increased during an emergency caesarean delivery.

Tacrolimus, azathioprine, ciclosporin and prednisolone are generally considered safe in pregnancy and for the breastfed infant and should be continued with dose adjustment as necessary. Screening for gestational diabetes (GDM) is necessary with prednisolone and tacrolimus. Current opinion is that the use of mycophenolate and sirolimus should be avoided in transplant recipients considering pregnancy, and women should be switched to alternative regimes before pregnancy; a period of 3–6 months' stability on a new medication regime prior to pregnancy is advised.

Diabetes mellitus

Diabetes may complicate a pregnancy either because a woman has type 1 or type 2 diabetes mellitus before pregnancy or because impaired glucose tolerance develops during the course of her pregnancy (GDM).

Prepregnancy counselling

The aim of prepregnancy counselling is to achieve the best possible glycaemic control before pregnancy and to educate diabetic women about the implications of pregnancy. Preparation for pregnancy works best if the health care providers delivering care to women outside of pregnancy are able to provide information to help women optimize their diabetes and other medications before they embark on a pregnancy. Advice includes:

- Optimization of glycaemic control to achieve an HbA1c of <42 mmol/mol without inducing hypoglycaemia.
- High-dose folic acid (5 mg daily) to reduce the risk of neural tube defects.
- Planning periconception adjustments to other medications such as statins and angiotensin-converting enzyme (ACE) inhibitors before pregnancy.

Poor glycaemic control is associated with a significantly increased risk of congenital anomalies, particularly neural tube defects and cardiac anomalies. The most critical period for the embryo is therefore the period of organogenesis, which occurs in the first 42 days of pregnancy, and this is often before the pregnancy is medically confirmed. The level of HbA1c in early pregnancy also correlates with the risk of early fetal loss. An HbA1c of >85 mmol/mol is associated with a fetal loss during pregnancy of around 30%. Prepregnancy care is associated with reduced rates of congenital malformation. In the preconception period, diabetes therapy should be intensified and adequate contraception encouraged until glucose control is good. Targets for therapy prepregnancy are premeal glucose levels of 4–7 mmol/l. Improved glycaemic control may be achieved with newer insulin delivery systems such as continuous subcutaneous insulin infusion pumps and glucose sensors.

Diabetic vascular complications are common in women of reproductive age and women with significant retinopathy, nephropathy and/or neuropathy benefit from multidisciplinary team review prior to pregnancy. It is important that a plan for medication adjustment is made and women are counselled regarding the additional potential complications associated with diabetic microvascular disease. This is particularly important for women with nephropathy, which is associated with a significantly increased risk of complications arising in pregnancy that would necessitate preterm delivery as for women with other types of renal disease (80% chance if 125–180 µmol/l; 75% chance if 180–220 µmol/l; and 60% chance if >220 µmol/l). There is also a risk that retinopathy can progress in pregnancy and during the postpartum period.

Maternal and fetal complications of types 1 and 2 diabetes mellitus

Congenital abnormality is an important cause of mortality and morbidity in diabetic pregnancies and is seen 2–4 times more often than in pregnancies without diabetes, with a threefold excess of cardiac and neural tube defects. In addition to structural malformations, fetal macrosomia is a frequent complication associated with maternal diabetes and frequently contributes to a traumatic birth and shoulder dystocia. Accelerated growth patterns are typically seen in the late second and third trimesters and are attributable to poorly controlled diabetes in the majority of cases. Stillbirth, particularly in the third trimester, remains too common in pregnancies complicated by maternal diabetes, being five times higher than in the general population. Concerns regarding fetal wellbeing, particularly in the presence of fetal macrosomia, frequently prompt early term delivery in women with diabetes, which in turn increases the likelihood of neonatal unit admission and reduces breastfeeding rates.

In general, maternal morbidity in diabetic pregnancies is related to the severity of diabetic-related vascular disease preceding the pregnancy. The risk of pre-eclampsia is increased threefold in women with diabetes, and particularly in those with underlying microvascular disease. All women with diabetes should be offered low-dose aspirin from 12 weeks' gestation to reduce the risk of pre-eclampsia. Women with diabetic retinopathy are at risk of progression of the disease and should be kept under careful surveillance (retinal screening at booking, 16–20 weeks' and 28 weeks' gestation). Other possible complications include an increased incidence of infection, severe hyperglycaemia or hypoglycaemia, diabetic ketoacidosis and the complications that may arise from the increased operative delivery rate.

Management of types 1 and 2 diabetes in pregnancy

Women with diabetes should be managed throughout their pregnancy by a multidisciplinary team involving diabetic specialist midwives and nurses, a dietician, an obstetrician and a physician. The primary goal of the team is to support the woman and her family during the pregnancy to safely optimize glycaemic control. Blood glucose monitoring is encouraged 7 times a day (before and 1 hour after meals) with targets of <5.3 mmol/l and 1-hour postprandial levels of <7.8 mmol/l. If not given before pregnancy, women require additional support and education regarding diet, use of oral hypoglycaemic agents such as metformin where appropriate, insulin adjustments for hyperglycaemia and management of hypoglycaemia, which is much more common and potentially very dangerous in pregnancy, particularly in women with reduced hypoglycaemic awareness.

Insulin resistance increases dramatically over the course of pregnancy and therefore women with type 1 and type 2 diabetes are usually required to increase their dose of insulin or metformin during the second half of pregnancy.

A plan for the pregnancy should be set out in early pregnancy and should include renal and retinal screening, fetal surveillance and a plan for delivery. Women with diabetes should be offered a fetal anomaly scan at 19–20 weeks with an assessment of the cardiac outflow tracts. Serial growth scans are also recommended to assess fetal growth and diagnose macrosomia and polyhydramnios. If antenatal corticosteroids are indicated, additional insulin therapy is required to maintain normoglycaemia, often requiring inpatient admission. Timing and mode of delivery should be determined on an individual basis. In general, provided the pregnancy has gone well, the aim would be to achieve a vaginal delivery at between 38 and 39 weeks. However, the development of macrosomia or maternal complications such as pre-eclampsia, together with the rate of failed induction, is such that the caesarean section rate amongst diabetic women often is as high as 50%. For women with type 1 diabetes and those with type 2 diabetes requiring insulin, a sliding scale of insulin and glucose should be commenced in labour, and maternal blood glucose levels maintained at 4–7 mmol/l to reduce risk of neonatal hypoglycaemia. Insulin requirements return to prepregnancy levels immediately following delivery and insulin doses should be adjusted accordingly. Women should be informed of the increased risk of hypoglycaemia in the postnatal period, particularly if they are breastfeeding.

Effects of pregnancy on diabetes

- Nausea and vomiting, particularly in early pregnancy.
- Greater importance of tight glucose control.
- Increase in insulin dose requirements in the second half of pregnancy.
- Increased risk of severe hypoglycaemia.
- Risk of deterioration of pre-existing retinopathy.
- Risk of deterioration of established nephropathy.

Effects of diabetes on pregnancy

- Increased risk of miscarriage.
- Risk of congenital malformation.
- Risk of macrosomia.
- Increased risk of pre-eclampsia.
- Increased risk of stillbirth.
- Increased risk of infection.
- Increased operative delivery rate.

Gestational diabetes

GDM complicates 10–15% of pregnancies depending on the diagnostic criteria used. Screening for diabetes in pregnancy is designed to detect previously undiagnosed type 2 diabetes and diabetes developing during pregnancy. Women who develop GDM are at increased risk of type 2 diabetes in later life, and education about diet and lifestyle during pregnancy can have important implications for future health. No single screening method has been shown to be perfect in terms of sensitivity and specificity for GDM. Screening is generally targeted at high-risk groups (women from an ethnic group with high rates of type 2 diabetes, a family history of type 2 diabetes, maternal obesity and a previous large for gestational age infant). Screening involves a glucose tolerance test, sometimes preceded by a glucose challenge test, but different diagnostic criteria are used in different hospitals. The UK National Institute for Health and Care Excellence (NICE) guidelines (2015) recommend a diagnosis of GDM with a fasting glucose ≥5.6 mmol/l and/or a 2 hour (post-75 g glucose load) of 7.8 mmol/l. The WHO guidelines (2013) recommend a diagnosis with a fasting glucose of 5.1 mmol/l and/or a 1 hour (post 75 g glucose load) of 10.0 mmol/l or 2 hour of 8.5 mmol/l. The principles of management during pregnancy are the same as for women with pre-existing diabetes. Women are educated regarding the risks associated with fetal macrosomia (increased operative delivery, shoulder dystocia, neonatal unit admission) and are encouraged to maintain capillary blood (fingerprick) glucose levels <5.3 mmol/l before meals and postprandial levels <7.8 mmol/l 1 hour after meals. Women unable to achieve this level of glycaemic control with changes to diet and lifestyle are treated with metformin and/or insulin as necessary. Treatment of GDM has been demonstrated to reduce the frequency of infants born large for gestational age.

One of the most important components of the management of women who develop GDM is the exclusion of type 2 diabetes after pregnancy. Screening with a fasting glucose or HbA1c should be offered 6–13 weeks after childbirth.

Factors associated with poor pregnancy outcome in diabetes

- Maternal social deprivation.
- No folic acid intake prepregnancy.
- Suboptimal approach of the woman to managing her diabetes.
- Suboptimal preconception care.
- Suboptimal glycaemic control at any stage.
- Suboptimal maternity care during pregnancy.
- Suboptimal fetal surveillance of big babies.

Other endocrinology disorders

Thyroid disease

Thyroid disease is common in women of childbearing age. Many of the symptoms of thyroid disease, such as heat intolerance, constipation, fatigue, palpitations and weight gain, resemble those of normal pregnancy and therefore new presentations of thyroid disease can be difficult to detect during pregnancy. Physiological changes of pregnancy, including plasma volume expansion, increased thyroid binding globulin production and relative iodine deficiency, also mean that thyroid hormone reference ranges for non-pregnant women are not useful in pregnancy. Free thyroxine 4 (fT4), free T3 (fT3) and thyroid-stimulating hormone (TSH) should be analyzed when assessing thyroid function in pregnancy, and total T3 and T4 not used. There is a fall in TSH and a rise in fT4 concentrations in the first trimester of normal pregnancy, followed by a fall in fT4 concentration with advancing gestation.

Hypothyroidism

Hypothyroidism is found in around 1% of pregnant women. Worldwide, the commonest cause of hypothyroidism is iodine deficiency, but this is rarely seen in the developed world, where autoimmune Hashimoto's thyroiditis is more common. Women diagnosed with hypothyroidism should continue thyroid replacement therapy during pregnancy and biochemical euthyroidism is the aim (TSH <4 mmol/l). Thyroid function tests should be performed serially in each trimester, or more often if dose adjustments are required. From the fetal perspective, maternal T4 levels are most important in the first trimester of pregnancy, where suboptimal replacement therapy is associated with developmental delay and pregnancy loss in some studies. Corrected hypothyroidism does not seem to influence pregnancy outcome or complications.

Hyperthyroidism

Autoimmune thyrotoxicosis (Graves' disease) affects around 2 per 1,000 pregnancies and has usually been diagnosed before pregnancy. Other causes of hyperthyroidism (5% overall) include toxic adenoma, subacute thyroiditis and toxic multinodular goitre. Symptoms include tremor, sweating, insomnia, hyperactivity and anxiety. Signs include goitre, Graves' ophthalmopathy, tachycardia, hypertension with a wide pulse pressure, weight loss and pretibial myxoedema. Treatment during pregnancy should be drug therapy, aiming to maintain maternal fT3 and fT4 levels in the high/normal range. Radioactive iodine is contraindicated because it completely obliterates the fetal thyroid gland. Treatment options include carbimazole or propylthiouracil (PTU) using the lowest acceptable dose, as high doses cross the placenta and may cause fetal hypothyroidism. Both drugs can also cause agranulocytosis, therefore regular checks of maternal white cell count are necessary. Beta-blockers can be used initially before the antithyroid drugs take effect. Thyroid surgery is rarely considered in pregnancy, but can be performed if a retrosternal goitre is causing upper airways obstruction due to tracheal compression, or if there is a suspicion of malignancy or failed medical therapy.

Uncontrolled thyrotoxicosis is associated with increased risks of miscarriage, preterm delivery and FGR. Thyroid function therefore needs to be closely monitored and many women can reduce their dose of medication, with almost one-third able to stop treatment in pregnancy. Doses usually need to be readjusted postpartum to prevent a relapse. TSH receptor stimulating antibodies cross the placenta and the risk of fetal Graves' disease after 20 weeks is proportional to their level, although still very low overall, as <10% of Graves' disease is associated with high levels of antibodies. Babies born to women with positive antibody titres should be reviewed after birth by the neonatology team to exclude thyroid dysfunction associated with maternal antibody passage.

Thyroid storm

A thyroid storm is a life-threatening event that arises in those with underlying thyroid disease, and can be fatal in 20–50% of untreated cases. It is usually the result of either undertreatment or infection, but it may be associated with labour and it can mimic imminent eclampsia. The diagnosis is made on clinical grounds with laboratory confirmation of hyperthyroidism. Features include excessive sweating, pyrexia, tachycardia, atrial fibrillation, hypertension, hyperglycaemia, vomiting, agitation and cardiac failure. Treatment is with PTU and high-dose corticosteroids, while beta-blockers are used to block the peripheral effect of thyroxine and supportive care with rehydration is also required.

Parathyroid disease

Hyperparathyroidism is caused by parathyroid hyperplasia or adenomas, which may be difficult to detect, and leads to hypercalcaemia due to elevated levels of parathyroid hormone (PTH). If diagnosed before pregnancy, the ideal treatment is surgical removal. However, if suspected in pregnancy, parathyroidectomy may still be indicated in severe cases, with mild hyperparathyroidism managed conservatively through hydration and a low calcium diet. The risks to the mother are from hypercalcaemic crises and complications such as acute pancreatitis, while fetal risks include increased rates of miscarriage, intrauterine death, preterm labour and neonatal tetany in untreated cases.

Hypoparathyroidism may be caused by autoimmune disease but is more commonly a complication of thyroid surgery. It is diagnosed by finding low serum calcium and low PTH levels. Untreated, it is associated with increased risks of second trimester miscarriage and fetal hypocalcaemia, resulting in bone demineralization and neonatal rickets. The aim of treatment is to maintain normocalcaemia through vitamin D and oral calcium supplements, with regular monitoring of calcium and albumin levels during pregnancy.

Pituitary tumours in pregnancy

Hyperprolactinaemia is an important cause of infertility and amenorrhoea, and is most often due to a benign pituitary microadenoma. The diagnosis is confirmed with a combination of measurement of the prolactin level and computed tomography (CT) or magnetic resonance imaging (MRI) scanning of the pituitary fossa. In 80% of cases it is treated with a dopamine agonist (bromocriptine or cabergoline), which causes the tumour to reduce in size. Larger tumours may require surgery or radiotherapy, which is best undertaken before pregnancy.

The pituitary gland enlarges by 50% during pregnancy, but it is rare for microadenomas to cause problems. Serial prolactin levels are unhelpful for monitoring tumour growth in pregnancy. Bromocriptine and cabergoline are usually stopped in pregnancy, and visual fields and relevant symptoms such as frontal headache are monitored. If there is evidence of tumour growth during pregnancy, bromocriptine or cabergoline should be recommenced, and appropriate neuroimaging arranged. In women with macroadenomas (>1 cm), it is advisable to continue with dopamine agonists because of the risk of the tumour enlarging under oestrogen stimulation.

Adrenal disease

Cushing's syndrome

Cushing's syndrome is rare in pregnancy as most affected women are infertile. It is characterized by increased glucocorticoid production, usually due to hypersecretion of adrenocorticotrophic hormone (ACTH) from a pituitary tumour. However, in pregnancy, adrenal causes (tumours) are more common. Diagnosis is difficult because many of the symptoms – striae, weight gain, weakness, glucose intolerance and hypertension – mimic normal pregnancy changes. If suspected, plasma cortisol levels should be measured (although levels increase in pregnancy) and adrenal imaging with ultrasound, CT or MRI should be used. There is a high incidence of pre-eclampsia, preterm delivery and stillbirth.

Conn's syndrome

Conn's syndrome is caused by an adrenal tumour producing excess aldosterone. While rare in pregnancy, it is considered one of the more common causes of secondary hypertension. Conn's syndrome usually presents with hypertension and hypokalaemia and is diagnosed by high aldosterone and low renin and enlargement of adrenals with CT scan or ultrasound.

Addison's disease

Addison's disease (adrenal insufficiency) is an autoimmune process associated with clinical symptoms of exhaustion, nausea, hypotension, hypoglycaemia and weight loss. The diagnosis is difficult to make in pregnancy because the cortisol levels, instead of being characteristically decreased, may be in the low–normal range due to the physiological increase in cortisol-binding globulin in pregnancy. Occasionally, the disease may present as a crisis, and treatment consists of glucocorticoid and fluid replacement. In diagnosed and adequately treated patients, the pregnancy usually continues normally. Replacement steroids should be continued in pregnancy and increased at times of stress such as hyperemesis and delivery.

Phaeochromocytoma

Phaeochromocytoma is a rare catecholamine-producing tumour, reported in 1 in 50,000 pregnancies. The tumours arise from the adrenal medulla in 90% of cases. In pregnancy, it may present as a hypertensive crisis and the symptoms may be similar to those of pre-eclampsia. A characteristic feature is paroxysmal hypertension, whereas the other symptoms of headaches, blurred vision, anxiety and convulsions may occur in pre-eclampsia. The diagnosis is confirmed by measurement of catecholamines in a 24-hour urine collection and in plasma, as well as by adrenal imaging. Treatment is by alpha- and beta-blockade with prazosin or phenoxybenzamine (alpha-blockers) and a beta-blocker (e.g. atenolol or propranolol), but surgical removal is the only cure. Caesarean section is the preferred mode of delivery, as it minimizes the likelihood of sudden increases in catecholamines associated with vaginal delivery. Maternal and perinatal mortality is greatly increased, especially if the diagnosis is not made before pregnancy.

Heart disease

Prepregnancy counselling

Most women with heart disease will be aware of their condition prior to becoming pregnant. Ideally, these women should be fully assessed by an obstetrician and cardiologist before embarking on a pregnancy and the maternal and fetal risks carefully explained. A plan to optimize medication should be made and if there is a possibility that the heart disease will require surgical correction, it is recommended that this should be undertaken before a pregnancy.

Issues in prepregnancy counselling of women with heart disease

- Risk of maternal death.
- Possible reduction of maternal life expectancy.
- Effects of pregnancy on cardiac disease.
- Mortality associated with high-risk conditions.
- Risk of fetus developing congenital heart disease.
- Risk of preterm labour and FGR.
- Need for frequent hospital attendance and possible admission.
- Intensive maternal and fetal monitoring during labour.
- Other options – contraception, adoption, surrogacy.
- Timing of pregnancy.

Antenatal management

Experienced physicians and obstetricians should manage pregnant women with significant heart disease in a joint obstetric/cardiac clinic. Continuity of care makes the detection of subtle changes in maternal wellbeing more likely. In trying to distinguish between 'normal' symptoms of pregnancy and impending cardiac failure, it is important to ask the pregnant woman if she has noted any breathlessness, particularly at night, any change in her heart rate or rhythm, any increased tiredness or a reduction in exercise tolerance (*Table 10.3*). Routine physical examination should include pulse rate, blood pressure, jugular venous pressure, heart sounds, ankle and sacral oedema and presence of basal crepitations.

Table 10.3 Stages of heart failure – New York Heart Association (NYHA) classification

Class	Patient symptoms
1 Mild	No limitation of physical activity. Ordinary physical activity does not precipitate fatigue, palpitations, dyspnoea, angina
2 Mild	Slight limitation of physical activity. Comfortable at rest, but ordinary physical activity results in fatigue, palpitation or dyspnoea
3 Moderate	Marked limitation of physical activity. Comfortable at rest, but less than ordinary activity causes fatigue, palpitation or dyspnoea
4 Severe	Unable to carry out any physical activity without discomfort. Symptoms of cardiac insufficiency at rest. If any physical activity is undertaken, discomfort is increased

Table 10.4 Toronto risk markers for maternal cardiac events

	Markers
1	Prior episode of heart failure, arrhythmia, or stroke
2	NYHA Class >II or cyanosis
3	Left heart obstruction
4	Reduced left ventricular function (EF <40%)

0 predictors: risk of cardiac event is 5%
1 predictor: risk of cardiac event is 37%
>1 predictors: risk of cardiac event is 75%

EF, ejection fraction; NYHA, New York Heart Association.

Most women will remain well during the antenatal period and outpatient management is usually possible, although women should be advised to have a low threshold for reducing their normal physical activities (*Tables 10.3, 10.4*). Echocardiography is non-invasive and useful in its ability to serially assess function and valves, and an echocardiogram at the booking visit and at around 28 weeks' gestation is usual. Any signs of deteriorating cardiac status should be carefully investigated and treated.

Anticoagulation is essential in patients with congenital heart disease who have pulmonary hypertension (PH) or artificial valve replacements, and in those in or at risk of atrial fibrillation. The use of anticoagulants during pregnancy is a complicated issue because warfarin is teratogenic if used in the first trimester, and is linked with fetal intracranial haemorrhage in the third trimester. Low-molecular-weight heparin is often used as an alternative to warfarin, especially in the first and third trimester, and can be titrated using factor Xa levels.

High-risk cardiac conditions

- Systemic ventricular dysfunction (ejection fraction <30%, NYHA Class III–IV).
- Pulmonary hypertension.
- Cyanotic congenital heart disease.
- Aortic pathology (dilated aortic root >4 cm, Marfan syndrome).
- Ischaemic heart disease.
- Left heart obstructive lesions (aortic, mitral stenosis).
- Prosthetic heart valves (metal).
- Previous peripartum cardiomyopathy.

Fetal risks of maternal cardiac disease

- Recurrence (congenital heart disease).
- Maternal cyanosis (fetal hypoxia).
- Iatrogenic prematurity.
- FGR.
- Effects of maternal drugs (teratogenesis, growth restriction, fetal loss).

Management of labour and delivery

In most cases the aim of management is to await the onset of spontaneous labour, as this will minimize the risk of intervention and maximize the chances of a normal delivery. Induction of labour should be considered for the usual obstetric indications and in very high-risk women, to ensure that delivery occurs at a reasonably predictable time when all the relevant personnel are present or available. Epidural anaesthesia is often recommended, as this reduces the pain-related stress and, thereby, some of the demand on cardiac function. However, regional anaesthesia

is not without some risk to both the mother and baby in some cardiac conditions, principally because of the potential complication of maternal hypotension. The input of a senior anaesthetist to formulate and document an anaesthetic management plan and minimize the procedure-related risks is essential. Prophylactic antibiotics should be given to any woman with a structural heart defect to reduce the risk of bacterial endocarditis. Depending on the severity of the condition, other forms of monitoring may be appropriate during labour, including oxygen saturation and continuous arterial blood pressure monitoring.

Assuming normal progress in labour, the second stage may deliberately be kept short, with an elective forceps or ventouse delivery if normal delivery does not occur readily. This reduces maternal effort and the requirement for increased cardiac output. Caesarean section should only be performed in situations where the maternal condition is considered too unstable to tolerate the physiological demands of labour. Caesarean delivery is associated with an increased risk of haemorrhage, thrombosis and infection, conditions that are likely to be much less well tolerated in women with cardiac disease. Postpartum haemorrhage in particular can lead to major cardiovascular instability. Ergometrine may be associated with intense vasoconstriction, hypertension and heart failure, and therefore active management of the third stage is usually with Syntocinon™ (synthetic oxytocin) alone. Syntocinon is a vasodilator and therefore should be given slowly to patients with significant heart disease, with low-dose infusions preferable. High-level maternal surveillance is required until the main haemodynamic changes following delivery have passed.

Management of labour in women with heart disease

- Avoid induction of labour if possible.
- Use prophylactic antibiotics.
- Ensure fluid balance.
- Avoid the supine position.
- Discuss regional/epidural anaesthesia/analgesia with senior anaesthetist.
- Keep the second stage short.
- Use Syntocinon judiciously.

Treatment of heart failure in pregnancy

The development of heart failure in pregnancy is dangerous, but the principles of treatment are the same as in the non-pregnant individual. The woman should be admitted and the diagnosis confirmed by clinical examination for signs of heart failure and by echocardiography confirming ventricular dysfunction. Drug therapy may include diuretics, vasodilators and digoxin. Oxygen and morphine may also be required. Arrhythmias also require urgent correction and drug therapy; for example, adenosine for supraventricular tachycardias. In all cases, assessment of fetal wellbeing is essential and should include fetal ultrasound to assess fetal growth and regular cardiotocography (CTG). If there is evidence of fetal compromise, premature delivery may be considered. Similarly, in cases of intractable cardiac failure, the risks to the mother of continuing the pregnancy and the risks to the fetus of premature delivery must be carefully balanced.

Risk factors for the development of heart failure in pregnancy

- Respiratory or urinary infections.
- Anaemia.
- Obesity.
- Corticosteroids.
- Tocolytics.
- Multiple gestation.
- Hypertension.
- Arrhythmias.
- Pain-related stress.
- Fluid overload.

Specific conditions

Ischaemic heart disease

Most pregnant women with myocardial infarction (MI) are >40 years with <1% are <35 years. The risk of MI during pregnancy is estimated at 1 in 10–15,000, and the peak incidence is in the third trimester, in parous women older than 35 years. The underlying pathology is frequently not atherosclerotic and coronary artery dissection is the primary cause in the postpartum period. Before the current practice of percutaneous transluminal coronary angioplasty (PTCA), mortality was reported as 20–37% for the mother and 17% for the fetus. PTCA is now considered acceptable but should still be only used when absolutely necessary, avoiding the time when the fetus is most susceptible to radiation (8–15 weeks). There is little experience with thrombolytic therapy in pregnancy, and although not apparently teratogenic, there are risks of fetal and maternal haemorrhage. The diagnosis of MI in pregnant women is often missed, and prompt diagnosis and therapy are necessary to reduce the high associated maternal and perinatal mortality.

Mitral and aortic stenosis

Obstructive lesions of the left heart are well-recognized risk factors for maternal morbidity and mortality, as they result in an inability to increase cardiac output to meet the demands of pregnancy. Aortic stenosis (AS) is usually congenital and mitral stenosis usually rheumatic in origin. For those with known mitral stenosis, 40% experience worsening symptoms in the pregnancy, with the average time of onset of pulmonary oedema at 30 weeks. The aim of treatment is to reduce the heart rate, achieved through bed rest, oxygen, beta-blockade and diuretic therapy. Balloon mitral valvotomy is the treatment of choice after delivery, but can be considered in pregnancy depending on the clinical condition and gestation. Maternal mortality is reported at 2% and the risk of an adverse fetal outcome is directly related to the severity of mitral stenosis. Pregnancy is usually well tolerated in women with isolated and mild and moderate AS, with normal exercise capacity and good ventricular function. However, the risk of maternal death in those with severe AS is reported as 17%, with fetal mortality of 30%. As with mitral stenosis, bed rest and medical treatment aims to reduce the heart rate to allow time for ventricular filling. If the woman's condition deteriorates before delivery is feasible, surgical intervention such as balloon or surgical aortic valvotomy can be considered, although there is less experience and success than with mitral stenosis.

Marfan syndrome

Marfan syndrome is an autosomal dominant connective tissue abnormality that may lead to mitral valve prolapse and aortic regurgitation, aortic root dilatation and aortic rupture or dissection. Pregnancy increases the risk of aortic rupture or dissection and has been associated with maternal mortality of up to 50% where there is marked aortic root dilatation. Echocardiography is the principal investigation, as it is able to determine the size of the aortic root, and should be performed serially throughout pregnancy, especially in women who enter pregnancy with an aortic root that is already dilated (>4 cm). Women with an aortic root <4 cm should be reassured that their risks are lower, and the risk of an adverse cardiac event is around 1%. A number of obstetric complications have also been described in women with Marfan syndrome: early pregnancy loss, preterm labour, cervical weakness, uterine inversion and postpartum haemorrhage.

Pulmonary hypertension

PH is characterized by an increase in the pulmonary vascular resistance resulting in an increased workload placed on the right side of the heart. The main symptoms are fatigue, breathlessness and syncope, and clinical signs are those of right heart failure. A median survival of <3 years from diagnosis has been reported. Specific treatments shown to improve symptoms and survival include endothelin blockers, such as bosentan, and phosphodiesterase inhibitors such as sildenafil.

In women with PH, pregnancy is associated with a high risk of maternal death. The demands of increasing blood volume and cardiac output may not be met by an already compromised right ventricle, and any decline in cardiac performance in pregnancy represents a life-threatening event. Women may deteriorate early (second trimester) or in the immediate postpartum period.

Close monitoring by a multidisciplinary team is crucial as the mortality of the condition remains high at 30–50%. Women with PH should be advised about the very significant risks of pregnancy. In women who choose to continue their pregnancy, targeted pulmonary vascular therapy is an option, with timely admission to hospital and delivery according to the progress of the woman and condition of the fetus.

Respiratory disease

Respiratory infection

The recent outbreaks of H1N1 and influenza A have increased the number of maternal deaths attributed to respiratory infection. According to the most recent report from the UK Confidential Enquiries into Maternal Deaths and Morbidity (2009–12), 1 in 11 pregnant women who died had influenza, and pregnancy should be considered a significant risk factor for the development of severe respiratory disease attributable to viral infection. All women in the UK are encouraged to have a seasonal flu vaccine in pregnancy and the importance of this in preventing serious morbidity and mortality cannot be over emphasized. Viral pneumonia follows a more complicated course in pregnancy and women often decompensate more quickly.

Prompt treatment and early involvement of respiratory and infectious disease specialists in addition to the intensive care is essential. Bacterial pneumonia should be treated using the same antibiotics as outside, with penicillin or cephalosporins usually the first choice, and erythromycin used if atypical organisms are suspected.

Pneumonia: warning signs

- Respiratory rate >30/minute.
- Hypoxaemia; pO_2 <7.9 kPa on room air.
- Acidosis; pH <7.3.
- Hypotension.
- Disseminated intravascular coagulation.
- Elevated blood urea.
- Evidence of multiple organ failure.

Asthma

The worldwide prevalence of asthma is increasing with 2–4% of pregnant women affected. Asthma is not consistently affected by pregnancy. However, prospective studies show that exacerbations of asthma are more likely to occur in women with severe asthma than mild asthma and that most episodes occur between 24 and 36 weeks of pregnancy.

There is evidence that proactive management of asthma-related symptoms and attacks during pregnancy decreases maternal and fetal morbidity. Asthma severity and suboptimal control are associated with adverse pregnancy outcomes. The effects of asthma on the fetus are still controversial and while systematic reviews report FGR is more common in women with symptomatic asthma than in non-asthmatic women, the historic increased risk of preterm delivery is not borne out by prospective studies. Prolonged maternal hypoxia can lead to FGR and ultimately to fetal brain injury. An association between hypertension and asthma has also been suggested, and although there is an increase in gestational hypertension, asthma does not seem to be a risk factor for pre-eclampsia. Labour and delivery are not usually affected by asthma and attacks are uncommon in labour. Parenteral steroid cover may be needed for those who are on regular steroids, regular medications should be continued throughout labour and bronchoconstrictors such as ergometrine or prostaglandin F2α should be avoided in women with severe asthma. Adequate hydration is important in labour, and regional anaesthesia is favoured over general to decrease the risk of bronchospasm, provide adequate pain relief and to reduce oxygen consumption and minute ventilation. The inheritance risk of asthma for the fetus ranges from 6% to 30%. Postpartum, there is no increased risk of exacerbations and those whose asthma deteriorated during pregnancy have usually returned to prepregnancy levels by 3 months after birth.

Features of severe life-threatening asthma

- Peak expiratory flow rate <35% of predicted.
- pO_2 <8 kPa.
- pCO_2 >4.6 kPa.
- Silent chest.
- Cyanosis.
- Bradycardia.
- Arrhythmia.
- Hypotension.
- Exhaustion.
- Confusion.

Many women with asthma are concerned about the effect of drugs on the fetus, and this can lead to inappropriate cessation of treatment in early pregnancy. However, it is safer to take asthma drugs in pregnancy than to leave asthma uncontrolled. Inhaled beta-sympathomimetics are safe, as is theophylline, although its metabolism is altered and drug levels need to be monitored. Long-acting β2 agonists like salmetrerol do not cause fetal malformation or FGR in prospective studies, and there is limited systemic absorption. Inhaled corticosteroids have been shown to be safe with no association with fetal malformations or perinatal morbidity in large studies and reviews. Oral corticosteroid use in the first trimester has been associated with an increased risk of fetal cleft lip or palate in epidemiological studies, but the increase in risk is small and not confirmed in other work. Data are reassuring on the safety of the leukotriene antagonist montelukast during pregnancy.

Management of asthma in pregnancy

- Pregnancy is a time to improve asthma care.
- Encourage smoking cessation.
- Ensure patient education regarding condition and adequate use of medications.
- Ensure optimal control and response to therapy throughout pregnancy.
- Manage exacerbations aggressively and avoid delays in treatment.
- Manage acute attacks as in non-pregnant individual.
- Offer a multidisciplinary team approach.

Cystic fibrosis

Cystic fibrosis (CF) is an inherited autosomal recessive condition, with a carrier frequency of around 1 in 25 in the general population. The abnormal gene controls the movement of salt in the body, and as a result the internal organs become clogged with thick mucus, leading to infections and chronic inflammation, particularly affecting the lungs, gut and pancreas. Life expectancy is increasing, with over half the current CF population expected to live over 35 years. Therefore, more women are surviving to an age at which pregnancy is possible, and the estimates of pregnancy rates among women with CF range from 5% to 10%.

Women with a higher FEV_1 (forced expiratory volume in 1 second) and higher body weight have been shown to be more likely to become pregnant. The live birth rate ranges from 70% to 90%, and the rate of spontaneous miscarriage is no different to the general population. However, the prematurity rate is around 25%, due to iatrogenic delivery where maternal health deteriorates, as well as a higher rate of spontaneous preterm labour. Maternal prognosis is poor if there is PH, infection with *Burkholderia cepacia*, if FEV_1 is <50% predicted or if there is chronic hypoxia (pO_2 <7.3 kPa). While pregnancy does not significantly shorten survival in women with CF, the long-term prognosis still needs consideration, as around 20% of mothers will not live for 10 years after delivery and 40% of those with poor lung function at the start of pregnancy will die in this time period.

Pregnant women with CF should be jointly managed between the obstetrician and a respiratory physician with expertise in CF, ideally in a specialist centre. Most women will have a daily physiotherapy regime and require prolonged antibiotic therapy and hospital admission during infective exacerbations. Close attention should be paid to maternal nutritional status and weight gain during pregnancy, with screening for GDM also indicated. Fetal growth and wellbeing should be monitored by serial ultrasound scans, as there is an association with FGR. It is also important to check the CF carrier status of the woman's partner, and the couple should be offered genetic counselling regarding the risks of the fetus having CF or being a carrier. Ideally, a vaginal delivery should be the aim in the absence of any other obstetric indications for caesarean section.

Sarcoidosis

Sarcoid is a non-caseating granulomatosis that may affect any organ, but principally affects the lung and skin. Complications include severe progressive lung problems with pulmonary fibrosis, hypoxaemia and PH, and these features are associated with a poor prognosis. Treatment is with corticosteroids. Sarcoidosis usually improves and is uncommonly diagnosed in pregnancy, although erythema

nodosum, which may occur in both normal pregnancy and in sarcoidosis, may cause diagnostic confusion. Pregnancy does not influence the long-term natural history of sarcoidosis.

Neurological disorders

Epilepsy

Approximately 30% of those with epilepsy are women in their childbearing years, which means 1 in 200–250 pregnancies occur in women with a history of epilepsy. Pregnancy has no consistent effect on epilepsy: some women will have an increased frequency of fits, others a decrease and some no difference. Nonetheless, there is a 10-fold increase in mortality among pregnant women with epilepsy, and 1 in 20 indirect maternal deaths occur in women with epilepsy. The principles of epilepsy management are that while the risks to pregnancy from seizures outweigh those from anticonvulsant medication, seizures should still be controlled with the minimum possible dose of the optimal drug.

Prepregnancy counselling in epilepsy

- Alter medication according to seizure frequency.
- Reduce to monotherapy where possible.
- Stress importance of compliance with medication.
- Preconceptional folic acid 5 mg.
- Explain risk of congenital malformation.
- Explain risk from recurrent seizures.

The principal concern related to epilepsy in pregnancy is the increased risk of congenital abnormality caused by anticonvulsant medications. All of these drugs are associated with a 2–3-fold increased risk of fetal abnormality (5–6%) compared with unexposed epileptic mothers. Pregnant women with epilepsy who do not take antiepilepsy drugs (AEDs) do not expose their offspring to an increased risk of congenital abnormalities. Polytherapy increases the risk of major congenital abnormality by about 3% for each additional AED. The major fetal abnormalities associated with anticonvulsant drugs (including sodium valproate, carbamazepine, phenytoin, phenobarbitone) are neural tube defects, facial clefts and cardiac defects. Many of these abnormalities are detectable by ultrasound and therefore all women should be offered detailed anomaly scanning. In addition, each drug is associated with a specific syndrome that includes developmental delay, nail hypoplasia, growth restriction and midface abnormalities. In the case of valproate, the likelihood of these effects is dose dependent (>1,000 mg/day) and it should be avoided in pregnant women, except when epilepsy cannot be controlled with other AEDs. Despite the risks of continuing anticonvulsants in pregnancy, failure to do so may lead to an increased frequency of epileptic seizures that may result in both maternal and fetal hypoxia. Therefore, women on multiple drug therapy should, wherever possible, be converted to monotherapy before pregnancy, and all epileptic women should be advised to start taking a 5 mg daily folic acid supplement prior to conception to reduce the risk of neural tube defects. In women who have been free of seizures for 2 years, consideration may be given prepregnancy to discontinuing medication.

Many factors contribute to altered drug metabolism in pregnancy and result in a fall in anticonvulsant drug levels. The reasons for increased fit frequency in pregnancy therefore include the effect of pregnancy on the metabolism of anticonvulsant drugs, as well as sleep deprivation or stress and poor compliance with medication. Monitoring of drug levels in pregnancy is difficult. An increase in dosage to combat the anticipated fall may lead to an increased fetal risk. In the majority of cases, provided there is no increase in frequency of seizures, the prenatal drug dosage can be continued. However, lamotrigine drug levels fall rapidly in pregnancy and in many cases this is associated with increased seizure activity, necessitating an increased dose. An increase in seizure frequency or a recurrence of seizures, especially in the context of subtherapeutic drug levels, should prompt an increase in dosage of all AEDs.

Delivery mode and timing is largely unaltered by epilepsy, unless there has been accelerated seizure frequency in pregnancy, and anticonvulsant medication should be continued during labour. Breastfeeding should be encouraged, although feeding is best avoided for a few hours after taking medication.

Information on safe handling of the neonate should be given to all epileptic mothers.

Causes of seizures in pregnancy

- Epilepsy.
- Eclampsia.
- Encephalitis or meningitis.
- Space-occupying lesions (e.g. tumour, tuberculoma).
- Cerebral vascular accident.
- Cerebral malaria or toxoplasmosis.
- Thrombotic thrombocytopaenic purpura.
- Drug and alcohol withdrawal.
- Toxic overdose.
- Metabolic abnormalities (e.g. hypoglycaemia).

Multiple sclerosis

Multiple sclerosis (MS) is a relapsing and remitting disease that causes disability through demyelination of nerves, leading to weakness, lack of coordination, numbness in the hands or feet, blurred vision, tremor, spasticity and voiding dysfunction. Like most autoimmune diseases, more women than men are affected, and two-thirds of MS patients are women. One in 1,000 pregnancies is estimated to occur in a woman with MS, and the onset of MS during pregnancy is unusual, with optic neuritis reported as the predominant symptom, usually postpartum. Pregnant women with MS are no more likely to experience complications in their pregnancy than those unaffected, nor are there increased risks of preterm delivery, FGR or congenital malformation. The course of MS during pregnancy changes – a lower relapse rate has been shown, while the rate of relapse rises significantly during the first 3 months postpartum. Interestingly, pregnancy after MS onset may be associated with a lower risk of progression of the condition. Certainly, pregnancy has no adverse effect on the progression of long-term disability.

Over the last 15 years the number of disease-modifying drugs (DMDs) that improve the long-term outcome of women with MS has increased. Given this relatively short time, experience of DMDs for MS has not yet built up to a level that allows reassuring prescribing. It is recommended that first-line treatments including glatiramer, interferon-beta, and dimethyl fumarate are stopped at conception. Steroids or intravenous immunoglobulin can be given to treat an acute relapse and should be used where clinically indicated. Delivery is not more complicated in MS patients and the mode of delivery should be decided using the usual obstetric criteria. Regional anaesthesia is not contraindicated and no effect on the subsequent risk of relapse has been found.

Migraine

Migraine is influenced by cyclical changes in the sex hormones, and attacks often occur during the menstrual period, attributed to a fall in oestrogen levels. Migraine often improves in pregnancy, with worsening of headaches occurring infrequently. Throughout pregnancy around 20% of pregnant women will experience migraine-like headaches, many of whom do not get migraines outwith pregnancy. Obstetric complications are not increased in migraine sufferers. Migraine during pregnancy should be treated with analgesics, antiemetics and, where possible, avoidance of factors that trigger the attack. Low-dose aspirin or beta-blockers may be used to prevent attacks.

Bell's palsy

The incidence of Bell's palsy is increased 10-fold during the third trimester of pregnancy. The outcome is generally good and complete recovery is the norm if the time of onset is within 2 weeks of delivery. The role of corticosteroids and antivirals is controversial but both can be used in pregnancy and they may hasten recovery if given with 24 hours of the onset of symptoms.

Haematological abnormalities

Haemoglobinopathies

Clinically significant variants of haemoglobin

- Sickle cell trait (HbAS).
- Sickle cell disease (HbSS).
- Sickle cell/haemoglobin C disease (HbSC).
- Sickle cell/beta thalassaemia.

Sickle cell anaemia

Sickle cell disease (SCD) is an autosomally inherited genetic condition, where abnormal haemoglobin (HbS) contains beta-globin chains with an amino acid substitution that results in it precipitating when in its reduced state. The red blood cells become sickle shaped and occlude small blood vessels. There is severe anaemia, chronic hyperbilirubinaemia, a predisposition to infection, vaso-occlusive complications including the acute chest syndrome, and CKD. PH is found in 30% of patients and is associated with a high mortality rate.

Advances in treatment of SCD have resulted in the average lifespan in the western world extending past 50 years, which means many more women with the condition are now becoming pregnant. Like other medical disorders, ideal management begins with prepregnancy optimization of maternal health and education about the risks in pregnancy. High-dose folate supplements (5 mg daily) are recommended and the majority of women are also managed from early pregnancy on low-dose aspirin (75 mg daily). Pregnancy is associated with an increased incidence of sickle cell crises that may result in episodes of severe pain, typically affecting the bones or chest. The acute chest syndrome may result from an initial uncomplicated crisis and is responsible for around 25% of all deaths in SCD. Crises in pregnancy may be precipitated by hypoxia, stress, infection and haemorrhage. Mothers are also at increased risk of miscarriage, pre-eclampsia, FGR and premature labour, with three times the risk of eclampsia compared to women without SCD. Thromboembolic events including cerebral vein thrombosis and deep venous thrombosis are implicated in the higher rates of maternal deaths reported in SCD.

Although sickle-cell haemoglobin C disease may cause only mild degrees of anaemia, it is associated with very severe crises that occur more often in pregnancy. In this condition, women are not as anaemic as those with SS disease and the severity of crises may be underestimated.

Sickle cell carriers have a 1:4 risk of having a baby with SCD if their partner also has sickle cell trait. Carriers are usually fit and well, but are at increased risk of urinary tract infection, and rarely suffer from crises.

Management of sickle cell crisis in pregnancy

- Prompt treatment.
- Adequate hydration.
- Oxygen.
- Analgesia.
- Screen for infection (urinary, respiratory).
- Antibiotics.
- Blood transfusion (leucocyte depleted and phenotype specific).
- Exchange transfusion.
- Prophylaxis against thrombosis (heparin).
- Fetal monitoring.

Thalassaemia

The thalassaemia syndromes are the commonest genetic blood disorders. The defect is a reduced production of normal haemoglobin and the syndromes are divided into alpha and beta types, depending on which globin chain is affected. In alpha-thalassaemia minor, there is a deletion of one of the two normal alpha genes required for haemoglobin production. Although the affected individual is chronically anaemic, this condition rarely produces obstetric complications except in cases of severe blood loss. It is important to screen the woman's partner for thalassaemia and to consider prenatal diagnosis; if he is also affected, there is a 1:4 chance of the fetus having alpha-thalassaemia major, which is lethal.

The beta-thalassaemias result from defects in the normal production of the beta chains. Beta-thalassaemia minor/trait is more commonly found in people from the East Mediterranean, but may also occur sporadically in other communities. Consequently, all pregnant women should be offered electrophoresis as part of the antenatal screening process. Beta-thalassaemia minor is not a problem antenatally, although women tend to be mildly anaemic and have a low mean corpuscular volume (MCV). Iron and folate supplements should be given and partners should also be screened. However, if both partners have beta-thalassaemia minor, there is a 1:4 chance the fetus could have beta-thalassaemia major, which is associated with profound anaemia in postnatal life.

Thrombocytopaenia

Thrombocytopaenia is defined as a platelet count $<150 \times 10^9/l$. Incidental or gestational thrombocytopaenia is common and is found in 7–8% of pregnant women. A modest drop in the platelet count to $100–150 \times 10^9/l$ is only very rarely associated with poor pregnancy outcomes. Bleeding is rarely a complication unless the count is $<50 \times 10^9/l$. However, the diagnosis of gestational thrombocytopaenia is a diagnosis of exclusion and can only be made when autoimmune and other causes have been excluded. It usually occurs in late pregnancy, with no prior history of thrombocytopaenia outside pregnancy and a normal platelet count recorded at the start of pregnancy. No intervention is required other than monitoring of the platelet count during and after pregnancy. There is no association with fetal thrombocytopaenia and spontaneous resolution occurs after delivery.

Causes of thrombocytopaenia in pregnancy

- Idiopathic:
  - increased consumption or destruction;
  - autoimmune;
  - antiphospholipid syndrome;
  - pre-eclampsia;
  - HELLP syndrome;
  - disseminated intravascular coagulation;
  - thrombotic thrombocytopaenic purpura;
  - hypersplenism.
- Decreased production:
  - sepsis;
  - HIV infection;
  - malignant marrow infiltration.

Autoimmune thrombocytopaenia

In immune thrombocytopaenic purpura (ITP), autoantibodies are produced against platelet surface antigens, leading to platelet destruction by the reticuloendothelial system. The incidence in pregnancy is around 1 in 5,000. The maternal platelet count may fall at any stage of pregnancy and can reach levels of $<50 \times 10^9/l$. Maternal haemorrhage at delivery is unlikely if the platelet count is $>50 \times 10^9/l$, and spontaneous bleeding during pregnancy very unlikely if the platelet count is >20 × 10⁹/l. There is a 5–10% chance of associated fetal thrombocytopaenia (<50 × 10⁹/l), which cannot be predicted using maternal counts or antibody tests.

Management in pregnancy should include serial monitoring of platelet count. If the count falls below 50 × 10⁹/l approaching 37 weeks' gestation, treatment should be considered. Corticosteroids (starting dose 40–60 mg prednisolone) act by suppressing platelet autoantibodies; however, high doses are often required to improve the platelet count, and long-term use is associated with weight gain, hypertension and diabetes. Corticosteroids also take 2–3 weeks to have a significant effect. Although more expensive, the use of intravenous immunoglobulin G (IgG) has been a major advance in the treatment of autoimmune thrombocytopaenia. IgG is the preferred option where a rapid platelet increase is required close to term, if the duration of treatment is likely to be prolonged or if unacceptably high maintenance doses of prednisolone are required. Vaginal delivery should be facilitated and regional anaesthesia avoided if the platelet count is <80 × 10⁹/l. Fetal blood sampling in labour and instrumental delivery by ventouse are best avoided because of the risk of fetal thrombocytopaenia. A cord blood sample must be collected for platelet counting, but the nadir of the neonatal platelet count occurs 2–5 days after delivery.

Bleeding disorders

Bleeding disorders during pregnancy and delivery

- Inherited:
  - vascular abnormalities;
  - platelet disorders;
  - coagulation disorders.
- Acquired:
  - thrombocytopaenia;
  - disseminated intravascular coagulation;
  - acquired coagulation disorders;
  - marrow disorders.

Inherited coagulation disorders

Von Willebrand disease, carriers of haemophilia A and B and factor XI deficiency account for over 90% of all women with inherited bleeding disorders.

Haemophilia A (FVIII deficiency) and haemophilia B (FIX deficiency) are X-linked defects with a prevalence of 1 in 10,000 and 1 in 100,000 respectively in the population. Carriers of haemophilia A or B usually have clotting factor activity about 50% of normal, but while factor VIIIC levels increase in pregnancy, factor IXC levels increase only slightly. Factor XI deficiency is a rare autosomal dominant bleeding disorder, where the bleeding risk does not relate to the severity of the factor deficiency. FXI levels do not rise significantly during pregnancy. Von Willebrand disease is the most common inherited bleeding disorder, with an estimated prevalence of 1%. It results from either a qualitative or quantitative defect in von Willebrand factor (VWF). The inheritance of von Willebrand disease is usually autosomal dominant and while increases in factor VIIIC and VWF antigen activity usually occur during normal pregnancy, they cannot be relied on to buffer the effects of the disease, particularly in severe cases.

Where possible, carriers of haemophilia and women with von Willebrand disease should be identified and counselled prior to pregnancy. Baseline coagulation factor assays should be performed as soon as pregnancy is confirmed and repeated in the third trimester. In haemophilia carriers, tests to confirm fetal sex should be offered, either by ultrasound or through sampling fetal deoxyribonucleic acid (DNA) in maternal blood, as this influences the use of interventions in labour.

Women with bleeding disorders are at significant risk of primary and secondary postpartum haemorrhage, and this risk can be minimized by appropriate prophylactic treatment.

Planning for delivery requires multidisciplinary input including a consultant haematologist, and is guided by the third trimester clotting factor levels, taking into account the woman's bleeding tendency. Women deemed to be at significant risk should have a care plan written that may include the use of factor concentrate, tranexamic acid or desmopressin (DDAVP) to cover labour and delivery. DDAVP can be administered intravenously to increase factors VIII and VWF in those known to be responders prepregnancy, and is most effective in haemophilia A carriers and type 1 von Willebrand disease.

In haemophilia carriers, epidurals may be permitted if the clotting factor is considered to be satisfactory. Invasive fetal monitoring, ventouse and rotational forceps should be avoided if there is a possibility that the fetus may be affected, and cord blood samples collected for coagulation tests.

Gastroenterology disorders

Peptic ulcer disease

Peptic ulceration is less common in pregnancy and pre-existing ulceration tends to improve, probably due to altered oestrogen levels and the improved maternal diet in pregnancy. Complications such as haemorrhage or perforation are rare. Treatment with antacids and common antiulcer medication (e.g. ranitidine, omeprazole) is safe. Pregnancy is not a contraindication to endoscopy.

Coeliac disease

Coeliac disease is a gluten-sensitive enteropathy with a prevalence of around 0.3–1% in the general population. It has been estimated that up to 1 in 70 pregnant women are affected by coeliac disease, but that many are undiagnosed. Untreated coeliac disease is associated with high rates of spontaneous miscarriage and other adverse pregnancy outcomes such as FGR. Once a gluten-free diet is established, women with coeliac disease can expect a healthy pregnancy outcome. Awareness that they are predisposed to other autoimmune diseases is the only other consideration.

Inflammatory bowel disease

The majority of patients with inflammatory bowel disease (IBD), which includes ulcerative colitis and Crohn's disease, are diagnosed during their reproductive years (incidence 3 per 1,000 pregnancies). Women with IBD have reduced fertility rates compared with the general population. Pregnancy does not usually alter the course of IBD, but new-onset IBD, uncontrolled disease activity at conception and previous bowel resection increase the risk of an adverse pregnancy outcome. Similarly, disease flare during pregnancy is more likely if the disease is active at the time of conception. Pregnant women with either ulcerative colitis or Crohn's disease have been shown to have similar rates of disease exacerbation, although flares in the first trimester and postpartum are more common in disease.

Supplementation with high-dose folic acid (5 mg daily) is recommended and supplementation with other vitamins is indicated according to measured deficiencies. Women with IBD have an increased rate of delivery by caesarean section, preterm labour and small for gestational age offspring. Caesarean section is indicated for the usual obstetric indications, and also if there is active perianal disease in Crohn's and usually if there is an ileoanal pouch.

The use of medication during conception and pregnancy is a cause of concern for many patients with IBD. Methotrexate is contraindicated, but the majority of other medications used to induce or maintain remission, including 5-aminosalicylates, azothiaprine, ciclosporin and corticosteroids, are low risk. Experience with anti-inflammatory monoclonal antibodies is growing and increasing evidence suggests agents like infliximab are low risk in the first two trimesters of pregnancy. A relapse of IBD in pregnancy may be treated with steroid tablets, intramuscular injection or enemas.

Pancreatitis

Pancreatitis is uncommon in pregnancy. The clinical presentation combines nausea and vomiting with severe epigastric pain, and attacks usually occur in the third trimester of pregnancy. The commonest cause of pancreatitis in pregnancy is gallstones, followed by alcohol, with hypertriglyceridemia and hyperparathyroidism much rarer causes. Management is supportive, with a small percentage of women developing chemical peritonitis associated with cardiac, renal and gastrointestinal complications, necessitating intensive care.

Liver disease

Viral hepatitis

Viral hepatitis is the commonest cause of jaundice in pregnancy worldwide. Acute viral hepatitis in the first trimester of pregnancy is associated with a higher rate of spontaneous miscarriage. The clinical features of hepatitis are no different to the non-pregnant patient, with the exception of hepatitis E infection and herpes simplex hepatitis. Hepatitis E is more likely to lead to fulminant hepatic failure in pregnancy, and is more common in primagravida and in the third trimester. There is also a significant association with obstetric complications such as preterm delivery, FGR and stillbirth. In underdeveloped countries, 20% of women infected in the third trimester die of fulminant hepatitis. Herpes simplex hepatitis is rare. While complications are common and associated perinatal mortality high, antiviral agents such as aciclovir have dramatically improved outcomes.

The incidence of hepatitis A in pregnancy is around 1 in 1,000 and fetal transmission is extremely rare. Acute hepatitis B infection occurs in 1–2 per 1,000 pregnancies and 1.5% of pregnant women are chronic carriers. There is no evidence that hepatitis B is any more common in pregnancy. The prevalence of hepatitis C in pregnant women is estimated at 1–2%. Hepatitis C infection is also associated with several adverse pregnancy outcomes, such as preterm rupture of membranes and GDM, as well as adverse neonatal outcomes, including low birthweight and neonatal unit admission (*Table 10.5* and see Chapter 11, Perinatal infections).

Autoimmune hepatitis

Autoimmune hepatitis (chronic active hepatitis) is characterized by progressive hepatic parenchymal destruction, eventually leading to cirrhosis. It is diagnosed on liver biopsy and in association with antismooth muscle antibodies and antinuclear antibodies. Its course in pregnancy is variable, with flares reported throughout gestation and postpartum. High fetal loss rates (around 20%) have been reported when autoimmune hepatitis is active during pregnancy. Immunosuppressive therapy should be continued during pregnancy according to disease activity.

Gallstones

The prevalence of gallstones in pregnancy is around 19% in multiparous women and 8% in nulliparous women. However, acute cholecystitis is much less common, occurring in around 0.1% of pregnant women. The aetiology of increased biliary sludge and gallstones in pregnancy is multifactorial. Increased oestrogen levels lead to increased cholesterol secretion and supersaturation of bile, and increased progesterone levels cause a decrease in small intestinal motility. Conservative medical management is recommended initially, especially during the first and third trimesters, in which surgical intervention may confer a risk of miscarriage or premature labour, respectively. Medical management involves intravenous fluids, correction of electrolytes, bowel rest, pain management and broad-spectrum antibiotics. However, relapse rates (40–90%) are high during pregnancy and surgical intervention may be warranted, preferentially performed (open or laparoscopic cholecystectomy) in the second trimester.

Primary biliary cirrhosis

Primary biliary cirrhosis (PBC) is an autoimmune disorder characterized by progressive destruction

Table 10.5 Viral hepatitis in pregnancy

	Hepatitis A	Hepatitis B	Hepatitis C	Hepatitis D ('delta')	Hepatitis E	Hepatitis G
Transmission	Faecal–oral	Parenteral Mucosal Sexual	Parenteral Mucosal Sexual	Parenteral	Faecal–oral	Parenteral
Chronic disease	None	2–6% adults	80%	70–80%	None	Rare
Fetal transmission	Rare	20–30%	5–10%	Cases reported	No cases reported	No cases reported
Vaccination	Safe in pregnancy	Safe in pregnancy	None available	Safe in pregnancy	None available	None available

of intrahepatic bile ducts, which ultimately leads to portal hypertension and hepatic failure. PBC is usually associated with reduced fertility and repeated pregnancy loss, with worsening liver function historically reported in pregnancy. More recent series suggest that women maintained on ursodeoxycholic acid (UDCA) tolerate pregnancy well, with no deterioration in liver function, but a risk of flare postpartum is reported.

Cirrhosis

Cirrhosis is very rare in pregnancy, as it is usually a complication of older people and because it leads to hormonal and metabolic alterations that are associated with anovulation. Women with a diagnosis of cirrhosis are usually advised to avoid pregnancy. However, cases have been reported, usually in association with portal hypertension. Bleeding from oesophageal varices has been reported in 25% of pregnant women with cirrhosis, and therefore all pregnant women with cirrhosis should be screened using endoscopy from the second trimester. Other complications include hepatic failure, encephalopathy, jaundice and malnutrition.

Connective tissue disease

Systemic lupus erythematosus

Systemic lupus erythematosus (SLE) is a chronic autoimmune inflammatory disease. SLE affects approximately 1 in 1000 people in the UK. It is six times more common in women, particularly of black Caribbean ethnicity. It may cause disease in any organ system, but principally it affects the joints (90%), skin (80%), lungs, nervous system, kidneys and heart. SLE may be diagnosed prenatally or may be suspected for the first time during pregnancy or postpartum, usually as a result of complications. The diagnosis is suggested by the finding of a positive assay for antinuclear antibodies (ANAs), while the presence of antibodies to double-stranded DNA is the most specific for SLE. If 4 of the 11 criteria in the American College of Rheumatology (ACR) classification system for SLE are present serially or simultaneously, a person is said to have SLE.

ACR criteria for classification of SLE

- Malar rash.
- Discoid rash.
- Photosensitivity.
- Oral ulcers.
- Non-erosive arthritis.
- Pleuritis or pericarditis.
- Renal disorder.
- Neurological disorder.
- Haematological disorder.
- Immunological disorder.
- Positive ANA.

SLE is characterized by periods of disease activity, flares and remissions. Pregnancy increases the risk of flares, but these also become more difficult to diagnose accurately due to coincident pregnancy symptoms. Flares are more common in the late second and third trimester, and are no more severe than in non-pregnancy. Active disease at the time of conception or new onset SLE in pregnancy both increase the chance of a flare. SLE is associated with significant risks of miscarriage, fetal death, pre-eclampsia, preterm delivery and FGR. Women with lupus nephritis are at greatest risk of these adverse outcomes, although pregnancy does not seem to alter renal function in the long term. Pregnancy outcome is also adversely affected by pre-existing hypertension and the presence of antiphospholipid antibodies.

Differentiation of SLE flare from pre-eclampsia

Pre-eclampsia and SLE
- Hypertension.
- Proteinuria.
- Thrombocytopaenia.
- Renal impairment.

SLE
- Rising anti-DNA titre.
- Fall in complement levels.
- No increase in serum uric acid.
- No abnormal liver function.

The term antiphospholipid syndrome (APS) is used to describe the association of anticardiolipin antibodies (aCL) and/or lupus anticoagulant (LA), with the typical clinical features of arterial or venous thrombosis, fetal loss after 10 weeks' gestation, three or more miscarriages at less than 10 weeks' gestation or delivery before 34 weeks' gestation due to FGR or pre-eclampsia. Importantly, a diagnosis of APS requires that the positive antibody titres must be present on two occasions, 3 months apart. APS may be primary or found in association with SLE.

Classification criteria for APS

Clinical

- Thrombosis:
  - venous;
  - arterial.
- Pregnancy morbidity:
  - fetal death >10 weeks;
  - preterm birth <35 weeks due to severe pre-eclampsia or growth restriction;
  - 3 or more unexplained miscarriages <10 weeks.

Laboratory

- aCL IgG and/or IgM:
  - medium/high titre;
  - 2 occasions, 8 weeks apart.
- LA:
  - 2 occasions, 8 weeks apart.

Due to these significant risks, pregnant women with SLE and APS require intensive monitoring for both maternal and fetal indications and should be prescribed low-dose aspirin to start by 12 weeks' gestation. The mother should book early to multidisciplinary care and be seen frequently. Baseline renal studies, including a 24-hour urine collection for protein, should be performed. Blood pressure should be monitored closely because of the increased risk of pre-eclampsia. Serial ultrasonography is performed to assess fetal growth, umbilical artery Doppler and liquor volume. If antenatal treatment is required for SLE, steroids, azathioprine, sulfasalazine and hydroxychloroquine may be given safely. NSAIDs can be given until week 32

of pregnancy. In women with APS who have suffered repeated pregnancy loss or severe obstetric complications, the combined use of low-dose aspirin and low-molecular-weight heparin has been shown to reduce the pregnancy loss rate.

Finally, 30% of mothers with SLE also have anti-Ro/La antibodies, which cross the placenta and can cause the clinical syndromes neonatal lupus and congenital heart block. The risk of neonatal lupus is around 5%, rising to 25% if a previous child was affected. It manifests as cutaneous lesions 2–3 weeks after birth, disappearing spontaneously without scarring within 6 months. The risk of congenital heart block is around 2%. It appears *in utero*, is detected at 18–20 weeks' gestation, is permanent and difficult to treat and is associated with a 20% rate of perinatal mortality. Of those who survive, over 50% need pacemakers in early infancy. There is a 16% recurrence risk in subsequent pregnancies.

Rheumatoid arthritis

Rheumatoid arthritis (RA) is a chronic inflammatory autoimmune disease affecting primarily the synovial joints. It affects more women than men, and around 1 in 1,000 pregnancies is affected. Most women with RA (75%) experience improvement during pregnancy but only 16% enter complete remission from symptoms of the disease. Of those who improve, 90% suffer a flare postpartum. Unlike other connective tissue diseases, no adverse effects of RA on pregnancy are reported, and there are no increases in pregnancy loss rates. The main concern of RA patients is the safety of medication used to control the disease. If paracetamol-based analgesics are insufficient, corticosteroids are preferred to NSAIDs, although the latter can be used up to 32 weeks' gestation if needed. Azathiaprine and hydroxychloroquine can be used in pregnancy. Mode of delivery is determined by the usual obstetric indications, except where severe RA limits hip abduction and vaginal delivery is not possible.

Scleroderma

Scleroderma is a very rare autoimmune disorder that may present as either a localized cutaneous condition or systemic sclerosis, associated with Raynaud's phenomenon and characterized by progressive fibrosis of skin, oesophagus, lungs, heart and kidneys. No treatment has been shown to influence the course of scleroderma and treatment is usually symptomatic. Women with systemic sclerosis may deteriorate in pregnancy, although it is unclear if this is due to the pregnancy, and those with multiorgan involvement are often advised against pregnancy. The main risks are for those recently diagnosed with PH or with renal disease, where rapid deterioration is possible. There are associated adverse fetal outcomes, with increased rates of preterm delivery, pre-eclampsia, growth restriction and perinatal mortality. Finally, venous access, blood pressure monitoring and invasive monitoring may be difficult because of skin and blood vessel involvement.

Skin disease

Physiology

Many physiological changes affect skin during pregnancy. Increased pigmentation, especially on the face, areolae, axillae and abdominal midline, is common. Spider naevi affect the face, arms and upper torso, and broad pink linear striae (striae gravidarum) frequently appear over the lower abdomen and thighs. Pruritus without rash affects up to 20% of normal pregnancies, but liver function tests should always be performed to exclude obstetric cholestasis (see Chapter 6, Antenatal obstetric complications).

Pre-existing skin disease

Some pre-existing skin conditions such as eczema or acne worsen in pregnancy. Atopic eczema is a common pruritic skin condition affecting 1–5% of the general population and causes the commonest pregnancy rash. It can be treated with emollients and bath additives. Hand and nipple eczema are common postpartum. Acne usually improves in pregnancy, but can flare in the third trimester and acne rosacea often worsens. Oral or topical erythromycin can be used, but retinoids are contraindicated. Psoriasis affects 2% of the population and during pregnancy it remains unchanged in around 40% of patients, improves in another 40% and worsens in around 20%. Topical steroids can still be used, while methotrexate is contraindicated.

Specific dermatoses of pregnancy

Pemphigoid gestationis

Pemphigoid gestationis (PG) is a rare pruritic auto-immune bullous disorder, with an incidence of around 1 in 60,000 pregnancies. It most commonly presents in the late second or third trimester with lesions beginning on the abdomen 50% of the time and progressing to widespread clustered blisters, sparing the face. Diagnosis is made by the clinical appearance and by direct immunofluorescence. Once established, the disease runs a complex course with exacerbations and remissions, and flares postpartum in 75% of cases. Management aims to relieve pruritus and prevent new blister formation, and is achieved through the use of potent topical steroids and/or oral prednisolone. There is some association with preterm delivery and small for gestational age births, but no increase in pregnancy loss has been reported. PG recurs in most subsequent pregnancies.

Polymorphic eruption of pregnancy

Polymorphic eruption of pregnancy (PEP) is a self-limiting pruritic inflammatory disorder that usually presents in the third trimester and/or immediately postpartum. The estimated incidence is 1 in 160 pregnancies and 75% of affected pregnancies are primagravida. PEP often begins on the lower abdomen involving pregnancy striae, and extends to thighs, buttocks, legs and arms, while sparing the umbilicus and rarely involving face, hands and feet. In 70% of patients the lesions become confluent and widespread, resembling a toxic erythema. Symptomatic treatment is sufficient and pregnancies appear to be otherwise unaffected, with no tendency to recur.

Prurigo of pregnancy

Prurigo of pregnancy is a common pruritic disorder that occurs in 1 in 300 pregnancies, and presents as excoriated papules on extensor limbs, abdomen and shoulders. It is more common in women with a history of atopy. Prurigo usually starts at around 25–30 weeks of pregnancy and resolves after delivery, with no effect on the mother or baby. Treatment is symptomatic with topical steroids and emollients.

Pruritic folliculitis of pregnancy

Pruritic folliculitis (PF) is a pruritic follicular eruption, with papules and pustules that mainly affect the trunk, but can involve the limbs. It is similar in appearance to acne lesions and is sometimes considered a type of hormonally-induced acne. Its onset is usually in the second and third trimester, and it resolves weeks after delivery. Topical steroid treatment is effective.

KEY LEARNING POINTS

- Women with medical conditions that adversely affect pregnancy outcome should be offered prepregnancy counselling by appropriately experienced healthcare professionals.
- Women with medical problems that preclude safe pregnancy should be offered safe, effective and appropriate contraception.
- Asthma is the commonest chronic disease encountered in pregnancy.
- Eisenmenger's syndrome and PH are associated with a risk of maternal mortality of up to 50% in pregnancy.
- Women found to be hypertensive in the first half of pregnancy require investigation for possible underlying causes.
- Women with pre-existing hypertension are at increased risk of superimposed pre-eclampsia, FGR and placental abruption.
- Women who become pregnant with serum creatinine values above 124 µmol/l have an increased risk of accelerated decline in renal function and poor outcome of pregnancy.
- Pre-existing diabetes increases maternal and fetal obstetric morbidity.
- The incidence of fetal macrosomia in diabetes can be reduced through good blood glucose control.
- The risk of perinatal and maternal morbidity is increased in pregnancies complicated by sickle cell disease.
- The main issue for pregnant women with epilepsy relates to the teratogenic risk of anticonvulsant medication drugs.

Further reading

James DK, Steer PJ, WeinerCP, Gonik B (2011). *High Risk Pregnancy: Management Options*, Fourth Edition. ISBN 9781416059080.

Nelson-Piercy C (2015). *Handbook of Obstetric Medicine*, Fifth Edition. ISBN 9781482241921.

Williams D, Davison J (2008). Chronic kidney disease in pregnancy *BMJ* **336** (7637):211–15.

Self assessment

CASE HISTORY

A 36-year-old woman with a history of type 1 diabetes is referred to the diabetes pregnancy service as she is considering a pregnancy. She has mild retinopathy and has not had any previous pregnancies and does not currently take any regular medication in addition to her insulin. Her most recent HbA1c is 65 mmol/mol.

A   What medication should she start prior to trying for a pregnancy?

B   Is her diabetes satisfactorily controlled and should she be encouraged to delay pregnancy?

C   What important pregnancy complications should be discussed with her prior to her embarking on a pregnancy?

ANSWERS

A   Folic acid should be recommended to all women planning a pregnancy but a higher dose should be prescribed to women with diabetes in view of the increased risk of neural tube defects. She should be advised to take 5 mg daily for 3 months prior to pregnancy.

B   Her diabetes is not satisfactorily controlled as her HbA1c is above the target range (42 mmol/mol). She should be encouraged to test her blood sugars pre and post meals and make adjustments to her insulin, aiming to maintain her blood sugars between 4 and 7 mmol/l.

C   Prior to pregnancy it is useful to inform women of the need for additional surveillance required in pregnancies complicated by maternal diabetes. The increased risk of miscarriage, congenital anomalies and pregnancy complications such as pre-eclampsia and fetal macrosomia should be discussed. It should be emphasized that good glycaemic control significantly reduces the risk of all of these complications.

EMQ

A Nifedipine.
B Lamotrigine.
C Warfarin.
D Labetalol.
E Propylthiouracil.
F Cyclizine.

G Ramipril.
H Methyldopa.
I Domperidone.
K Atenolol.
L Salbutamol.

The items listed are commonly used pharmacological agents in medical conditions in pregnancy. For each description, choose the SINGLE most appropriate answer from the list of options. Each option may be used once, more than once or not at all.

1 An example of an ACE inhibitor; usually contraindicated in pregnancy.

2 An example of an antiepileptic drug commonly prescribed in pregnancy.

3 An antihypertensive medication that acts as a calcium-channel blocker.

4 Used for the treatment of asthma – usually as an inhaler.

ANSWERS

1G Ramipril is a commonly prescribed ACE inhibitor.

2B Lamotrigine is commonly prescribed in pregnancy.

3A Nifedipine is commonly used to treat hypertension in pregnancy.

4L Salbutamol inhalers should be continued in pregnancy for women with asthma.

SBA QUESTIONS

Choose the single best answer.

1 A woman with a history of Grave's disease who underwent partial thyroidectomy 5 years ago has had her thyroid function tested by her GP at 7 weeks of pregnancy. This shows the following:

TSH   8.6 IU/l   (normal 1–5)
T4   11.4 pmol/l   (normal 6–15)

The appropriate course of action is:

A Repeat thyroid function tests (TFTs) in 6 weeks.
B Repeat TFTs in 12 weeks.
C Commence carbimazole.
D Commence propylthiouracil.
E Commence thyroxine.

ANSWER

E Commence thyroxine. The TFT result is consistent with significant hypothyroidism, which should be treated in pregnancy with thyroxine replacement.

2 Warfarin is contraindicated in pregnancy. Which of the following abnormalities are commonly associated with warfarin use in the first trimester?

A Claw hand.
B Dextrocardia.
C Nasal hypoplasia.

D Neural tube defect.
E Renal agenesis.

ANSWER

C Nasal hypoplasia is a recognized teratogenic feature of warfarin therapy.

3 The administration of which drug in the first trimester of pregnancy is typically associated with neural tube defects?

   A   Enalapril.

   B   Lithium.

   C   Nitrofurantoin.

   D   Sodium valproate.

   E   Warfarin.

ANSWER

D Sodium valproate is associated with an increased risk of several different congenital anomalies; the risk of neural tube defects is particularly high with this medication, although this is reduced with high-dose folic acid.

JENNY E MYERS

LEARNING OBJECTIVES

- To understand the common viral and bacterial infections seen in pregnancy that have implications for the mother, fetus and infant.
- Learn which infections are included in routine pregnancy screening and the principles of their management.

- Learn the consequences of perinatal infection on the developing fetus.

Introduction

Viral and bacterial infections are very common in pregnancy and can have significant consequences for both the pregnant mother and her infant. For some infections, routine screening is offered in many health care settings. For other infections, testing and treatment are dictated by the stage of pregnancy and/or the severity of the maternal symptoms. Some infections are also associated with congenital abnormalities or direct consequences for fetal wellbeing.

This chapter provides some of the background to the commonly encountered and important infections, both bacterial and viral, that affect pregnancy.

The epidemiology of these infections is discussed in addition to the screening and diagnostic tests used in routine practice. Potential implications for the fetus and mother with possible treatment options are also discussed.

Infections causing congenital abnormalities

Rubella

Infective organism

Rubella virus is a togavirus spread by droplet transmission.

Prevalence

Rubella is still common in many developing countries and worldwide; more than 100,000 children every year are born with congenital rubella syndrome (CRS). Since the introduction of the mumps, measles and rubella vaccine (MMR), rubella is now a very uncommon infection in the UK; there were 42 documented cases in the UK in 2012. However, concerns regarding a link with the vaccine and autism in the 1990s has resulted in a significant increase in the number of susceptible pregnant women. An analysis of samples tested between 2004 and 2009 demonstrated a small but significant increase in those whose antibody levels fell below the threshold. Over the 6-year period the number of women found to be susceptible to rubella increased by 60% from 2.1 to 3.5%. Low antibody levels were particularly common among younger women who would have been eligible for MMR vaccination in the 1990s (14%) and in women from ethnic minorities.

Screening

Until recently (April 2016), screening was recommended in early pregnancy for immunity to rubella. However, as the prevalence of rubella has now reached such low levels in the UK, screening is no longer routinely offered. In many other countries where the vaccination programme is less established, screening may still be offered.

This is an unusual antenatal screening test as there is no effective intervention that can be implemented during the index pregnancy to reduce the risk of harm to that fetus, nor does it attempt to identify currently affected pregnancies. The aim of screening for rubella in pregnancy is to identify susceptible women so that postpartum vaccination may protect future pregnancies against rubella infection and its consequences.

For pregnant women who are screened and rubella antibody is not detected, rubella vaccination after pregnancy should be advised. Vaccination during pregnancy is contraindicated because of a theoretical risk that the vaccine itself could be teratogenic, as it is a live vaccine. No cases of CRS resulting from vaccination during pregnancy have been reported. However, women who are vaccinated postpartum should be advised to use contraception for 1 month.

Clinical features

Rubella infection is characterized by a febrile rash but is asymptomatic in the mother in 20–50% of cases. Features of CRS can include sensorineural deafness, congenital cataracts, blindness, encephalitis and endocrine problems.

The risk of congenital rubella infection reduces with gestation. If infection of the fetus does occur, the defects caused are also less severe with more advanced gestations. Congenital infection in the first 12 weeks of pregnancy among mothers with symptoms is over 80% and reduces to 25% at the end of the second trimester. Rubella defects occur in 100% of infants infected during the first 11 weeks of pregnancy, whereas primary rubella contracted between 16 and 20 weeks of gestation carries only a minimal risk of deafness. Rubella infection prior to the estimated date of conception or after 20 weeks' gestation carries no documented risk to the fetus.

Management

If infection during pregnancy is confirmed, the risk of CRS should be assessed depending on the gestation when infection occurred. If infection occurred prior to 16 weeks' gestation, termination of pregnancy should be offered. If the infection occurs later in pregnancy, the woman should be given appropriate information and reassured.

Syphilis

Infective organism

Syphilis is a sexually acquired infection caused by *Treponema pallidum*.

Prevalence

The incidence of infectious syphilis in England and Wales is low and appears to have reduced in women in the UK over the last decade, with around 250 cases per year. There has been an increase in the rates of infection in men (4,054 cases in 2014), thought to be predominantly in men with same sex partners.

In a national survey in 2010–11, over 1,900 pregnancies were identified with a positive screen for syphilis (0.15% screened UK pregnancies) with around 1,400 confirmed cases. One-quarter of these women had newly diagnosed infections, with 28% of women requiring treatment for the first time in pregnancy. Five children born to women requiring treatment had confirmed congenital syphilis. Among women with past or current syphilis infection, about half were white; 29% were born in the UK, 24% elsewhere in Europe and 23% in sub-Saharan Africa.

Clinical features

Primary syphilis may present as a painless genital ulcer 3–6 weeks after the infection is acquired (condylomata lata) (**Figure 11.1**). However, this may be on the cervix and go unnoticed.

Secondary manifestations occur 6 weeks to 6 months after infection and present as a maculopapular rash or lesions affecting the mucous membranes. Ultimately 20% of untreated patients will develop symptomatic cardiovascular tertiary syphilis and 5–10% will develop symptomatic neurosyphilis.

In pregnant women with early, untreated (primary or secondary) syphilis, 70–100% of infants will be infected and approximately 25% will be stillborn. Mother-to-child transmission of syphilis in pregnancy is associated with fetal growth restriction (FGR), fetal hydrops, congenital syphilis

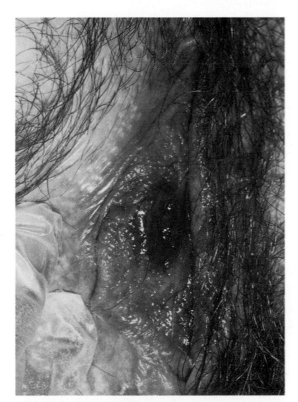

Figure 11.1 Primary syphilitic chancre. (Courtesy of Dr Raymond Maw, Royal Victoria Hospital, Belfast.)

(which may cause long-term disability), stillbirth, preterm birth and neonatal death. The risk of congenital transmission declines with increasing duration of maternal syphilis prior to pregnancy. Adequate treatment with benzathine penicillin markedly improves the outcome for the fetus.

Screening

Because treatment is so effective, routine antenatal screening for all pregnant women is recommended and the uptake for national screening in the UK is very high (>95%). The body's immune response to syphilis is the production non-specific and specific treponemal antibodies. These can be detected by serological tests. Non-treponemal tests detect non-specific treponemal antibodies and include the Venereal Diseases Research Laboratory (VDRL) and rapid plasma reagin (RPR) tests. Treponemal tests detect specific treponemal antibodies and include enzyme immunoassays (EIAs), *T. pallidum* haemagglutination assay (TPHA) and the fluorescent treponemal antibody-absorbed test (FTA-abs). EIA tests that detect immunoglobulin (Ig) G or IgG and IgM are rapidly replacing the VDRL and TPHA combination for syphilis screening in the UK. EIAs are over 98% sensitive and over 99% specific. Non-treponemal tests, on the other hand, may result in false negatives, particularly in very early or late syphilis, in patients with reinfection or those who are human immunodeficiency virus (HIV) positive. The VDRL may be falsely positive in women with lupus. Overall there is a 20% false-positive rate from screening tests; women should therefore be referred for expert assessment and diagnosis in a genitourinary medicine (GUM) clinic.

None of these serological tests will detect syphilis in its incubation stage, which may last for an average of 25 days.

Management

The initial step is to confirm the diagnosis and to test for any other sexually transmitted diseases. Once a diagnosis of syphilis is confirmed the GUM clinic will institute appropriate contact tracing of sexual partners. Older children may also need to be screened for congenital infection.

Parenteral penicillin has a 98% success rate for preventing congenital syphilis. A Jarish–Herxheimer reaction may occur with treatment as a result of release of proinflammatory cytokines in response to dying organisms. This presents as a worsening of symptoms, and fever for 12–24 hours after commencement of treatment. It may be associated with uterine contractions and fetal distress. Many clinicians therefore admit women at the time of commencement of treatment for monitoring.

If a woman is not treated during pregnancy her baby should be treated after delivery. An infected baby may be born without signs or symptoms of disease but if not treated immediately, may develop serious problems within a few weeks. Untreated babies often develop developmental delay, have seizures or die.

Toxoplasmosis

Infective organism

Toxoplasma gondii is a protozoan parasite found in cat faeces, soil or uncooked meat. Infection occurs by ingestion of the parasite from undercooked meat or from unwashed hands.

Prevalence

Around 350 cases of toxoplasmosis are reported in England and Wales each year, but the actual number of infections could be as high as 350,000 and estimates suggest up to one-third of people in the UK will be infected by toxoplasmosis at some point in their life. Congenital toxoplasmosis is rare in the UK, with estimates suggesting only around 1 in every 10,000–30,000 babies are born with the condition.

Screening

Only about 10 severely affected babies are diagnosed per year in the UK and for this reason the UK National Screening Committee stated in 2011 that screening for toxoplasmosis should not be offered routinely. There is a lack of evidence that antenatal screening and treatment reduces mother-to-child transmission or the complications associated with *T. gondii* infection. In the UK women should be advised about appropriate preventive measure such as avoiding eating rare or raw meat; avoiding handling cats and cat litter; and wearing gloves and washing hands when gardening or handling soil.

Even in France, where more women acquire infection during pregnancy and pregnant women are screened, the benefits of such a programme appear to be limited.

Clinical features

The initial infection is usually asymptomatic, or may be a glandular fever-like illness. Parasitaemia usually occurs within 3 weeks of infection. Therefore, congenital infection is only a significant risk if the mother acquires the infection during or immediately before pregnancy.

Infection during the first trimester of pregnancy is most likely to cause severe fetal damage (85%), but only 10% of infections are transmitted to the fetus at this gestation. In the third trimester 85% of infections are transmitted, but the risk of fetal damage decreases to around 10%.

Severely infected infants may have ventriculomegaly or microcephaly, chorioretinitis and cerebral calcification. These features may be detected on ultrasound scan. The majority of infected infants are asymptomatic at birth but develop sequelae several years later.

Management

The diagnosis of primary infection with toxoplasmosis during pregnancy is made by the Sabin Feldman dye test. Enzyme-linked immunosorbant assays (ELISAs) are available for IgM antibody. However, IgM may persist for months or even years, so often serial testing for rising titres is necessary. If suspicion of congenital toxoplasmosis has arisen because of an abnormal ultrasound scan of the fetus, an amniocentesis can be performed. Polymerase chain reaction (PCR) analysis of amniotic fluid is highly accurate for the identification of *T. gondii*.

Spiramycin treatment can be used in pregnancy (a 3-week course of 2–3 g per day). This reduces the incidence of transplacental infection but has not been shown to definitively reduce the incidence of clinical congenital disease. If toxoplasmosis is found to be the cause of abnormalities detected on ultrasound scan of the fetus, then termination of pregnancy can be offered.

Cytomegalovirus

Infective organism

Cytomegalovirus (CMV) is a deoxyribonucleic acid (DNA) herpes virus. It is transmitted by respiratory droplet transmission and is excreted in the urine.

Prevalence

It is a common virus in the UK and about 60% of women are seropositive for CMV when they become pregnant and consequently, approximately 40% are susceptible to infection, although there is also a risk associated with recurrent infection. In the UK, it is estimated that 1–2 in 200 infants will be born with congenital CMV. Of these, it is estimated that 13% will have problems at birth, such as hearing loss and learning difficulties, with a similar number being asymptomatic at birth but developing problems in later life.

Primary infection is more likely to cause symptomatic congenital CMV (40%) and long-term sequelae than reactivation of infection (1%). However, the high incidence of CMV seropositivity among pregnant women worldwide means that transplacental transmission during reactivated infection accounts for 30–50% of congenital infections.

Clinical features

Primary infection usually produces no symptoms or mild non-specific flu-like symptoms in the mother. The diagnosis is often made after abnormalities are seen in the fetus on ultrasound scan. The main features seen in an affected fetus are growth restriction, microcephaly, intracranial calcification (**Figure 11.2**), ventriculomegaly, ascites or hydrops.

There may not be any abnormalities detected on antenatal ultrasound, but affected infants may later be found to have neurological damage such as blindness,

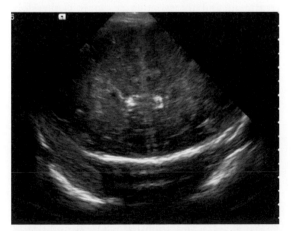

Figure 11.2 Ultrasound of a fetal brain demonstrating intracranial calcification secondary to CMV infection. (Courtesy of Dr Ed Johnstone, St Mary's Hospital, Manchester.)

deafness or developmental delay. The neonate can also be anaemic and thrombocytopaenic, with hepatosplenomegaly, jaundice and a purpural rash.

Management

A serological diagnosis of primary CMV can be made by demonstrating the development of CMV antibodies in a seronegative woman, who initially develops CMV IgM antibody and subsequently IgG antibody. Virology laboratories usually keep the blood sample taken in early pregnancy, so if infection is suspected a sample taken at the time of presentation can be compared with the initial booking sample to determine whether seroconversion has occurred. Since IgM can be secreted for several months, it is not sufficient to simply demonstrate IgM in a sample at the time of presentation; it has to be a new finding in a woman who was negative for IgM at the time of booking.

If there is a suspicion that the fetus may be infected amniotic fluid can be tested for the virus by PCR. Since the virus is excreted in fetal urine it can be found in amniotic fluid.

If abnormalities are detected on ultrasound and these are felt to be due to congenital CMV infection, termination of pregnancy should be discussed. A much more difficult situation is when CMV infection is known to have occurred, but the fetus appears normal on ultrasound, as there remains a 20% chance of neurological abnormality in this fetus.

Like other herpes viruses, CMV has the capacity to establish latency and be reactivated. After infection the virus is excreted for weeks or months by adults and for years by infants. It persists in the lymphocytes throughout life and can be transmitted by blood transfusion or transplantation. Reactivation occurs intermittently, with shedding in the genital urinary or respiratory tract.

Chickenpox

Infective organism

Chickenpox is caused by the varicella zoster virus (VZV), a herpes virus that is transmitted by droplet spread and direct personal contact.

Prevalence

In the UK, over 90% of individuals over 15 years of age are immune to chickenpox. Although contact with chickenpox is common in pregnancy, infection during pregnancy is uncommon, with an estimated prevalence of 3/1,000 pregnancies. Antenatal screening for chicken pox is not currently recommended in the UK, but women identified as being seronegative can consider vaccination either prepregnancy or in the postnatal period.

Clinical features

Non-immune pregnant women are more vulnerable to chickenpox and may develop a serious pneumonia, hepatitis or encephalitis. The mortality rate is approximately five times higher in pregnant women than in non-pregnant adults. Pneumonia occurs in about 10% of women with chickenpox and seems more severe at later gestations. It may also cause the fetal varicella syndrome (FVS) or varicella infection of the newborn.

Management

Women should be asked whether they have had chickenpox at the initial booking visit. If they have not had chickenpox, they should be advised to avoid contact with it during pregnancy, and if they accidentally come into contact with it should advise their doctor or midwife about the exposure as soon as possible.

When contact occurs with chickenpox, a careful history must be taken to confirm the significance of the contact (length of exposure and closeness of contact) and the susceptibility of the patient. Significant contact is defined as being in the same room as someone for 15 minutes or more, or face-to-face contact. Individuals with the virus are infectious for 48 hours prior to the appearance of the rash and until the vesicles crust over (usually 5 days).

Testing for immunity

If a woman reports that she has been in contact with chickenpox, she should have a blood test for confirmation of VZV immunity, by testing for VZV IgG. This can usually be performed within 24–48 hours and the virology laboratory may be able to use serum stored from the early pregnancy booking blood sample.

Management of the non-immune woman exposed to chickenpox

If immunity is not confirmed and there has been significant exposure, women should be given varicella zoster immunoglobulin (VZIG) as soon as possible. VZIG is effective when given up to 10 days after contact and may prevent or attenuate the disease. Women who have had exposure to chickenpox (regardless of whether or not they have received VZIG) should be asked to notify their doctor or midwife early if a rash develops.

Management of chickenpox in pregnancy

Women with chickenpox should avoid contact with other pregnant women and neonates until the lesions have crusted over. Current recommendations state that oral aciclovir 800 mg five times per day for 7 days should be prescribed for pregnant women with chickenpox if they present within 24 hours of the onset of the rash and if they are more than 20 weeks' gestation. Aciclovir should also be considered before 20 weeks' gestation. VZIG has no therapeutic benefit once chickenpox has developed. If the woman smokes cigarettes, has chronic lung disease, is taking corticosteroids or is in the latter half of pregnancy, a hospital assessment should be considered, even in the absence of complications.

Women hospitalized with varicella should be nursed in isolation from babies or potentially susceptible pregnant women or non-immune staff.

Delivery during the viraemic period may be extremely hazardous. The maternal risks are bleeding, thrombocytopaenia, disseminated intravascular coagulopathy and hepatitis. There is a high risk of varicella infection of the newborn with significant morbidity and mortality. Supportive treatment and intravenous aciclovir is therefore desirable, allowing resolution of the rash and transfer of protective antibodies from the mother to the fetus. However, delivery may be required in women to facilitate assisted ventilation in cases where varicella pneumonia is complicated by respiratory failure.

The fetus

Spontaneous miscarriage does not appear to be increased if chickenpox occurs in the first trimester. FVS is characterized by one or more of the following:

- Skin scarring in a dermatomal distribution.
- Eye defects (microphthalmia, chorioretinitis, cataracts).
- Hypoplasia of the limbs.

- Neurological abnormalities (microcephaly, cortical atrophy, mental restriction and dysfunction of bowel and bladder sphincters).

This only occurs in a minority of infected fetuses (approximately 1%). FVS has been reported as early as 3 weeks' and up to 28 weeks' gestation. The risk appears to be lower in the first trimester (0.55%). No case of FVS has been reported when maternal infection has occurred after 28 weeks.

If the mother has contracted chickenpox during pregnancy, referral to a fetal medicine specialist should be considered at 16–20 weeks or 5 weeks after infection for discussion and detailed ultrasound examination, when findings such as limb deformity, microcephaly, hydrocephalus, soft-tissue calcification and FGR can be detected. A time lag of at least 5 weeks after the primary infection is advised as it takes several weeks for these features to manifest.

Maternal infection around the time of delivery

If maternal infection occurs at term, there is a significant risk of varicella of the newborn. Elective delivery should normally be avoided until 5–7 days after the onset of maternal rash to allow for the passive transfer of antibodies from mother to the infant. Neonatal ophthalmic examination should be organized after birth.

If birth occurs within the 7-day period following the onset of the maternal rash, or if the mother develops the chickenpox rash within the 7-day period after birth, the neonate should be given VZIG. The infant should be monitored for signs of infection until 28 days after the onset of maternal infection.

Neonatal infection should be treated with aciclovir following discussion with a neonatologist and virologist. VZIG is of no benefit once neonatal chickenpox has developed.

Contact with shingles

Following the primary infection, the virus remains dormant in sensory nerve root ganglia but can be reactivated to cause a vesicular erythematous skin rash in a dermatomal distribution known as herpes zoster (HZ) or shingles. The risk of a pregnant woman acquiring infection from an individual with HZ in non-exposed sites (for example, thoracolumbar) is remote.

Other congenital infections associated with pregnancy loss and preterm birth

Parvovirus

Infective organism

Parvovirus B19 (PVB19) is a relatively common infection in pregnancy, and is transmitted through respiratory droplets.

Incidence

Immunity to PVB19 infection occurs in 50% of women of childbearing age and therefore 50% are susceptible to infection during pregnancy. It occurs most commonly in those pregnant women who work with young children, for example teachers.

Routine screening in pregnancy is not currently recommended as there are currently no agreed treatment or prevention methods to protect the baby from being infected.

Clinical features

In adults, many (20–25%) cases are asymptomatic or produce symptoms of a mild flu-like illness and/or arthropathy. In children it usually causes a characteristic rash (slapped cheek syndrome). There is a transplacental transmission rate of 17–33% and the fetus is most vulnerable if infected in the second trimester. In most fetuses infected with PVB19, there will be spontaneous resolution with no long-term consequences, but the infection can cause an aplastic anaemia.

The anaemic fetus may then become hydropic due to high output cardiac failure and liver congestion. This is the most common presentation during pregnancy and is seen on ultrasound scan. If a fetus is hydropic, the velocity of blood flow in the fetal middle cerebral artery can be measured. If the velocity is high, it is suggestive of anaemia, and PVB19 would be one of several differential diagnoses.

Management

The diagnosis is made by demonstrating seroconversion of the mother, who develops IgM antibodies to PVB19, having previously tested negative. Viral DNA amplifications, using PCR in maternal and fetal serum or amniotic fluid, is the most sensitive and accurate diagnostic test.

A hydropic fetus may recover spontaneously as the mother and fetus recover from the virus, or may require treatment by *in utero* transfusion.

Infection in the first 20 weeks of pregnancy can lead to hydrops fetalis and intrauterine death, as treatment by intrauterine transfusion is not possible at early gestations. Prior to 20 weeks the fetal loss rate is approximately 10%.

If the anaemia is treated by *in utero* transfusion, the fetus can make a complete recovery. Parvovirus does not cause neurological damage, and if the fetus survives the anaemia, the outcome is usually normal. After 20 weeks' gestation the fetal loss rate is estimated to be approximately 1%.

Listeria

Infective organism

Listeria monocytogenes is an aerobic and facultatively anaerobic motile gram-positive bacillus. It has an unusual life cycle with obligate intracellular replication. People with reduced cell-mediated immunity, and hence pregnant women, are therefore most at risk.

Incidence

The incidence of *L. monocytogenes* infection in pregnant women is around 18 times higher than in the non-pregnant population but is still rare, with rates of 1 in 8,000. Contaminated food is the usual source of infection. Usual sources include unpasteurized milk, ripened soft cheeses and pâté. It is therefore recommended that pregnant women should be offered information on how to reduce the risk of listeriosis by dietary modification. *L. monocytogenes* is not transmitted in hot cooked foods and does not multiply in the freezer. However, it survives and multiplies at refrigerator temperatures and hence can be transmitted in chilled foods (e.g. milk, soft cheese, prawns, pate).

Clinical features

Pregnant women with listeriosis most commonly suffer from a flu-like illness with fever and general malaise. About one-third of women may be asymptomatic. Transmission to the fetus may occur either via the ascending route through the cervix, or transplacentally secondary to maternal bacteraemia. Approximately 20% of affected pregnancies result in miscarriage or stillbirth. Premature delivery may occur in over 50%.

Neonates may have respiratory distress, fever, sepsis or neurological symptoms and the overall neonatal mortality rate has been estimated at 38%.

Management

The diagnosis of listeriosis depends on clinical suspicion and isolation of the organism from blood, vaginal swabs or the placenta. Meconium staining of the amniotic fluid in a preterm fetus may increase clinical suspicion for listeriosis.

For women with listeriosis during pregnancy, intravenous antibiotic treatment (ampicillin 2 g given every 6 hours) is indicated.

Malaria

Infective organisms

Although malaria can be caused by four species of malarial parasite (*Plasmodium falciparum*, *P. vivax*, *P. ovale* and *P. malariae*), the species that carries the worst prognosis for the mother and fetus, and the organism of greatest importance on a worldwide scale, is *P. falciparum*. This is a protozoan parasite transmitted by the female anopheline mosquito.

Incidence

Incidence varies depending on geographical location, but malaria is endemic in sub-Saharan Africa, South Asia and some parts of South America. It is estimated that one billion people worldwide carry parasites at any time, and 0.5–3 million people per year die from malaria. Pregnant women have an increased risk of malarial infection compared to their non-pregnant adult counterparts. The incidence of parasitaemia has been found to be higher in primiparous women (66%) than in multiparous women (21–29%).

In endemic areas, where many women are semi-immune, malarial parasites are often found in large numbers sequestrated in the placenta, even when blood films are negative. This may lead to the diagnosis being missed, unless there is a high index of suspicion and the placenta is examined appropriately.

Clinical features

Maternal effects include a cyclical spiking pyrexia, which may be associated with miscarriage and preterm labour. Severe anaemia may develop rapidly, but many women from endemic areas may also have other risk factors for severe anaemia. Hypoglycaemia is common and may be severe in pregnancy. Pulmonary oedema, due to abnormal capillary permeability, results in high mortality (approximately 50%). Haemolysis causes jaundice and renal failure.

Fetal effects include premature delivery and FGR. Placental sequestration of parasites is associated with abnormal uteroplacental Doppler wave forms and is also implicated in the higher rate of transmission of HIV. Coinfection with HIV is common in many of the areas where malaria is endemic, and vertical transmission of both malaria and HIV to the fetus seems to be commoner if the two infections coexist.

Management

If malaria is suspected, prompt symptomatic and supportive treatment with appropriate antimalarial therapy is important. The choice of antimalarial will vary, depending on local patterns of disease and drug resistance and expert advice should be sought. In endemic areas preventive strategies include the use of insecticide-treated bed nets and intermittent preventive treatment during pregnancy.

If women from non-endemic areas are planning to travel to endemic areas, they should only do so if absolutely necessary during their pregnancy. Insecticide sprays, mosquito nets, appropriate clothing to reduce the risk of mosquito bites and drug prophylaxis can all be used. Expert advice on which antimalarial is appropriate for the area is important. The risks of teratogenicity must be balanced against the serious risk of contracting malaria in pregnancy.

Infections acquired around the time of delivery with serious neonatal consequences

Herpes

Infective organism

Herpes simplex virus (HSV) is a double-stranded DNA virus. There are two viral types, HSV-1 and HSV-2. The majority of orolabial infections are caused by HSV-1. These infections are usually acquired during childhood through direct physical contact such as kissing. Genital herpes is a sexually transmitted infection and is most commonly caused by HSV-2 (**Figure 11.3**).

Incidence

Genital herpes is the most common ulcerative sexually-transmitted infection in the UK. There has been an increasing prevalence of anogenital herpes in the UK over the last decade with around 20,000 cases per year. Neonatal herpes is a viral infection with a high morbidity and mortality, and is most commonly acquired at or near the time of delivery due to contact with infected secretions. It is rare, with an estimated incidence of 5 per 100,000 live births.

Clinical features

Genital herpes presents as ulcerative lesions on the vulva, vagina or cervix. The woman may give a history of this being a recurrent problem, in which case the lesion is often less florid. A primary infection may be associated with systemic symptoms and may cause urinary retention.

Neonatal herpes may be caused by HSV-1 or HSV-2, as either viral type can cause genital herpes. Almost all cases of neonatal herpes occur as a result of direct

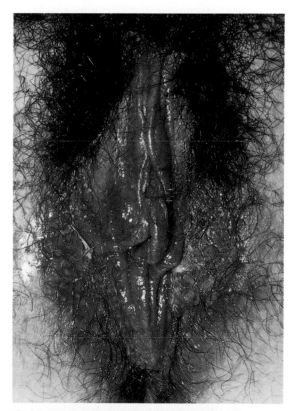

Figure 11.3 Primary genital herpes. (Courtesy of Dr Richard Lau, St George's Hospital, London.)

Table 11.1 Classification of neonatal herpes

	Death (in treated babies) %	Neurological morbidity %
Localized to skin, eye and/mouth	Rare	<2
Local central nervous system disease	6	70
Disseminated infection	30	17

contact with infected maternal secretions, although cases of postnatal transmission have been described.

Neonatal herpes is classified into three subgroups: disease localized to skin, eye and/mouth; local central nervous system (CNS) disease (encephalitis alone); and disseminated infection with multiple organ involvement (*Table 11.1*).

Factors influencing transmission include the type of maternal infection (primary or recurrent), the presence of transplacental maternal neutralizing antibodies, the duration of rupture of membranes before delivery, the use of fetal scalp electrodes and the mode of delivery. The risks are greatest when a woman acquires a new infection (primary genital herpes) in the third trimester, particularly within 6 weeks of delivery, as viral shedding may persist and the baby is likely to be born before the development of protective maternal antibodies. Very rarely, congenital herpes may occur as a result of transplacental intrauterine infection.

Management

Symptomatic genital herpes infections are confirmed by direct detection of HSV. A swab for viral detection should be used. Any woman with suspected first-episode genital herpes should be referred to a genitourinary physician, who will confirm the diagnosis by viral culture or PCR, advise on management and arrange a screen for other sexually transmitted infections. The use of aciclovir is recommended (400 mg three times daily) and is associated with a reduction in the duration and severity of symptoms and a decrease in the duration of viral shedding. It is well tolerated and considered safe in pregnancy.

It may be difficult to distinguish clinically between recurrent and primary genital HSV infections, as up to 15% of first-episode HSV infections are not true primary infections. For women presenting within 6 weeks of expected delivery, type-specific HSV antibody testing is advisable. The presence of antibodies of the same type as the HSV isolated from genital swabs would confirm this episode to be a recurrence rather than a primary infection and elective caesarean section would not be indicated to prevent neonatal transmission.

Primary infections

Providing that delivery does not ensue within the next 6 weeks, the pregnancy should be managed expectantly and vaginal delivery anticipated. There is no evidence that HSV acquired in pregnancy is associated with an increased incidence of congenital abnormalities. Following first or second trimester acquisition, suppressive aciclovir from 36 weeks of gestation reduces HSV lesions at term and hence the need for delivery by caesarean section.

Caesarean section should be the recommended mode of delivery for all women developing first-episode genital herpes in the third trimester, particularly those developing symptoms within 6 weeks of expected delivery, as the risk of neonatal transmission of HSV is very high at 41%. For women who opt for a vaginal birth, rupture of membranes should be avoided and invasive procedures, such as fetal scalp electrodes or fetal scalp pH measurement, should not be used. Intravenous aciclovir given intrapartum to the mother and subsequently to the neonate may be considered.

Recurrent episodes

A recurrent episode of genital herpes occurring during the antenatal period is not an indication for delivery by caesarean section. Women presenting with recurrent genital herpes lesions at the onset of labour should be advised that the risk to the baby of neonatal herpes is very small (1–3%). Daily suppressive aciclovir 400 mg three times daily should be considered from 36 weeks' gestation. Women with recurrent genital herpes lesions and confirmed rupture of membranes at term should be advised to have delivery expedited by the appropriate means. Invasive procedures in labour should be avoided for women with recurrent genital herpes lesions. The neonatologist should be informed of babies born to mothers with recurrent genital herpes lesions at the time of labour.

Group B streptococcus

Infective organism

Group B streptococcus (*Streptococcus agalactiae*) (GBS) is a gram-positive coccus frequently found as a vaginal commensal. It can cause sepsis in the neonate and transmission can occur from the time the membranes are ruptured until delivery.

Prevalence

GBS is recognized as the most frequent cause of severe early-onset (less than 7 days of age) infection in newborn infants. Approximately 21% of women in UK carry GBS as a commensal in the vagina. The background incidence of early-onset GBS disease in the UK is 0.5 in 1,000 births, which increases to 2.5 in 1,000 in women with GBS carriage confirmed in the current pregnancy.

The mortality from early-onset GBS disease in the UK is 6% in term infants and 18% in preterm infants. Even when treated appropriately, some infants will still die of early-onset disease, particularly when the disease is well established prior to birth.

Screening

Universal screening is carried out in the USA but this practice is not currently recommended in the UK. The incidence of early-onset GBS disease in the UK in the absence of systematic screening or widespread intrapartum antibiotic prophylaxis is similar to that seen in the USA after universal screening and intrapartum antibiotic prophylaxis, despite comparable vaginal carriage rates.

Clinical features

The mother will not have symptoms as GBS is a common vaginal commensal.

An infected neonate may demonstrate signs of neonatal sepsis including sudden collapse, tachypnoea, nasal flaring, poor tone, jaundice, etc.

Management

Antenatal

If GBS is detected incidentally, antenatal treatment is not recommended as it does not reduce the likelihood of GBS colonization at the time of delivery.

Intrapartum antibiotic prophylaxis

It is during labour that infection of the fetus/neonate occurs. Antibiotics (penicillin or clindamycin) given in labour are estimated to be 60–80% effective in reducing early-onset neonatal GBS infection.

The Royal College of Obstetricians and Gynaecologists (RCOG) therefore recommends that intrapartum antibiotic prophylaxis is discussed with women with the following risk factors, and that the argument for using prophylaxis is stronger if more than one risk factor is present, if the woman has had a previous baby with neonatal GBS or if GBS bacteruria is detected, as this is associated with a higher risk of neonatal disease.

Risk factors requiring prophylaxis for GBS

- Intrapartum fever (>38°C).
- Prolonged rupture of membranes greater than 18 hours.
- Prematurity less than 37 weeks.
- Previous infant with GBS.
- Incidental detection of GBS in current pregnancy.
- GBS bacteruria.

Approximately 15% of all UK pregnancies have one or more of the risk factors and using this strategy, 25% of women will receive intrapartum antibiotics with 50–69% reduction in early-onset GBS infection in the neonate. Therefore, 5,882 women need to be treated to prevent one neonatal death.

It is recommended that intravenous penicillin 3 g be given as soon as possible after the onset of labour (or after development of a risk factor) and 1.5 g four-hourly until delivery. Clindamycin 900 mg should be given intravenously 8-hourly to those allergic to penicillin.

There is no good evidence to support the administration of intrapartum antibiotic prophylaxis to women in whom GBS carriage was detected in a previous pregnancy. If chorioamnionitis is suspected, broad-spectrum antibiotic therapy including an agent active against GBS should replace GBS-specific antibiotic prophylaxis. Women undergoing planned caesarean delivery in the absence of labour or membrane rupture do not require antibiotic prophylaxis for GBS, regardless of GBS colonization status. The risk of neonatal GBS disease is extremely low in this circumstance.

The neonate

Many infants with early-onset GBS disease have symptoms at or soon after birth. Neonatal sepsis can progress rapidly to death. Whether they received intrapartum antibiotics or not, any newborn infant with clinical signs compatible with infection should be treated promptly with broad-spectrum antibiotics, which provide cover against early-onset GBS disease and other common pathogens. Blood cultures should always be obtained before antibiotic treatment is commenced, and cerebrospinal fluid (CSF) cultures should be considered. Randomized controlled trials have not provided a sufficient evidence base for clear treatment recommendations in well, newborn infants whose mothers had risk factors for GBS. Some clinicians will recommend treatment of the infants, while others will prefer to observe them because the balance of risks and benefits of treatment is uncertain. Each hospital will have its own guideline.

Chlamydia

Infective organism

Chlamydia trachomatis is an obligate intracellular organism.

Prevalence

Chlamydia is the commonest sexually transmitted organism in the UK and USA. Between 1 in 8–10 men and women who are sexually active and under 25 years old screen positive for chlamydia and there are over 120,000 cases diagnosed in women per year in the UK. In the UK an opportunistic chlamydia screening programme for under 25 year olds has been initiated. While it is not a routine antenatal screening test in the UK, NICE recommends that all women booking for antenatal care, who are younger than 25 years, are informed of the National Screening Programme.

Clinical features

Chlamydia is frequently asymptomatic in the pregnant woman. Infection with chlamydia is associated with preterm rupture of membranes, preterm delivery and low birthweight. Transmission to the fetus occurs at the time of delivery and can cause conjunctivitis and pneumonia.

Management

Treatment with azithromycin or erythromycin is recommended. Tetracyclines such as doxycycline should be avoided if possible during pregnancy. Appropriate contact tracing can be arranged via a GUM clinic.

Gonorrhoea

Infective organism

Neisseria gonorrhoeae is a gram-negative diplococcus.

Prevalence

The prevalence of gonorrhoea in pregnancy varies with the population studied. In the UK it is the second most common bacterial sexually-transmitted disease, with around 8,000 cases per year in women.

Clinical features

Gonococcal infection in women is frequently asymptomatic, or women may present with a mucopurulent discharge or dysuria. Rarely disseminated gonorrhoea may cause low-grade fever, a rash and polyarthritis. There is an increased risk of coinfection with chlamydia and an increased risk of preterm rupture of membranes and preterm birth. Transmission to the fetus occurs at the time of delivery and can cause ophthalmia neonatorum.

Management

Bacteriological swabs should be taken and specific swabs/testing for concomitant infection with chlamydia should also be undertaken. Cephalosporins are effective against gonococcus, but empirical treatment for chlamydia should also be considered. Appropriate contact tracing can be arranged via a GUM clinic.

Perinatal infections causing long-term disease

Human immunodeficiency virus

Infective organism

The HIV virus is a ribonucleic acid (RNA) retrovirus transmitted through sexual contact; blood and blood products; shared needles for IV drug users;

or vertical (mother to child) transmission, which mainly occurs in the late third trimester, during labour, delivery or breast feeding.

Prevalence

In 2014, the HIV prevalence was 1.5 per 1,000 women screened in the UK. Prevalence in London was 3.5 per 1,000 and in the rest of England was 0.7–1.6 per 1,000. The majority of HIV-positive pregnant women are black African, with 43.7 per 1,000 living with HIV in the UK in 2014 compared to 0.7 per 1,000 non-black African women.

Screening

Routine antenatal screening has increased detection rates and new treatments have dramatically increased life expectancy.

In the UK, all pregnant women should be offered screening for HIV early in pregnancy because appropriate antenatal interventions can reduce maternal-to-child transmission of HIV infection from 25–30% to less than 2%. Care needs to be taken to ensure that the woman understands the reasons for screening, and that appropriate interventions would be of benefit to her baby. She should also consider the consequences of a positive result prior to embarking on screening, but be reassured about confidentiality and support, should this be the case. A positive HIV antibody test result should be given to the woman in person by an appropriately trained health professional; this may be a specialist nurse, midwife, HIV physician or obstetrician. The issue of disclosure of the HIV diagnosis to her partner should be handled with sensitivity and she should be reassured that her confidentiality will be respected.

Some women remain at risk of becoming infected with HIV during their pregnancy. These women should be offered repeat testing during pregnancy. Rapid HIV tests should be offered to women who present for labour unbooked.

Clinical features

Infection with HIV begins with an asymptomatic stage with gradual compromise of immune function eventually leading to acquired immunodeficiency syndrome (AIDS). The time between HIV infection and development of AIDS ranges from a few months to as long as 17 years in untreated patients.

Management

The principal risks of mother to child (vertical) transmission are related to maternal plasma viral load, obstetric factors and infant feeding.

Interventions to reduce the risk of HIV transmission can reduce the risk of vertical transmission from 25–30% to less than 2%. These include (*Table 11.2*):

- Antiretroviral therapy, given antenatally and intrapartum to the mother and to the neonate for the first 4–6 weeks of life.

- Delivery by elective caesarean section in the presence of a high viral load.

- Avoidance of breastfeeding.

Table 11.2 Risk factors for vertical transmission of HIV

Increased risk of transmission	Reduced risk of transmission
Advanced maternal HIV disease	
High maternal plasma viral load	
Low CD4 lymphocyte counts	Low or undetectable viral counts at time of delivery
Prolonged rupture of membranes	Antiretroviral therapy
Chorioamnionitis	Delivery by caesarean section
Preterm delivery	
Coexisting viral infections (e.g. herpes, hepatitis C)	
Breastfeeding doubles transmission rate	Exclusive formula feeding

In the UK, where there is unrestricted access to interventions in pregnancy, the transmission rate has been estimated at 0.57%.

All women who are HIV positive should be advised to take antiretroviral therapy during pregnancy and at delivery. The optimal regime is determined by an HIV physician on a case-by-case basis. The decision to start, modify or stop antiretroviral therapy should be undertaken by an HIV physician. The choice of treatment and the gestation at which it is commenced will depend on whether the woman needs treatment for her own health or simply to prevent vertical transmission. It also depends on her viral load, viral resistance and whether the woman agrees to delivery by caesarean section.

Women who do NOT require HIV treatment for their own health should be offered antiretroviral therapy to prevent mother-to-child transmission. For these women antiretroviral therapy is usually commenced between 28 and 32 weeks' gestation and should be continued intrapartum. A maternal sample for plasma viral load should be taken at delivery. Antiretroviral therapy is usually discontinued soon after delivery but the precise time of discontinuation should be planned by the HIV physician.

A planned vaginal delivery is an option for women who have a viral load below 50 copies/ml at 36 weeks' gestation. Historically, it has been routine obstetric practice to avoid obstetric intervention in these women (amniotomy, use of fetal scalp electrodes, fetal blood sampling, instrumental delivery). However, a more recent review of the evidence suggests that in women with an undetectable viral load (<50 copies/ml), there is no evidence to support an increased risk of vertical transmission associated with these interventions. A caesarean delivery is recommended if a woman is taking azidothymidine (AZT), also known as zidovudine (ZDV), monotherapy or if viral load is above 50 copies/ml at or beyond 36 weeks' gestation. A caesarean delivery should also be recommended for women with hepatitis C coinfection as the risk of transmission is higher.

Women with a high viral load (>1,000 copies/ml) at the time of delivery should be given IV AZT if they are undergoing a planned caesarean section or present with spontaneous rupture of membranes.

Management of infants

The cord should be clamped as early as possible after delivery and the baby should be bathed immediately after the birth.

In the UK, where safe infant feeding alternatives are available, all women who are HIV positive should be advised not to breastfeed their babies as this increases the risk of mother-to-child transmission.

All infants born to women who are HIV positive should be treated with antiretroviral therapy from birth. AZT is usually administered orally to the neonate for 4–6 weeks, unless the mother started antiretroviral therapy late in pregnancy. Highly active antiretroviral therapy (HAART) may be considered for neonates of mothers who started antiretroviral therapy late in pregnancy.

Maternal antibodies crossing the placenta are detectable in most neonates of mother who are HIV positive. This means that neonates test positive for HIV antibodies. For this reason, direct viral amplification by PCR is used for the diagnosis of infant infections. Typically, tests are carried out at birth, then at 3 weeks, 6 weeks and 6 months.

 KEY LEARNING POINTS

- The prevalence of HIV is around 2 per 1,000 maternities in the UK; the majority of infected women are non-British born.
- Antiretroviral therapy is recommended in pregnancy and the choice, dosing and timing of therapy should be planned by an HIV physician.
- Successful treatment with viral suppression therapy can reduce the viral load to <50 copies/ml in most cases.
- Planned vaginal delivery is recommended (in the absence of other obstetric contraindications) in women with an undetectable viral load (<50 copies/ml) at or beyond 36 weeks' gestation.
- Planned caesarean section delivery should be offered to women with a high viral load in late pregnancy.
- Infants born to women with HIV should be treated with antiretroviral medications and follow routine newborn vaccination programmes.
- Women with HIV (regardless of viral load at delivery) should be advised against breastfeeding where safe alternatives are available.

Hepatitis B

Infective organism

The hepatitis B virus (HBV) is a DNA virus that is transmitted mainly in blood, but also in other body fluids such as saliva, semen and vaginal fluid. Drug users who share needles are at high risk. In some areas in the world (e.g. China), chronic hepatitis B is prevalent and vertical transmission is very common.

Prevalence

Two billion people worldwide are infected with HBV. More than 350 million have chronic (lifelong) infections.

In the UK, approximately 1 in 1,000 people are thought to have the virus. The prevalence of hepatitis B surface antigen (HBsAg) in pregnant women in the UK has been found to range from 0.5% to 1%. There is wide variation in prevalence among different ethnic groups, and oriental women in particular appear to have a higher prevalence of HBsAg.

Screening

Serological screening for HBV should be offered to pregnant women so that effective postnatal intervention can be offered to infected women to decrease the risk of mother-to-child transmission.

As many as 85% of babies born to mothers who are positive for the hepatitis e antigen (eAg) will become HBsAg carriers and subsequently become chronic carriers, compared with 31% of babies who are born to mothers who are eAg negative. It has been estimated that chronic carriers of HBsAg are 22 times more likely to die from hepatocellular carcinoma or cirrhosis than non-carriers.

Mother-to-child transmission of HBV is approximately 95% preventable through administration of vaccine and Ig to the baby at birth. To prevent mother-to-child transmission, all pregnant women who are carriers of HBV need to be identified. Because of the high proportion of cases of mother-to-child transmission that can be prevented through vaccination and immunization, the UK National Screening Committee recommends that all pregnant women be screened for HBV.

Clinical features

Hepatitis B is a virus that infects the liver, but many people with hepatitis B viral infection have no symptoms. The HBV has an incubation period of 6 weeks to 6 months.

Management

Women who screen positive for hepatitis B should be referred to a hepatologist for ongoing monitoring for the long-term consequences of chronic infection, for example hepatocellular carcinoma.

To prevent vertical transmission of hepatitis B, a combination of hepatitis B Ig and hepatitis B vaccine may be given. Virology laboratories will usually advise on the appropriate regime. The combined treatment provides better therapy than either alone. The passive Ig provides immediate protection against any virus transmitted to the baby from contact with blood during delivery, and should be given immediately after delivery. The active vaccine provides ongoing protection from subsequent exposure in the household. The active vaccine is given in three doses: at birth, at 1 month and at 6 months of age.

Hepatitis C

Infective organism

The hepatitis C virus (HCV) is a RNA virus. Acquisition of the virus occurs predominantly through infected blood products and injection of drugs. It can also occur with tattooing and body piercing. Mother-to-child transmission can occur due to contact with infected maternal blood around the time of delivery, and the risk is higher in those coinfected with HIV. Sexual transmission is extremely rare.

Prevalence

In the UK the overall antenatal prevalence has been estimated to be around 1%, with regional variation. The risk of mother-to-child transmission is estimated to lie between 3% and 5% and it is estimated that 70 births each year are infected with HCV as a result of mother-to-child transmission in the UK. The risk of mother-to-child transmission of HCV increases with increasing maternal viral load.

Screening

Current recommendations are that pregnant women should not be offered routine screening for HCV. This is because there is a lack of evidence-based effective interventions for the treatment of HCV in pregnancy, and a lack of evidence about which interventions reduce vertical transmission of HCV from mother to child.

Clinical features

HCV is a major public health concern due to its long-term consequences on health. It is one of the major causes of liver cirrhosis, hepatocellular carcinoma and liver failure. Following initial infection only 20% of women will have hepatic symptoms, 80% being asymptomatic. The majority of pregnant women with hepatitis C will not have reached the phase of having the chronic disease, and may well be unaware that they are infected.

Management

Testing for HCV in the UK involves detection of anti-HCV antibodies in serum with subsequent confirmatory testing by PCR for the virus, if a positive result is obtained. Upon confirmation of a positive test, a woman should be offered post-test counselling and referral to a hepatologist for management and treatment of her infection.

In non-pregnant adults, interferon and ribavirin can be used to treat hepatitis C infection, but these are contraindicated in pregnancy.

There is no strong evidence regarding mode of delivery in women with hepatitis C. Consensus groups therefore do not recommend elective caesarean section for all hepatitis C women, although it is recommended if the woman is also HIV positive.

New developments

In recent years a non-invasive method has been developed to diagnose and monitor fetal anaemia. This is done by using Doppler ultrasound to measure the velocity of blood flow in the fetal middle cerebral artery. Faster flow is indicative of fetal anaemia. This has improved the diagnosis and management of fetuses infected with parvovirus, as the main effect of this infection is anaemia.

Antiretroviral HIV therapies have been developed and research has focussed on which therapies are more appropriate for different groups of women.

Hepatitis B vaccination programmes are being extended worldwide. In some countries, such as Taiwan, this has already resulted in lower transmission rates and a reduction in childhood hepatocellular carcinoma.

Further research is needed into the treatment of hepatitis C in pregnancy with antiviral agents, and into the most appropriate mode of delivery in women with hepatitis C. The development of a hepatitis C vaccination would confer long-term health benefits.

KEY LEARNING POINTS

- Screening for infections in pregnancy is associated with a reduction in the burden of some long-term viral conditions – particularly HIV and hepatitis B.
- Active management of HIV infection in pregnancy dramatically reduces the risk of vertical transmission.
- Most treatments for infections are suitable for use in pregnancy (with a small number of exceptions) and treatment should not be withheld just because a woman is pregnant.
- A small number of infections can cause congenital anomalies in the fetus that can be picked up on antenatal ultrasound.

Further reading

Fetal anomaly screening programme. https://www.gov.uk/government/uploads/system/uploads/attachment_data/file/421650/FASP_Standards_April_2015_final_2_.pdf.

National Institute for Health and Care Excellence. Antenatal care. Available at http://www.nice.org.uk/guidance/qs22 (last accessed 01.02.2016).

Royal College of Obstetricians and Gynaecologists Clinical Guidelines. https://www.rcog.org.uk/guidelines.

The British HIV Association guidelines for the management of HIV infection. http://www.bhiva.org/documents/Guidelines/Pregnancy/2012/BHIVA-Pregnancy-guidelines-update-2014.pdf.

The Infectious Diseases in Pregnancy Screening (IDPS) Programme. UK National Screening Committee. September 2010. https://www.gov.uk/government/uploads/system/uploads/attachment_data/file/384721/IDPS_programme_standards_Revised_Final.pdf.

Self assessment

CASE HISTORY

A 26-year-old nursery worker attends the antenatal clinic complaining of reduced fetal movements at 28 weeks' gestation having been in contact with slapped cheek syndrome 6 weeks previously. She has an ultrasound scan performed that shows fetal ascites (**Figure 11.4**).

A What is the likely diagnosis and how might this be confirmed?

B What Doppler ultrasound test should be performed on the baby?

C What therapy could be considered for the fetus that may improve the outcome?

ANSWERS

A The diagnosis is likely to be acute parvovirus infection. This can be confirmed with a maternal blood test confirming IgM and/or new IgG antibodies. In addition, amniotic fluid can be tested for parvovirus by PCR.

B A middle cerebral artery Doppler can be performed (**Figure 11.5**), which may confirm fetal anaemia caused by aplastic anaemia.

C If the fetus is confirmed to be anaemic, intrauterine blood transfusion can be considered. This can potentially prolong the pregnancy until the fetus has recovered or has reached a gestation where it is safe to consider birth.

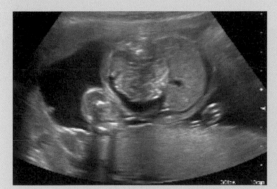

Figure 11.4 Fetal ascites. (Courtesy of Dr Ed Johnstone, St Mary's Hospital, Manchester.)

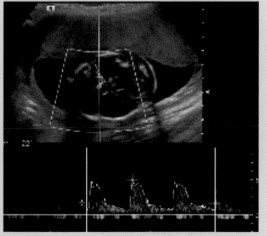

Figure 11.5 Middle cerebral Doppler to test for fetal anaemia. (Courtesy of Dr Ed Johnstone, St Mary's Hospital, Manchester.)

EMQ

A Aciclovir.
B Ampicillin.
C Azithromycin.
D Cefotaxime.

E Doxycycline.
F HAART.
G Penicillin.
H Zidovudine.

For each description, choose the SINGLE most appropriate answer from the list of options. Each option may be used once, more than once or not at all.

1 Treatment for syphilis in pregnancy that pre-vents 98% of congenital infections.

2 Treatment to prevent neonatal infection with GBS infection.

3 Treatment to reduce the vertical transmission of HIV virus from 28 weeks' gestation.

4 Treatment for primary genital herpes infection in pregnancy.

ANSWERS

1G Parenteral penicillin (IV and IM) is the standard treatment for syphilis in pregnancy.

2G Penicillin in the form of IV benzylpenicillin is given to women in whom GBS infection has been isolated in the antenatal period.

3F HAART should be prescribed (where possible) to women with HIV in the third trimester.

4A Aciclovir is the standard treatment for genital herpes.

SBA QUESTIONS

Choose the single best answer.

1 An antenatal patient tests positive for syphilis using the VDRL screening test. Which of the following is a definitive test for syphilis?

A Cholesterol-lecithin – cardiolipin antigen test.
B FTA-abs test.
C PCR.
D RPR test.
E Ziehl–Neelsen stain.

ANSWER

B The VDRL is a nontreponemal serological screening for syphilis. The basis of the test is that an anti-body produced by a patient with syphilis reacts with an extract of ox heart (diphosphatidyl glycerol). It therefore detects anti-cardiolipin antibodies (IgG, IgM or IgA), visualized through foaming of the test tube fluid, or 'flocculation'.

   The RPR test uses the same antigen as the VDRL, but in that test it has been bound to several other molecules including a carbon particle to allow visualization of the flocculation reaction without the need of a microscope. Both tests are used as screening tests and have a false-positive rate, so anyone who screens positive must have a definitive diagnostic test such as the FTA-abs test. This test uses antibodies specific for the *Treponema pallidum* species.

   The Ziehl–Neelsen stain is a bacteriological stain used to identify acid-fast organisms, mainly mycobacteria. PCR is a technique used in molecular biology to amplify a single copy or a few copies of a piece of DNA.

2 A nursery nurse who is 18 weeks pregnant rings to say that children at her nursery have been diagnosed with slapped cheek syndrome. Which of the following antibodies would be evidence of a recent infection?

A IgA to parvovirus.
B IgG to CMV.
C IgG to parvovirus.
D IgM to CMV.
E IgM to parvovirus

ANSWER

E Slapped cheek syndrome or disease (also known as erythema infectiosum or fifth disease) is caused by infection with parvovirus B19. A recent infection is characterized by the presence of IgM to parvovirus, whereas a previous infection would be characterized by IgG antibodies.

3 Which class of white cells are preferentially depleted by HIV?

A CD4.
B CD8.
C CD16.
D CD25.
E CD68.

ANSWER

A CD4 (cluster of differentiation 4) is a glycoprotein found on the surface of immune cells such as T helper cells, monocytes, macrophages and dendritic cells. HIV infection leads to a progressive reduction in the number of T cells expressing CD4.

4 A woman presents with an ulcerated lesion on a vulva and urinary retention. What is the most likely cause?

A Candida.
B HPV.
C HSV.
D Syphilis.
E *Trichomonas vaginalis.*

ANSWER

C Candida is a yeast infection that typically presents with a white, non-offensive vaginal discharge and vaginal irritation. *Trichomonas vaginalis* is a flagellated protozoan parasite and infection typically presents with an offensive vaginal discharge and irritation. Syphilis presents with a painless ulcer or chancre, and HPV infection may present with genital warts. HSV causes genital herpes and typically presents with painful ulcers and urinary retention.

Labour: normal and abnormal

DEIRDRE J MURPHY

LEARNING OBJECTIVES

- To understand the maternal and fetal anatomy relevant to labour and delivery.
- To understand the physiological principles of labour and delivery.
- To understand the contributors to normal labour and its management.
- To understand the contributors to abnormal labour and its management.
- To introduce the social, psychological and governance elements of labour and delivery.

Introduction

Labour or human parturition is the physiological process that results in birth of a baby, delivery of the placenta and the signal for lactation to begin. At a human level it is a major life event for the woman and her partner that heralds the start of parenting. In terms of providing care to a woman in labour, attention must be paid to safety and clinical outcomes but also to her emotional wellbeing and the desire for a fulfilling birth experience. Normal labour requires observation and support and falls within the expertise of midwifery care. Abnormal labour must be recognized and acted upon, and requires a multidisciplinary team including a midwife, obstetrician, anaesthetist and neonatologist. While most labours result in a positive outcome, some labours result in tragedy and each health care team needs to have the skill set to care for women and their families through all types of outcome.

Health professionals who manage labour must have an understanding of the anatomy and physiology of the mother and fetus, what distinguishes a normal from an abnormal labour, when it is appropriate to intervene, how to intervene safely and how to support the woman and her partner through unexpected labour events. The first important step is to recognize when labour has started. Labour is then divided into three stages: the first stage begins with diagnosis of the onset of labour and is complete when full cervical dilatation has been reached; the second stage begins with full cervical dilatation and ends with birth of the baby; and the third stage begins with birth of the baby and ends with complete delivery of the placenta and membranes. Complications can occur during any of the three stages and can be divided into maternal and fetal-neonatal complications.

An understanding of the physiological and anatomical principles involved in normal and abnormal labour is best summarized using the '3 Ps', which are the powers, the passages and the passenger. The 'powers' refers to forces, firstly the contractions of the uterine muscle that result in passage of the fetus through the birth canal, and secondly the maternal effort of pushing in the second stage of labour. The 'passages' refers to the birth canal itself, which is made up of the bony pelvis, the muscles of the pelvic floor and the soft tissues of the perineum. The 'passenger' refers to the fetus in terms of its size (small, average, large), presentation (that part of the fetus entering the pelvis first, e.g. vertex of head, face, brow or breech) and position (orientation of the presenting part in relation to the maternal public symphysis, e.g. occipito-anterior, occipito-posterior). When the 3Ps are favourable, normal labour is likely to ensue, resulting in an unassisted or spontaneous vaginal birth.

When any of the 3Ps are unfavourable, labour is likely to be abnormal, resulting in the need for intervention and with that, an increased risk of morbidity or mortality. It is important that labour and its outcomes are audited locally, nationally and internationally, to ensure that the best outcomes are achieved and that lessons are learned where adverse events occur. Priorities, choices and outcomes are very different depending on whether a woman gives birth in a developed or developing-world setting. Even within well-resourced settings there can be marked differences in the perspectives of women and their care providers, reflected in differences in place of birth, choice of care provider, analgesia use, mode of delivery and outcomes for mothers and babies. Labour and childbirth has physical, psychological, social, cultural and political dimensions, which makes it a very interesting area to work in.

Maternal and fetal anatomy

The maternal pelvis

The pelvic inlet

The pelvic inlet or brim is bounded anteriorly by the upper border of the symphysis pubis (the joint separating the two pubic bones), laterally by the upper margin of the pubic bone, the ileopectineal line and the ala of the sacrum, and posteriorly by the promontory of the sacrum (**Figure 12.1**). The normal transverse diameter in this plane is 13.5 cm and is wider than the anterior–posterior (A–P) diameter, which is normally 11.0 cm (**Figure 12.2**).

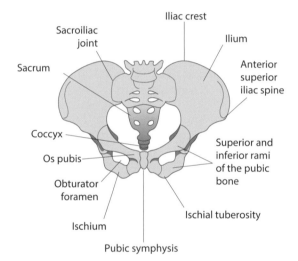

Figure 12.1 The bony pelvis.

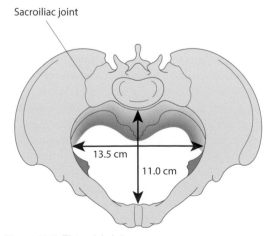

Figure 12.2 The pelvic brim.

The fetal head typically enters the pelvis orientated in a transverse position in keeping with the wider transverse diameter. The angle of the inlet is normally 60° to the horizontal in the erect position, but in Afro-Caribbean women this angle may be as much as 90°. This increased angle may delay the head entering and descending through the pelvis during labour compared to labour in Caucasian women.

The midpelvis

The midpelvis, also known as the midcavity, can be described as an area bounded anteriorly by the middle of the symphysis pubis, laterally by the pubic bones, the obturator fascia and the inner aspect of the ischial bone and spines, and posteriorly by the junction of the second and third sections of the sacrum. The midpelvis is almost round, as the transverse and anterior diameters are similar at 12 cm. The ischial spines are palpable vaginally and are used as important landmarks for two purposes:

- To assess the descent of the presenting part on vaginal examination (e.g. station zero is at the level of the ischial spines, −1 is 1 cm above the spines and +1 is 1 cm below the spines).

- To provide a local anaesthetic pudendal nerve block. The pudendal nerve passes behind and below the ischial spine on each side. A pudendal nerve block may be used for a vacuum or forceps-assisted delivery.

Station zero is an important landmark clinically because instrumental delivery can only be performed if the fetal head has reached the level of the ischial spines or below.

The pelvic outlet

The pelvic outlet is bounded anteriorly by the lower margin of the symphysis pubis, laterally by the descending ramus of the pubic bone, the ischial tuberosity and the sacrotuberous ligament, and posteriorly by the last piece of the sacrum. The AP diameter of the pelvic outlet is 13.5 cm and the transverse diameter is 11 cm (**Figures 12.3, 12.4**). Therefore, the transverse is the widest diameter at the inlet, but at the outlet it is the AP diameter, and the fetal head must rotate from a transverse to an AP position as it passes through the pelvis. Typically, this happens in the midpelvis where the transverse and AP diameters are similar. In addition, the pelvic axis describes an imaginary curved line, a path that the

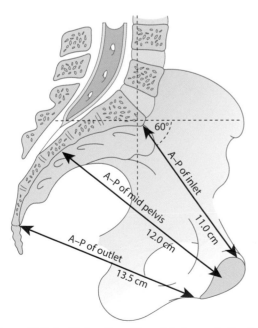

Figure 12.3 Sagittal section of the pelvis demonstrating the anterior–posterior (A–P) diameters of the inlet and outlet.

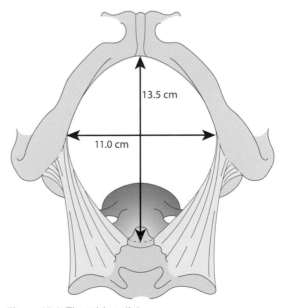

Figure 12.4 The pelvic outlet.

centre of the fetal head must take during its passage through the pelvis, from entry at the inlet, descent and rotation in the midpelvis and exit at the outlet. Recognizing the important features of the maternal pelvis is central to understanding the mechanism of labour.

Pelvic shape

The pelvic measurements described above are average values and relate to bony points. Maternal stature, ethnicity, previous pelvic fractures and metabolic bone disease, such as rickets, may all be associated with measurements less than the population average. Furthermore, as the pelvic ligaments at the pubic ramus and the sacroiliac joints loosen towards the end of the third trimester, the pelvis becomes more flexible and these diameters may increase during labour. It is also possible to enhance the pelvic dimensions with more favourable maternal positions in labour (e.g. squatting or kneeling). It is now uncommon to perform X-rays or computed tomography (CT) or magnetic resonance imaging (MRI) of the pelvis to measure the pelvic dimensions because they have, on the whole, proven to be of little clinical use in predicting the outcome of labour. A variety of pelvic shapes are described, and these may contribute to difficulties encountered in labour. The gynaecoid pelvis is the most favourable for labour, and also the most common (**Figure 12.5**). Other pelvic shapes are shown in **Figures 12.6–12.8**. An android-type pelvis is said to predispose to failure of rotation and deep transverse arrest and the anthropoid shape encourages an occipito-posterior (OP) position. A platypelloid pelvis is also associated with an increased risk of obstructed labour due to failure of the head to engage, rotate or descend.

The pelvic floor

This is formed by the two levator ani muscles which, with their fascia, form a musculofascial gutter during the second stage of labour (**Figure 12.9**). The configuration of the bony pelvis together with the gutter-shaped pelvic floor muscles encourage the

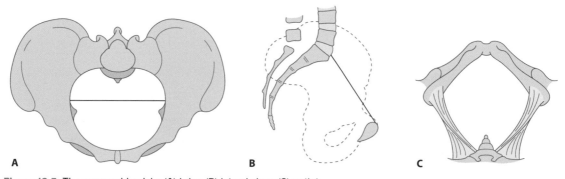

Figure 12.5 The gynaecoid pelvis: (**A**) brim; (**B**) lateral view; (**C**) outlet.

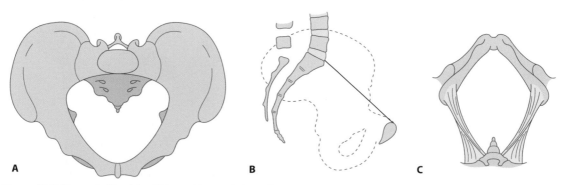

Figure 12.6 The android pelvis: (**A**) brim; (**B**) lateral view; (**C**) outlet.

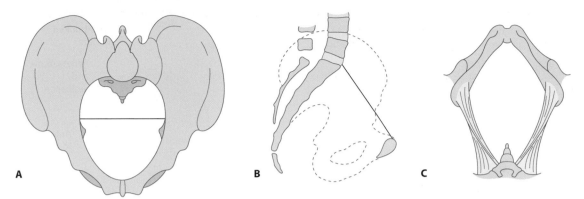

Figure 12.7 The anthropoid pelvis: (**A**) brim; (**B**) lateral view; (**C**) outlet.

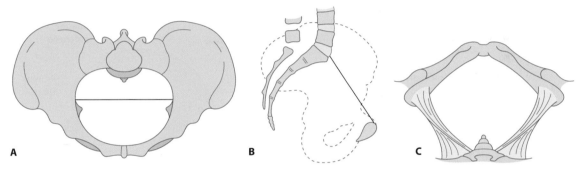

Figure 12.8 The platypelloid pelvis: (**A**) brim; (**B**) lateral view; (**C**) outlet.

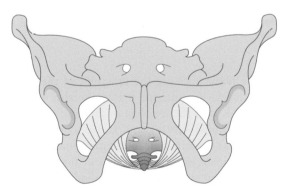

Figure 12.9 The musculofascial gutter of the levator sling.

fetal head to flex and rotate as it descends through the midpelvis towards the pelvic outlet.

The perineum

The final obstacle to be overcome by the fetus during labour is the perineum. The perineal body is a condensation of fibrous and muscular tissue lying between the vagina and the anus (**Figure 12.10**). It receives attachments of the posterior ends of the bulbo-cavernous muscles, the medial ends of the superficial and deep transverse perineal muscles and the anterior fibres of the external anal sphincter. The perineum is taut and relatively resistant in the nulliparous woman, and pushing can be prolonged. Vaginal birth may result in tearing of the perineum and pelvic floor muscles or an episiotomy (surgical cut) may be required. The perineum is stretchy and less resistant in multiparous women, resulting in faster labour and a higher probability of delivering with an intact perineum.

The fetal skull

The skull bones, sutures and fontanelles

The fetal skull is made up of the vault, the face and the base. The sutures are the lines formed where the individual bony plates of the skull meet one another. At the time of labour, the sutures

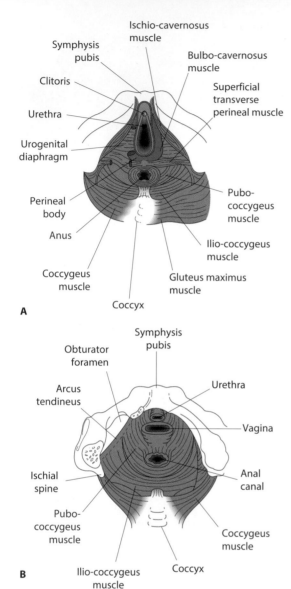

Figure 12.10 The perineum, perineal body and pelvic floor from below, showing superficial (**A**) and deeper (**B**) views. The pelvic floor muscles are made up of the levator ani (pubo-coccygeus and ilio-coccygeus).

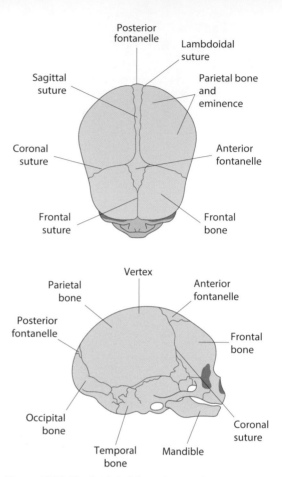

Figure 12.11 The fetal skull from the superior and lateral views.

joining the bones of the vault are soft, unossified membranes, whereas the sutures of the fetal face and the skull base are firmly united (**Figure 12.11**). The vault of the skull is composed of the parietal bones and parts of the occipital, frontal and temporal bones. Between these bones there are four membranous sutures: the sagittal, frontal, coronal and lambdoidal sutures.

The fontanelles are the junctions of the various sutures. The anterior fontanelle, also known as bregma, is at the junction of the sagittal, frontal and coronal sutures, and is diamond shaped. On vaginal examination four suture lines can be felt. The posterior fontanelle lies at the junction of the sagittal suture and the lambdoidal sutures between the two parietal bones and the occipital bone, and is smaller and triangular shaped. On vaginal examination three suture lines can be felt. The fact that the sutures are not fixed is important for labour. It allows the bones to move together and even to overlap. The parietal bones usually slide over the frontal and occipital bones. Furthermore, the bones themselves are compressible. Together, these characteristics of the fetal skull allow a process called 'moulding' to occur, which reduces the

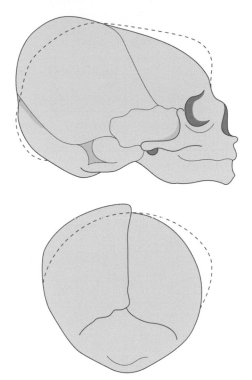

Figure 12.12 Schematic representation of moulding of the fetal skull.

diameters of the fetal head and encourages progress through the bony pelvis, while still protecting the underlying brain (**Figure 12.12**). However, severe moulding, or moulding early in labour, can be a sign of obstructed labour due to a fetal malposition (failure of the head to rotate) or cephalopelvic disproportion (a mismatch between the size of the fetal head and maternal pelvis). The area of the fetal skull bounded by the two parietal eminences and the anterior and posterior fontanelles is termed the 'vertex'. In normal labour the vertex of the fetal head is the presenting part and the posterior fontanelle (indicating the occiput) is used to define the position of the fetal head in relation to the pubic symphysis. The anatomical differences between the anterior and posterior fontanelles on vaginal examination facilitate correct diagnosis of the fetal head position in labour. The occipito-anterior (OA) position is the most favourable for a spontaneous vaginal birth. The occipito-transverse (OT) position or OP position is a malposition and may result in prolonged labour, instrumental delivery or caesarean section.

The diameters of the skull

The fetal head is ovoid in shape. The attitude of the fetal head refers to the degree of flexion and extension at the upper cervical spine. Different longitudinal diameters are presented to the pelvis in labour depending on the attitude of the fetal head (**Figures 12.13, 12.14**). The longitudinal diameter that presents with a flexed attitude of the fetal head (chin on the chest) is the suboccipito-bregmatic diameter. This is usually 9.5 cm and is measured from beneath the occiput (suboccipital) to the centre of the anterior fontanelle (bregma). The longitudinal diameter that presents in a less well-flexed head, such as is found in an OP position, is the suboccipito-frontal diameter. It is measured from the suboccipital region to the prominence of the forehead and measures 10 cm.

With further extension of the head, the occipito-frontal diameter presents (deflexed OP). This is measured from the root of the nose to the posterior fontanelle and is 11.5 cm. The greatest longitudinal diameter that may present is the mento-vertical, which is taken from the chin to the furthest point of the vertex and measures 13 cm. This is known as a brow presentation and it is usually too large to pass through the normal pelvis. Extension of the fetal head beyond this point results in a smaller diameter. The submento-bregmatic diameter is measured from below the chin to the anterior fontanelle and is 9.5 cm. This is termed a face presentation. A face presentation can deliver vaginally when the chin is anterior (mento-anterior position).

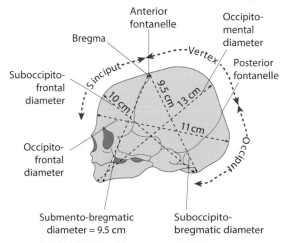

Figure 12.13 The diameters of the fetal skull.

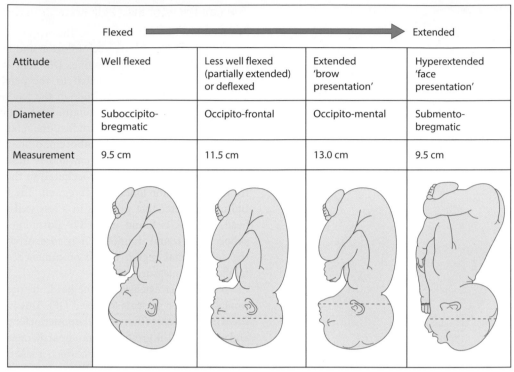

	Flexed $\longrightarrow$ Extended			
Attitude	Well flexed	Less well flexed (partially extended) or deflexed	Extended 'brow presentation'	Hyperextended 'face presentation'
Diameter	Suboccipito-bregmatic	Occipito-frontal	Occipito-mental	Submento-bregmatic
Measurement	9.5 cm	11.5 cm	13.0 cm	9.5 cm

Figure 12.14 The effect of fetal attitude on the presenting diameter.

KEY LEARNING POINTS

- The pelvic inlet is wider in the transverse than in the AP diameter.
- The pelvic outlet is wider in the AP than in the transverse diameter.
- The ischial spines are located in the midpelvis and denote station zero.
- The fetal head enters the pelvis in a transverse position, rotates in the midpelvis and delivers in an AP position.
- Pelvic dimensions may increase during labour due to pelvic ligament laxity.
- The shape of the pelvis and pelvic floor muscles aid flexion and rotation of the fetal head.
- The sutures and fontanelles are used to assess the position and attitude of the fetal head.
- Moulding of the skull bones during labour reduces the measurements of the fetal head.
- A fetus in a flexed OA position with a gynaecoid pelvis is most favourable for vaginal birth.
- Perineal tissues offer resistance to delivery especially in a nulliparous woman.

Physiology of labour

The mechanisms underlying human parturition are not fully understood and differ from other animal models that have been studied. In particular, the process that initiates labour is poorly understood. There are a number of important elements. The cervix, which is initially long, firm, and closed, with a protective mucus plug, must soften, shorten, thin out (effacement) and dilate for labour to progress. The uterus must change from a state of relaxation to an active state of regular, strong, frequent contractions to facilitate transit of the fetus through the birth canal. Each contraction must be followed by a resting phase in order to maintain placental blood flow and adequate perfusion of the fetus. The pressure of the presenting part on the pelvic floor muscles as the fetus descends from the midpelvis to the pelvic outlet produces a maternal urge to push, enhanced further by stretching of the perineum.

The onset of labour occurs when the factors that inhibit contractions and maintain a closed cervix diminish and are overtaken by the actions of factors that do the opposite. Both mother and fetus appear to contribute to this process.

The uterus

Myometrial cells of the uterus contain filaments of actin and myosin, which interact and bring about contractions in response to an increase in intracellular calcium. Prostaglandins and oxytocin increase intracellular free calcium ions, whereas beta-adrenergic compounds and calcium-channel blockers do the opposite. Separation of the actin and myosin filaments brings about relaxation of the myocyte; however, unlike any other muscle cell of the body, this actin–myosin interaction occurs along the full length of the filaments so that a degree of shortening occurs with each successive interaction. This progressive shortening of the uterine smooth muscle cells is called retraction and occurs in the cells of the upper part of the uterus. The result of this retraction process is the development of the thicker, actively contracting 'upper segment'. At the same time, the lower segment of the uterus becomes thinner and more stretched. Eventually, this results in the cervix being 'taken up' (effacement) into the lower segment of the uterus so forming a continuum with the lower uterine segment (**Figure 12.15**). The cervix effaces

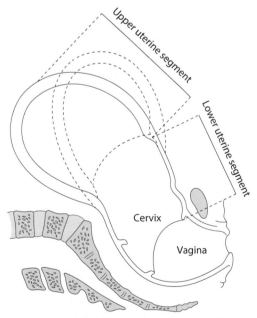

Figure 12.15 The thick upper segment and the thin lower segment of the uterus at the end of the first stage of labour. The dotted lines indicate the position assumed by the uterus during contraction.

and then dilates, and the fetus descends in response to this directional force.

It is essential that the myocytes of the uterus contract in a coordinated way. Individual myometrial cells are laid down in a mesh of collagen. There is cell-to-cell communication by means of gap junctions, which facilitate the passage of various products of metabolism and electrical current between cells. These gap junctions are absent for most of the pregnancy but appear in significant numbers at term. Gap junctions increase in size and number with the progress of labour and allow greater coordination of myocyte activity. Prostaglandins stimulate their formation, while beta-adrenergic compounds are thought to do the opposite. A uterine pacemaker from which contractions originate probably exists but has not been demonstrated histologically.

Uterine contractions are involuntary in nature and there is relatively little extrauterine neuronal control. The frequency of contractions may vary during labour and with parity. Throughout the majority of labour, they occur at intervals of 2–4 minutes and are described in terms of the frequency within a 10-minute period (i.e. 2 in 10 increasing to 4–5 in 10 in advanced labour). Their duration also varies during labour, from 30 to 60 seconds or occasionally longer. The frequency of contractions can be recorded on a cardiotocograph (CTG) using a pressure transducer (tocodynamometer) positioned on the abdomen at the fundus of the uterus. The intensity or amplitude of the intrauterine pressure generated with each contraction averages between 30 and 60 mmHg.

The cervix

The cervix contains myocytes and fibroblasts separated by a 'ground substance' made up of extracellular matrix molecules. Interactions between collagen, fibronectin and dermatan sulphate (a proteoglycan) during the earlier stages of pregnancy keep the cervix firm and closed. Contractions at this point do not bring about effacement or dilatation. Under the influence of prostaglandins, and other humoral mediators, there is an increase in proteolytic activity and a reduction in collagen and elastin. Interleukins bring about a proinflammatory change with a significant invasion by neutrophils. Dermatan sulphate is replaced by the more hydrophilic hyaluronic acid, which results in an increase in water content of the cervix. This causes cervical softening or 'ripening', so that contractions, when they begin, can bring about the processes of effacement and dilatation.

Hormonal factors

Progesterone maintains uterine relaxation by suppressing prostaglandin production, inhibiting communication between myometrial cells and preventing oxytocin release. Oestrogen opposes the action of progesterone. Prior to labour, there is a reduction in progesterone receptors and an increase in the concentration of oestrogen relative to progesterone. Prostaglandin synthesis by the chorion and the decidua is enhanced, leading to an increase in calcium influx into the myometrial cells. This change in the hormonal milieu also increases gap junction formation between individual myometrial cells, creating a functional syncytium, which is necessary for coordinated uterine activity. The production of corticotrophin-releasing hormone (CRH) by the placenta increases in concentration towards term and potentiates the action of prostaglandins and oxytocin on myometrial contractility. The fetal pituitary secretes oxytocin and the fetal adrenal gland produces cortisol, which stimulates the conversion of progesterone to oestrogen.

It is unclear which of these hormonal changes actually initiates labour. As labour becomes established, the output of oxytocin increases through the 'Fergusson reflex'. Pressure from the fetal presenting part against the cervix is relayed via a reflex arc involving the spinal cord and results in increased oxytocin release from the maternal posterior pituitary.

Normal labour

Diagnosis of labour

The onset of labour can be defined as the presence of strong regular painful contractions resulting in progressive cervical change. Therefore, a diagnosis of labour strictly speaking requires more than one vaginal examination after an interval and is made in retrospect. In practice, the diagnosis is suspected when a woman presents with contraction-like pains, and

is confirmed when the midwife performs a vaginal examination that reveals effacement and dilatation of the cervix. Loss of a 'show' (a blood-stained plug of mucus passed from the cervix) or spontaneous rupture of the membranes (SROM) does not define the onset of labour, although these events may occur around the same time. Labour can be well established before either of these events occurs, and both may precede labour by many days. Although much is understood about the physiology of labour in humans, the initiating process is still unclear. It is certainly true, however, that the uterus and cervix undergo a number of changes in preparation for labour, which start a number of weeks before its onset.

Stages of labour

Labour can be divided into three stages. The definitions of these stages rely predominantly on anatomical criteria, and in real terms the moment of transition from first to second stage may not be apparent. The important events when labour is normal are the diagnosis of labour and the maternal urge to push, which usually corresponds with full dilatation of the cervix and the baby's head resting on the perineum. Defining the three stages of labour becomes more relevant if labour is not progressing normally. The average duration of a first labour is 8 hours, and that of a subsequent labour 5 hours. First labour rarely lasts more than 18 hours, and second and subsequent labours not usually more than 12 hours.

First stage

This describes the time from the diagnosis of labour to full dilatation of the cervix (10 cm). The first stage of labour can be divided into two phases. The 'latent phase' is the time between the onset of regular painful contractions and 3–4 cm cervical dilatation. During this time, the cervix becomes 'fully effaced'. Effacement is a process by which the cervix shortens in length as it becomes incorporated into the lower segment of the uterus. The process of effacement may begin during the weeks preceding the onset of labour, but will be complete by the end of the latent phase. Effacement and dilatation should be thought of as consecutive events in the nulliparous woman, but they may occur simultaneously in the multiparous woman. Dilatation is expressed in centimetres from 0 to 10 cm. The duration of the latent phase is variable, and time limits are arbitrary. However, it usually lasts between 3 and 8 hours, being shorter in multiparous women.

The second phase of the first stage of labour is called the 'active phase' and describes the time between the end of the latent phase (3–4 cm dilatation) and full cervical dilatation (10 cm). It is also variable in length, usually lasting between 2 and 6 hours, shorter in multiparous women. Cervical dilatation during the active phase occurs typically at 1 cm/hour or more in a normal labour (again, an arbitrary value), but is only considered abnormal if it occurs at less than 1 cm in 2 hours.

Second stage

This describes the time from full dilatation of the cervix to delivery of the fetus or fetuses. The second stage of labour may also be subdivided into two phases. The 'passive phase' describes the time between full dilatation and the onset of involuntary expulsive contractions. There is no maternal urge to push and the fetal head is still relatively high in the pelvis. The second phase is called the 'active second stage'. There is a maternal urge to push because the fetal head is low (often visible), causing a reflex need to 'bear down'. In a normal labour, the second stage is often diagnosed at this late point because the maternal urge to push prompts the midwife to perform a vaginal examination. If a woman never reaches a point of involuntary pushing, the active second stage is said to begin when she starts making voluntary pushing efforts directed by her midwife. Conventionally, a normal active second stage should last no longer than 2 hours in a nulliparous woman and 1 hour in women who delivered vaginally before. Again, these definitions are fairly arbitrary, but there is evidence that a second stage of labour lasting more than 3 hours is associated with increased maternal and fetal morbidity. Use of epidural anaesthesia will influence the length and management of the second stage of labour. A passive second stage of 1 or 2 hours is usually recommended to allow the head to rotate and descend prior to active pushing.

Third stage

This is the time from delivery of the fetus or fetuses until complete delivery of the placenta(e) and membranes. The placenta is usually delivered within a few minutes of the birth of the baby. A third stage lasting more than 30 minutes is defined as abnormal, unless the woman has opted for 'physiological management' (see below under Management of third stage), in which case it is reasonable to extend this definition to 60 minutes.

The duration of labour

There is no ideal length of labour for all women but morbidity increases when labour is too fast (precipitous) or two slow (prolonged). From a psychological perspective, the morale of most women starts to deteriorate after 6 hours in labour, and after 12 hours the rate of deterioration accelerates. There is a greater incidence of fetal hypoxia and need for operative delivery associated with longer labours. It is difficult to define prolonged labour, but it would be reasonable to suggest that labour lasting longer than 12 hours in nulliparous women and 8 hours in multiparous women should be regarded as prolonged. Precipitous labour is defined as expulsion of the fetus within less than 3 hours of the onset of regular contractions.

The mechanism of labour

This refers to the series of changes in position and attitude that the fetus undergoes during its passage through the birth canal. It is described here for the vertex presentation and the gynaecoid pelvis. The relation of the fetal head and body to the maternal pelvis changes as the fetus descends through the pelvis. This is essential so that the optimal diameters of the fetal skull are present at each stage of the descent.

 VIDEO 12.1

The mechanism of a spontaneous vaginal delivery: http://www.routledgetextbooks.com/textbooks/tenteachers/obstetricsv12.1.php

Engagement

The fetal head normally enters the pelvis in the transverse position or some minor variant of this, taking advantage of the widest pelvic diameter. Engagement is said to have occurred when the widest part of the presenting part has passed successfully through the inlet. Engagement has occurred in the vast majority of nulliparous women prior to labour, usually by 37 weeks' gestation, but not so for the majority of multiparous women. The number of fifths of the fetal head palpable abdominally is used to describe whether engagement has taken place. If more than two-fifths of the fetal head is palpable abdominally, the head is not yet engaged.

Descent

Descent of the fetal head is needed before flexion, internal rotation and extension can occur (**Figure 12.16**). During the first stage and passive phase of the second stage of labour, descent of the fetus occurs as a result of uterine contractions. In the active phase of the second stage of labour, descent of the fetus is assisted by voluntary efforts of the mother using her abdominal muscles and the Valsalva manoeuvre ('pushing').

Flexion

The fetal head is not always completely flexed when it enters the pelvis. As the head descends into the narrower midpelvis, flexion occurs. This passive movement occurs, in part, due to the surrounding structures and is important in reducing the presenting diameter of the fetal head.

Internal rotation

If the head is well flexed, the occiput will be the leading point, and on reaching the sloping gutter of the levator ani muscles it will be encouraged to rotate anteriorly so that the sagittal suture now lies in the AP diameter of the pelvic outlet (i.e. the widest diameter). If the fetus has engaged in the OP position,

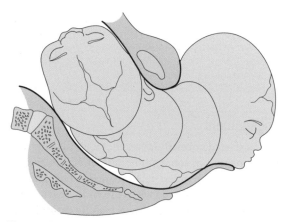

Figure 12.16 Descent and flexion of the head followed by internal rotation and ending of the head by extension.

internal rotation can occur from an OP position to an OA position. This long internal rotation may explain the increased duration of labour associated with OP position. Alternatively, an OP position may persist, resulting in a 'face to pubes' delivery. Furthermore, the persistent OP position may be associated with extension of the fetal head and a resulting increase in the diameter presented to the pelvic outlet. This may lead to obstructed labour and the need for instrumental delivery or even caesarean section.

Extension

Following completion of internal rotation, the occiput is beneath the symphysis pubis and the bregma is near the lower border of the sacrum. The well-flexed head now extends and the occiput escapes from underneath the symphysis pubis and distends the vulva. This is known as 'crowning' of the head. The head extends further and the occiput underneath the symphysis pubis acts as a fulcrum point as the bregma, face and chin appear in succession over the posterior vaginal opening and perineal body. This extension process, if controlled, reduces the risk of perineal trauma. However, the soft tissues of the perineum offer resistance, and some degree of tearing occurs in the majority of first births.

Restitution

When the head is delivering, the occiput is directly anterior. As soon as it crosses the perineum, the head aligns itself with the shoulders, which have entered the pelvis in the oblique position. This slight rotation of the occiput through one-eighth of the circle is called 'restitution'.

External rotation

In order to be delivered, the shoulders have to rotate into the direct AP plane (remember, the widest diameter at the outlet). When this occurs, the occiput rotates through a further one-eighth of a circle to the transverse position. This is called external rotation (**Figure 12.17**).

Delivery of the shoulders and fetal body

When restitution and external rotation have occurred, the shoulders will be in the AP position. The anterior shoulder is under the symphysis pubis and delivers first, and the posterior shoulder delivers subsequently. Although this process may occur

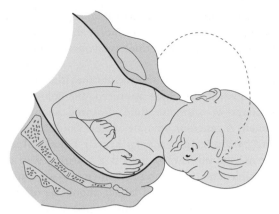

Figure 12.17 External rotation of the head after delivery as the anterior shoulder rotates forward to pass under the suprapubic arch.

without assistance, traction is often exerted by gently pulling the fetal head in a downward direction along the axis of the pelvis to help release the anterior shoulder from beneath the pubic symphysis.

Normally the rest of the fetal body is delivered easily, with the posterior shoulder guided over the perineum by gentle upward traction in the opposite direction, so delivering the baby on to the maternal abdomen.

Management of normal labour

Women are advised to contact their local labour suite or their community midwife if they think their waters may have broken (SROM) or when their contractions are occurring every 5 minutes or more. It is important to recognize that women have very different thresholds for seeking advice and reassurance. The need for pain relief may result in admission to hospital before either of these two criteria is reached. Whether at home or in hospital, the attending midwife will then make an assessment of the situation based on the history and on clinical examination, and the preferences of the woman.

History

A detailed history should be taken including past obstetric history, history of the current pregnancy, relevant medical history and events leading up to hospital attendance.

Admission history

- Previous births and size of previous babies.
- Previous caesarean section.
- Onset, frequency, duration and perception of strength of the contractions.
- Whether membranes have ruptured and, if so, colour and amount of amniotic fluid lost.
- Presence of abnormal vaginal discharge or bleeding.
- Recent activity of the fetus (fetal movement).
- Medical or obstetric issues of note (e.g. diabetes, hypertension, fetal growth restriction [FGR]).
- Any special requirements (e.g. an interpreter or particular emotional/psychological needs).
- Maternal expectations of labour and delivery?
- Birth preferences or a birth plan?

General examination

It is important to identify women who have a raised body mass index (BMI), as this may complicate the management of labour. The temperature, pulse and blood pressure must be recorded and a sample of urine tested for protein, blood, ketones, glucose and nitrates.

Abdominal examination

After the initial inspection for scars indicating previous surgery, it is important to determine the lie of the fetus (longitudinal, transverse or oblique) and the nature of the presenting part (cephalic or breech). If it is a cephalic presentation, the degree of engagement must be determined in terms of fifths palpable abdominally. A head that remains high (five-fifths palpable) and unengaged (more than two-fifths palpable) is a poor prognostic sign for successful vaginal delivery. If there is any doubt as to the presentation or if the head is high, an ultrasound scan should be performed to confirm the presenting part or the reason for the high head (e.g. OP position, deflexed head, placenta praevia, fibroid, etc).

Abdominal examination also includes an assessment of the contractions; this takes time (at least 10 minutes) and is done by palpating the uterus directly, not by looking at the tocograph. The tocograph provides reliable information on the frequency, regularity and duration of contractions, but not the strength (see below).

Vaginal examination

The purpose and technique of vaginal examination is explained to the woman and her consent must be obtained. Most women find vaginal examinations uncomfortable and every effort should be made to maintain the woman's dignity and privacy. The index and middle fingers are passed to the top of the vagina and the cervix. The cervix is examined for position, length and effacement, consistency, dilatation and application to the presenting part. The length of the cervix at 36 weeks' gestation is about 3 cm. It gradually shortens by the process of effacement and may still be uneffaced in early labour. The dilatation is estimated digitally in centimetres. At about 4 cm of dilatation, the cervix should be fully effaced. Providing the cervix is at least 4 cm dilated, it should be possible to determine both the position and the station of the presenting part. When no cervix can be felt, this means the cervix is fully dilated (10 cm).

A vaginal examination also allows assessment of the fetal head position, station, attitude and the presence of caput or moulding. In normal labour, the vertex will be presenting and the position can be determined by locating the occiput. The occiput is identified by feeling for the triangular posterior fontanelle and the three suture lines. Failure to feel the posterior fontanelle may be because the head is deflexed (abnormal attitude), the occiput is posterior (malposition) or there is so much caput and moulding that the sutures cannot be felt. All of these indicate the possibility of a prolonged labour or a degree of mechanical obstruction. Normally, the occiput will be transverse (OT position) or anterior (OA position). Relating the leading part of the head to the ischial spines will give an estimation of the station. This vaginal assessment of station should always be taken together with assessment of the degree of engagement by abdominal palpation. If the head is fully engaged (zero-fifth palpable) at or below the ischial spines (0 to +1 cm or more) and the occiput is anterior (OA), the outlook is favourable for vaginal delivery.

The condition of the membranes should also be noted. If they have ruptured, the colour and amount of amniotic fluid draining should be noted. A generous amount of clear fluid is a good prognostic feature; scanty, heavily blood-stained or meconium-stained fluid is a warning sign of possible fetal compromise. Women who are found not to be in established labour should be offered appropriate analgesia and support. Most can safely go home, to return when the contractions increase in strength and frequency.

The admission history and examination provide an initial screen for abnormal labour and increased maternal/fetal risk. If all features are normal and reassuring, the woman will remain under midwifery care. If there are risk factors identified, medical involvement in the form of the on-call obstetric team may be appropriate. Women in labour should have their pulse measured hourly and their temperature and blood pressure every 4 hours. The frequency of contractions should be recorded every 30 minutes and a vaginal examination performed every 4 hours (unless other factors suggest it needs to be repeated on a different time-frame). It should be noted when the woman voids urine, and this should be tested for ketones and protein. Women who chose epidural analgesia may need to be catheterized. Once the second stage is reached, the blood pressure and pulse should be performed hourly, and vaginal examinations offered every hour also.

Fetal assessment in labour

A healthy term fetus is usually able to withstand the demands of a normal labour. However, with each contraction, placental blood flow and oxygen transfer are temporarily interrupted and a fetus that is compromised before labour starts will become increasingly so. Insufficient oxygen delivery to the fetus causes a switch from aerobic to anaerobic metabolism and results in the generation of lactic acid and hydrogen ions. In excess, these saturate the buffering systems of the fetus and cause a metabolic acidosis, which if prolonged and severe, can cause neuronal damage and permanent neurological injury, even intrapartum fetal death. Hypoxia and acidosis cause a characteristic change in the fetal heart rate (FHR) pattern, which can be detected by auscultation and the CTG. Meconium (fetal stool) is often passed by a healthy fetus at or after term as a result of maturation of the gastrointestinal tract; in this scenario, it is usually thin and a very dark green or brown colour. However, it may also be expelled from a fetus exposed to marked intrauterine hypoxia or acidosis; in this scenario, it is often thicker and much brighter green in colour.

Fetal assessment options in labour

- Inspection of amniotic fluid – fresh meconium staining, absence of fluid, and heavy blood-stained fluid or bleeding are markers of potential fetal compromise.
- Intermittent auscultation of the fetal heart using a Pinard stethoscope or a hand-held Doppler ultrasound.
- Continuous external electronic fetal monitoring (EFM) using CTG.
- Continuous internal electronic fetal monitoring using a fetal scalp electrode (FSE) and CTG.
- Fetal scalp blood sampling (FBS).

The FHR should be auscultated with a Pinard stethoscope, or by using a hand-held Doppler device, early on in the initial assessment. It should be listened to for at least 1 minute immediately after a contraction. This should be repeated every 15 minutes during the first stage of labour and at least every 5 minutes in the second stage. The practice of performing an 'admission CTG' on all women is no longer recommended; however, a CTG should be performed if there are issues that might complicate labour and delivery. Most of these women will also be advised to have continuous EFM throughout labour, using the CTG. Women who begin labour with intermittent auscultation will be advised to change to continuous EFM if any complications occur during labour.

Indications for continuous EFM

- Significant meconium staining of the amniotic fluid.
- Abnormal FHR detected by intermittent auscultation.
- Maternal pyrexia (temperature ≥38.0°C or ≥37.5°C on two occasions).
- Fresh vaginal bleeding.
- Augmentation of contractions with an oxytocin infusion.
- Maternal request.

The quality of a CTG recording is sometimes poor because of the fetal position, or maternal obesity. A FSE may overcome this problem. It is fixed onto the skin of the fetal scalp and picks up the FHR directly. It rarely causes any harm to the fetus but requires a certain degree of cervical dilatation to be applied and for the membranes to be ruptured if they have remained intact. It is contraindicated in the presence of significant maternal infection (e.g. HIV or hepatitis C).

The interpretation of the FHR pattern on a CTG is discussed in Chapter 4, Assessment of fetal wellbeing. In brief, features of a normal FHR pattern include a baseline heart rate of between 110 and 160 bpm (averaged over a 20 minute interval or more), variability of between 5 and 25 bpm (variation in the FHR above and below the baseline), accelerations (a transient increase in FHR of at least 15 bpm lasting at least 15 seconds) and the absence of decelerations (transient decrease in the FHR of 15 bpm or more). Interpreting the CTG in labour is somewhat different to that of an antenatal CTG, particularly in the second stage. The absence of accelerations is of uncertain significance during labour, and the presence of early or variable decelerations (contemporaneous with contractions) later on in labour is extremely common and not usually a sign of significant fetal compromise.

Each feature of the CTG (baseline rate, variability, accelerations and decelerations) should be assessed each time a CTG is reviewed. Each feature can be described as 'reassuring', 'non-reassuring' or 'abnormal' according to certain strict nationally

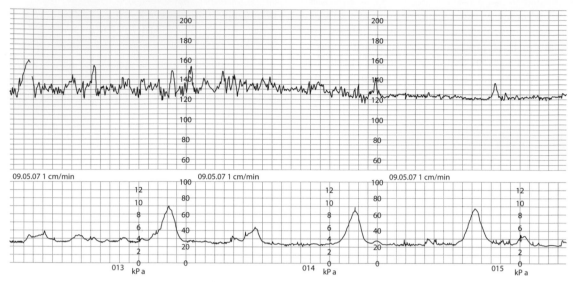

Figure 12.18 A normal cardiotocograph (CTG), showing a baseline fetal heart rate of approximately 120 bpm, frequent accelerations, baseline variability of 10–15 bpm and no decelerations. The uterus is contracting approximately once every 5 minutes.

agreed definitions outlined in the National Institute for Health and Care Excellence (NICE) guideline on intrapartum management. If all four features are reassuring, then the CTG is classified as 'normal' (**Figure 12.18**). If one feature is non-reassuring (and the other three are reassuring), then the CTG is classified as 'suspicious'. If there are two or more non-reassuring features, or any one abnormal feature, then the CTG is 'pathological'. Any reversible causes must be considered and addressed (e.g. dehydration, mother lying flat) and if it persists, further assessment of the fetus is necessary with FBS. If this is not possible or safe, then the baby should be delivered without delay. Unfortunately, the CTG can be difficult to interpret and it carries a significant false-positive rate (i.e. it often raises the possibility of fetal compromise when in fact the fetus is still in good condition). In order that the use of the CTG does not lead to unnecessary intervention, FBS may be performed during labour to measure fetal pH and base excess directly (see below under Management of possible fetal compromise). Often, these results are normal even when the CTG is abnormal and labour can continue with close monitoring. The use of EFM, only introduced in the 1970s, has been controversial and its value in 'low-risk' labour is doubtful. Education and training are crucial in the proper use of all equipment. Unfortunately, these

devices were introduced widely before CTG recordings and their outcomes were fully evaluated. There is little doubt that babies' lives have been saved by the use of EFM, but its use also contributed to the rise in caesarean section and instrumental delivery rates and has led to reduced mobility in labour and increased parental anxiety. This remains a challenge.

The partogram

The introduction of a graphic record of labour in the form of a partogram has been an important development. This record allows an instant visual assessment of the progress of labour based on the rate of cervical dilatation compared with an expected norm, according to the parity of the woman, so that slow progress can be recognized early and appropriate actions taken to correct it where possible. Other key observations are entered on to the chart, including the frequency and strength of contractions, the descent of the head in fifths palpable and station, the amount and colour of the amniotic fluid draining and basic observations of maternal wellbeing, such as blood pressure, heart rate and temperature (**Figure 12.19**).

A line can be drawn on the partogram at the end of the latent phase demonstrating progress of

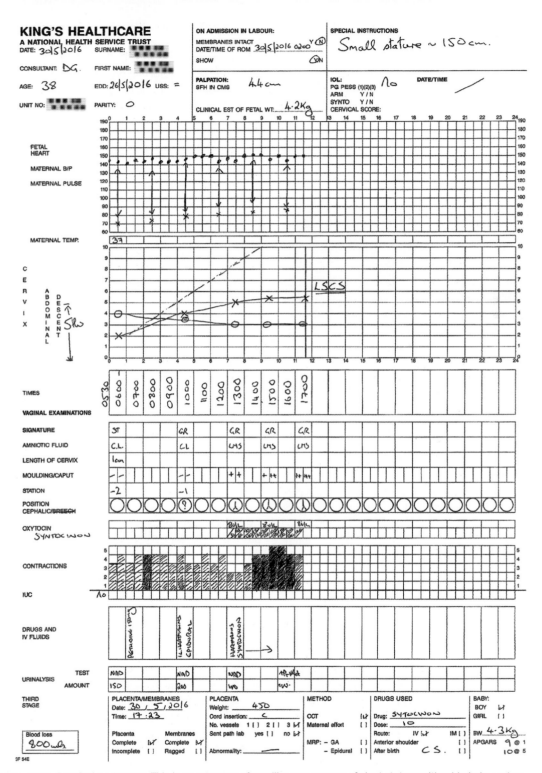

Figure 12.19 A typical partogram. This is a partogram of a nulliparous woman of short stature with a big baby and an augmented labour. The labour culminates with an emergency caesarean section for cephalopelvic disproportion.

1 cm dilatation per hour. Another line ('the action line') can be drawn parallel and 4 hours to the right of it. If the plot of actual cervical dilatation reaches the action line, indicating slow progress, then consideration should be given to a number of different measures that aim to improve progress (see below). Progress can also be considered slow if the cervix dilates at less than 1 cm every 2 hours.

Management during first stage

> ### KEY LEARNING POINTS
>
> Management of first stage of labour:
>
> - First stage of labour is the interval from diagnosis of labour to full dilatation of the cervix.
> - One-to-one midwifery care should be provided.
> - Additional emotional support from a birth partner should be encouraged.
> - Obstetric and anaesthetic care should be available as required.
> - Maternal and fetal wellbeing should be monitored.
> - Vaginal examinations are performed 4 hourly or as clinically indicated.
> - Progress of labour is monitored using a partogram with timely intervention if abnormal.
> - Appropriate pain relief should be provided consistent with the woman's wishes.
> - Ensure adequate hydration and light diet to prevent ketosis.

Women who are in the latent phase of labour should be encouraged to mobilize and should be managed away from the labour suite where possible. Indeed, they may well go home, to return later when the contractions are stronger or more frequent. Encouragement and reassurance are extremely important. Intervention during this phase is best avoided unless there are identified risk factors. Simple analgesics are preferred over nitrous oxide gas and epidurals. There is no reason to restrict eating and drinking, although lighter foods and clear fluids may be better tolerated. Vaginal examinations are usually performed every 4 hours to determine when the active phase has been reached (approximately 4 cm dilatation and full effacement). Thereafter, the timing of examinations should be decided by the midwife in consultation with the woman. Four-hourly

is standard practice; however, this frequency may be increased if the midwife thinks that progress is unusually slow or fast or if there are fetal concerns. The lower limit of normal progress is 1 cm dilatation every 2 hours once the active phase has been reached. Descent of the presenting part through the pelvis is another crucial component of progress and should be recorded at each vaginal examination. Full dilatation may be reached, but if descent is inadequate, vaginal delivery will not occur.

During the first stage, the membranes may be intact, may have ruptured spontaneously or may be ruptured artificially. Generally speaking, if the membranes are intact, it is not necessary to rupture them if the progress of labour is satisfactory.

Maternal and fetal observations are carried out as described previously and recorded on the partogram. Women should receive one-to-one care (i.e. from a dedicated midwife) and should not be left alone for any significant period of time once labour has established. They should be able to choose birth partners themselves and should be able to adopt whatever positions they find most comfortable. Mobility during labour is encouraged and it is likely that standing upright encourages progress. Unfortunately, many women adopt a supine position (lying down), especially if there is a need for continuous EFM (i.e. the CTG). Women may drink during established labour and those who are becoming dehydrated may benefit from intravenous fluids to prevent ketosis, which can impair uterine contractility. Light diet is acceptable if there is no obvious risk factor for needing a general anaesthetic and if the woman has not had pethidine or diamorphine for pain relief, which can cause vomiting. Shaving and enemas are unnecessary and antacids need only be given to women with risk factors for complications, or to those who have had opioid analgesia. A variety of methods of pain relief are available, depending on the location of the birth, and these are discussed below under Pain relief in labour.

'Active management of labour' was a collection of interventions that was routinely recommended to nulliparous women to maximize the chances of a normal birth. It included one-to-one midwifery care, 2-hourly vaginal examinations, early artificial rupture of membranes and use of oxytocin augmentation if progress fell more than 2 hours behind the schedule of 1 cm dilatation per hour. A variety of studies failed to show any obvious benefit of active management, except that derived from one-to-one care, the only component now recommended for all women in normal labour.

Management during second stage

If the labour has been normal, the first sign of the second stage is likely to be an urge to push experienced by the mother. Full dilatation of the cervix should be confirmed by a vaginal examination if the head is not visible. The woman will get an expulsive reflex with each contraction, and will generally take a deep breath, hold it, and strain down (the Valsalva manoeuvre). Women will be guided by their own urge to push; however, the midwife has an important role to play, with advice, support and reassurance if progress is poor. Women should be discouraged from lying supine, or semi-supine, and should adopt any other position that they find comfortable. Lying in the left lateral position, squatting and 'all fours' are particularly effective options. Maternal and fetal surveillance intensifies in the second stage, as described previously. The development of fetal acidaemia may accelerate, and maternal exhaustion and ketosis increase in line with the duration of active pushing. Use of regional analgesia (epidural or spinal) may interfere with the normal urge to push, and the second stage is more often diagnosed on a routine scheduled vaginal examination. Pushing is usually delayed for at least 1 hour and up to 2 hours if an epidural is *in situ* (the 'passive second stage'). However, in all cases the baby should be delivered within 4 hours of reaching full dilatation.

Descent and delivery of the head

The progress of descent of the head can be judged by watching the perineum. At first, there is a slight general bulge as the woman bears down. When the head stretches the perineum, the anus will begin to open and soon after this the baby's head will be seen at the vulva at the height of each contraction. Between contractions, the elastic tone of the perineal muscles will push the head back into the pelvic cavity. The perineal body and vulva will become more and more stretched, until eventually the head is low enough to pass forwards under the subpubic arch. When the head no longer recedes between contractions it is described as crowning. This indicates that it has passed through the pelvic floor, and delivery is imminent. Vaginal and perineal tears are common consequences of vaginal birth, particularly during first deliveries. The 'hands-on' approach has been very popular. As crowning occurs, the hands of the accoucheur are used to flex the fetal head and guard the perineum. The belief is that controlling the speed of delivery of the fetal head will limit maternal soft-tissue damage; however, there is little evidence to support this practice over the alternative 'hands-off' approach. Once the head has crowned, the woman should be discouraged from bearing down by telling her to take rapid, shallow breaths ('panting').

An episiotomy is a surgical cut, performed with scissors, which extends from the vaginal fourchette in a mediolateral direction, usually to the right, through the perineum and incorporating the lower vaginal wall (see Chapter 13, Operative delivery). It is performed during most instrumental births (ventouse or forceps) or to hasten delivery if there is suspected fetal compromise (e.g. fetal bradycardia). It will only accelerate the birth if the head has passed through the pelvic floor, so should not be performed too early. It does not help prevent more severe perineal injury involving the anal sphincter and its routine use in normal labour was abandoned some time ago. Effective analgesia is required, and this will usually be with infiltration of local anaesthetic if the woman does not have an epidural.

Delivery of the shoulders and rest of the body

Once the fetal head is born, a check is made to see whether the cord is wound tightly around the neck, thereby making delivery of the body difficult. If this is the case, the cord may need to be clamped and divided before delivery of the rest of the body. With the next contraction, there is restitution and external rotation of the head and the shoulders can be delivered. To aid delivery of the shoulders, there should be gentle traction on the head downwards and forwards until the anterior shoulder appears beneath the pubis. The head is then lifted gradually until the posterior shoulder appears over the perineum and the baby is then swept upwards to deliver the body and legs. If the infant is large and traction is necessary to deliver the body, it should be applied to the shoulders only, and not to the head. Shoulder dystocia (difficulty in delivering the shoulders) is discussed in Chapter 14, Obstetric emergencies.

Immediate care of the neonate

After the baby is born, it lies between the mother's legs or is delivered directly on to the maternal abdomen. The baby will usually take its first breath within seconds. There is no need for immediate clamping of the cord, and indeed about 80 ml of blood will be transferred from the placenta to the baby before cord pulsations cease, reducing the chances of later neonatal anaemia and iron deficiency. The baby's head should be kept dependent to allow mucus in the respiratory tract to drain, and oropharyngeal suction should only be applied if really necessary. After clamping and cutting the cord, the baby should have an Apgar score calculated at 1 minute of age (see Chapter 16, The neonate), which is then repeated at 5 minutes. Immediate skin-to-skin contact between mother and baby will help bonding, and promote the further release of oxytocin, which will encourage uterine contractions. The baby should be dried and covered with a warm blanket or towel, maintaining this contact. Initiation of breastfeeding should be encouraged within the first hour of life, and routine newborn measurements of head circumference, birthweight and temperature are usually performed soon after this hour has elapsed. Before being taken from the delivery room, the first dose of vitamin K should be given (if parental consent has been given) and the infant should have a general examination for abnormalities and a wrist label attached for identification.

Management of third stage

The third stage is the interval between delivery of the baby and the complete expulsion of the placenta and membranes. This normally takes between 5 and 10 minutes and is considered prolonged after 30 minutes, unless a physiological approach is preferred.

Separation of the placenta occurs because of the reduction of volume of the uterus due to uterine contraction and the retraction (shortening) of the lattice-like arrangement of the myometrial muscle fibres. A cleavage plane develops within the decidua basalis and the separated placenta lies free in the lower segment of the uterine cavity. Management of the third stage can be described as 'active' or 'physiological'.

Signs of placental separation

- Apparent lengthening of the cord.
- A small gush of blood from the placental bed.
- Rising of the uterine fundus to above the umbilicus (**Figure 12.20**).
- Uterine contraction resulting in firm globular feel on palpation.

Active management of the third stage

- Intramuscular injection of 10 IU oxytocin, given as the anterior shoulder of the baby is delivered, or immediately after delivery of the baby.
- Early clamping and cutting of the umbilical cord.
- Controlled cord traction (**Figure 12.21**).

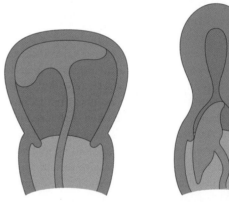

Figure 12.20 Signs of separation and descent of the placenta. After separation, the uterine upper segment rises up and feels more rounded.

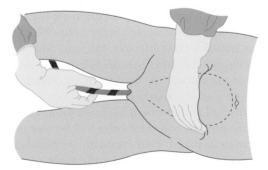

Figure 12.21 Delivering the placenta by controlled cord traction.

Active management

Active management of the third stage should be recommended to all women because high-quality evidence shows that it reduces the incidence of post-partum haemorrhage (PPH) from 15% to 5%. When the signs of placental separation are recognized, controlled cord traction is used to expedite delivery of the placenta. When a contraction is felt, the left hand should be moved suprapubically and the fundus elevated with the palm facing towards the mother. At the same time, the right hand should grasp the cord and exert steady traction so that the placenta separates and is delivered gently, care being taken to peel off all the membranes, usually with a twisting motion. Uterine inversion is a rare complication, which may occur if the uterus is not adequately controlled with the left hand and excessive traction is exerted on the cord in the absence of complete separation and a uterine contraction (see Chapter 14, Obstetric emergencies).

In approximately 2% of cases, the placenta will not be expelled by this method. If no bleeding occurs, a further attempt at controlled cord traction should be made after 10 minutes. If this fails, the placenta is 'retained' and will require manual removal under general or regional anaesthesia in the operating theatre. It is now recognized that a modified approach to active management of the third stage may be preferable with delayed cord clamping for between 1 and 3 minutes. This approach allows autotransfusion of placental blood to the neonate while maintaining the benefit of a reduced risk of PPH. It is of particular importance in preterm birth.

Physiological management

Physiological management of the third stage is where the placenta is delivered by maternal effort and no uterotonic drugs are given to assist this process. It is associated with heavier bleeding, but women who are not at undue risk of PPH should be supported if they choose this option. In the event of haemorrhage (estimated blood loss >500 ml) or if the placenta remains undelivered after 60 minutes of physiological management, active management should be recommended.

After completion of the third stage, the placenta should be inspected for missing cotyledons or a succenturiate lobe. If these are suspected, examination under anaesthesia and manual removal of placental tissue (MROP) should be arranged, because in this situation the risk of PPH is high. Finally, the vulva of the mother should be inspected for any tears or lacerations. Minor tears do not require suturing, but tears extending into the perineal muscles (or, indeed, an episiotomy) will require careful repair (see Chapter 13, Operative delivery).

KEY LEARNING POINTS

Features of normal labour:

- Spontaneous onset at 37–42 weeks' gestation.
- Singleton pregnancy.
- Cephalic vertex presentation.
- No artificial interventions.
- Cervical dilatation of at least 1 cm every 2 hours in the active phase of first stage.
- Active second stage no more than 2 hours in primiparous and 60 minutes in multiparous woman.
- Spontaneous vaginal delivery.
- Third stage lasting no more than 30 minutes with active management.

Abnormal labour

Labour becomes abnormal when there is poor progress (as evidenced by a delay in cervical dilatation or descent of the presenting part) and/or the fetus shows signs of compromise. Also, if there is a fetal malpresentation, a multiple pregnancy, a uterine scar or if labour has been induced, labour cannot be considered normal. Progress in labour is dependent on the '3 Ps' as described previously (powers, passages, passenger). Abnormalities in one or more of these factors can slow the normal progress of labour. Plotting the findings of serial vaginal examinations on the partogram will help to highlight poor progress during the first and second stages of labour.

Patterns of abnormal progress in labour

The use of a partogram to plot the progress of labour improves the detection of poor progress. Three patterns of abnormal labour are commonly described (**Figure 12.22**).

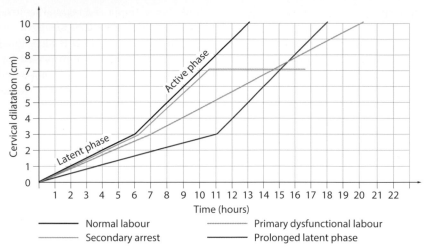

Figure 12.22 Abnormalities of the partogram

Prolonged latent phase occurs when the latent phase is longer than the arbitrary time limits discussed previously. It is more common in primiparous women and probably results from a delay in the chemical processes that occur within the cervix that soften it and allow effacement. Prolonged latent phase can be extremely frustrating and tiring for the woman. However, intervention in the form of artificial rupture of membranes (ARM) or oxytocin infusion will increase the likelihood of poor progress later in the labour and the need for caesarean birth. It is best managed away from the labour suite with simple analgesics, mobilization and reassurance. The partogram should not be commenced until the latent phase of labour is complete.

'Primary arrest' is the term used to describe poor progress in the active first stage of labour (<2 cm cervical dilatation/4 hours) and is also more common in primiparous women. It is most commonly caused by inefficient uterine contractions, but can also result from cephalopelvic disproportion (CPD), malposition and malpresentation of the fetus. 'Secondary arrest' occurs when progress in the active first stage is initially good but then slows or stops altogether, typically after 7 cm dilatation. Although inefficient uterine contractions may be the cause, fetal malposition, malpresentation and CPD feature more commonly than in primary arrest. 'Arrest in the second stage of labour' (not to be confused with 'secondary arrest') occurs when delivery is not imminent after the usual interval of pushing in the second stage

of labour. This may be due to inefficient uterine activity, malposition, malpresentation, CPD or a resistant perineum. In some cases it may be due to maternal exhaustion, fear or pain.

Management of abnormal labour

Poor progress in the first stage of labour

Poor progress in the first stage of labour has been defined as cervical dilatation of less than 2 cm in 4 hours, usually associated with failure of descent and rotation of the fetal head. It may relate to the powers, the passages or the passenger.

Dysfunctional uterine activity ('powers')

This is the most common cause of poor progress in labour. It is more common in primigravidae and in older women and is characterized by weak, irregular and infrequent contractions. The assessment of uterine contractions is most commonly carried out by clinical examination and by using external uterine tocography. Intrauterine pressure catheters are available and these do give a more accurate measurement of the pressure being generated by the contractions, but they are invasive and rarely necessary. A frequency of four to five contractions per 10 minutes is usually considered ideal. Fewer contractions than this does not necessarily mean progress will be slow, but more frequent examinations may be indicated to detect poor progress earlier. When poor progress in labour is suspected, it is usual to recommend repeat vaginal examination at 2 hours rather than 4 hours after the last. If delay is confirmed, the woman should be offered ARM and, if there is still poor progress in a further 2 hours, advice should be sought from an obstetrician regarding the use of an oxytocin infusion to augment the contractions. The infusion is commenced at a slow rate initially and increased every 30 minutes, according to a well-defined protocol. Continuous EFM is necessary as excessively frequent strong contractions may cause fetal compromise (**Figure 12.23**). Women should be offered an epidural before oxytocin is started, along with ongoing hydration and emotional support.

Multiparous women are less likely to experience poor progress in labour secondary to dysfunctional uterine activity. Extreme caution must be exercised when making this diagnosis in a multiparous woman where an alternative explanation, such as malposition or malpresentation or obstructed labour due to CPD, is more likely. An obstetrician must be closely involved in the assessment of such a woman and the decision to augment with oxytocin must be considered very carefully.

Excessive uterine contractions in a truly obstructed labour may result in uterine rupture in a multiparous woman, a complication that is extremely rare in primiparous women. Augmentation with oxytocin is contraindicated if there are concerns regarding the condition of the fetus.

If progress fails to occur despite 4–6 hours of augmentation with oxytocin, a caesarean section will usually be recommended.

Cephalopelvic disproportion ('passages' and 'passenger')

CPD implies anatomical disproportion between the fetal head and maternal pelvis. It can be due to a large head, small pelvis or a combination of the two relative to each other. Women of short stature (<1.60 m) with a large baby in their first pregnancy are potential candidates to develop this problem. The pelvis may be unusually small because of previous fracture or metabolic bone disease. Rarely, a fetal anomaly will contribute to CPD. Obstructive hydrocephalus may cause macrocephaly (abnormally large fetal head), and fetal thyroid and neck tumours may cause extension at the fetal neck. Relative CPD is more common and occurs with malposition of the fetal head. The OP position is associated with deflexion of the fetal head and presents a larger skull diameter to the maternal pelvis (**Figures 12.14, 12.24**). Oxytocin can be given carefully to a primigravida with mild

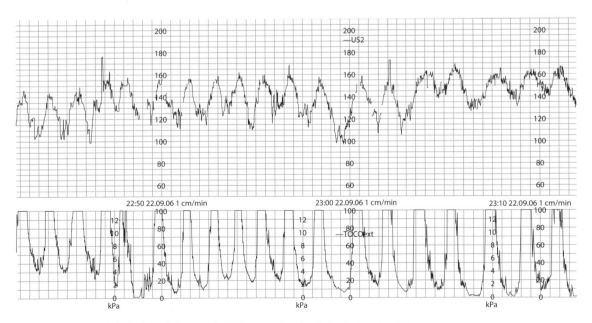

Figure 12.23 A pathological cardiotocograph (CTG) secondary to uterine hyperstimulation.

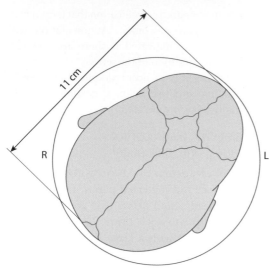

Figure 12.24 Vaginal palpation of the head in the right occipito-posterior position. The circle represents the pelvic cavity, with a diameter of 12 cm. The head is poorly flexed so that the anterior fontanelle is easily felt.

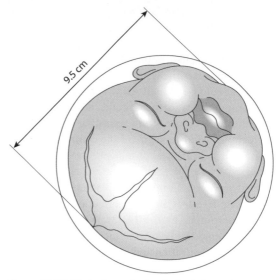

Figure 12.25 Vaginal examination in the left mento-anterior position. The circle represents the pelvic cavity, with a diameter of 12 cm.

to moderate CPD as long as the CTG is normal. Relative disproportion may be overcome if the malposition is corrected (i.e. rotation to a flexed OA position). Oxytocin must never be used in a multiparous woman where CPD is suspected.

Findings suggestive of CPD

- Fetal head is not engaged.
- Progress is slow or arrests despite efficient uterine contractions.
- Vaginal examination shows severe moulding and caput formation.
- Head is poorly applied to the cervix.
- Haematuria.

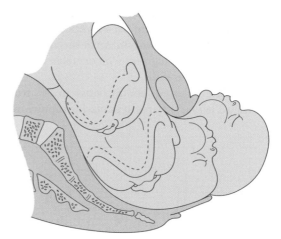

Figure 12.26 The mechanism of labour with a face presentation. The head descends with increasing extension. The chin reaches the pelvic floor and undergoes forward rotation. The head is born by flexion.

Malpresentation (the 'passenger')

A firm application of the fetal presenting part on to the cervix is necessary for good progress in labour. A face presentation (**Figures 12.25, 12.26**) may apply poorly to the cervix and the resulting progress in labour may be poor, although vaginal birth is still possible. Brow presentation is associated with the mento-vertical diameter presenting, which is simply too large to fit through the bony pelvis unless flexion

occurs or there is hyperextension to a face presentation (**Figures 12.27, 12.28**). Brow presentation therefore often manifests as poor progress in the first stage, often in a multiparous woman. Shoulder presentations cannot deliver vaginally and once again poor progress will occur. Malpresentations are more common in women of high parity and carry a risk of uterine rupture if labour is allowed to continue without progress.

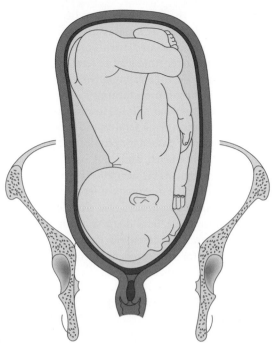

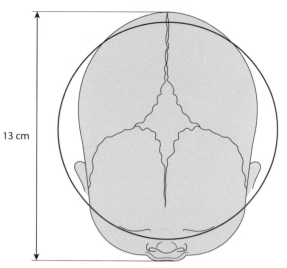

Figure 12.28 Vaginal examination with brow presentation. The circle represents the pelvic cavity, with a diameter of 12 cm. The mento-vertical diameter of 13 cm is too large to permit engagement of the head.

Figure 12.27 Brow presentation. The head is above the pelvic brim and not engaged. The mento-vertical diameter of the head is trying to engage in the transverse diameter at the brim.

Abnormalities of the birth canal ('passages')

The bony pelvis may cause delay in the progress of labour as discussed above (CPD). Abnormalities of the uterus and cervix can also delay labour. Unsuspected fibroids in the lower uterine segment can prevent descent of the fetal head. Delay can also be caused by 'cervical dystocia', a term used to describe a non-compliant cervix that effaces but fails to dilate because of severe scarring or rigidity, usually as a result of previous cervical surgery such as a cone biopsy. Caesarean section may be necessary.

Poor progress in the second stage of labour

Birth of the baby is expected to take place within 3 hours of the start of the active second stage (pushing) in nulliparous women and 2 hours in parous women. Delay is diagnosed if delivery is not imminent after 2 hours of pushing in a nulliparous labour and 1 hour for a parous woman. The causes of second stage delay can again be classified as

abnormalities of the powers, the passages and the passenger. Secondary dysfunctional uterine activity ('powers') is a common cause of second stage delay, and may be exacerbated by epidural analgesia. Having achieved full dilatation, the uterine contractions may become weak and ineffectual and this is sometimes associated with maternal dehydration and ketosis. If no mechanical problem is anticipated and the woman is primiparous, the treatment is with rehydration and intravenous oxytocin. If the woman is multiparous, a full clinical assessment should be performed by a skilled obstetrician prior to considering oxytocin due to the risks described above.

Delay in the second stage can occur because of a narrow midpelvis (android pelvis), which prevents internal rotation of the fetal head ('passages'). This may result in arrest of descent of the fetal head at the level of the ischial spines in the transverse position, a condition called deep transverse arrest (**Figure 12.29**). It may also occur due to a resistant perineum, particularly in a nulliparous woman.

Delay can also occur because of a persistent OP position of the fetal head ('passenger'). In this situation, the head will either have to undergo a long rotation to OA or be delivered in the OP position (i.e. face to pubes). By the time delay in the second stage of labour has been diagnosed, the NICE guidelines

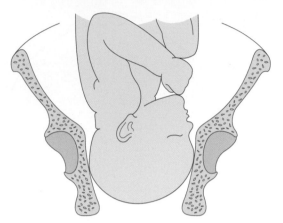

Figure 12.29 Deep transverse arrest of the head.

recommend that oxytocin should not be started. Inefficient uterine activity therefore needs to be corrected proactively at the beginning of the second stage.

Instrumental vaginal birth should be considered for prolonged second stage if the safety criteria have been fulfilled (see Chapter 13, Operative delivery). This may be performed in the labour room or may be more safely carried out as a 'trial' in theatre with easy recourse to caesarean delivery if the attempt is unsuccessful. If the safety criteria for instrumental vaginal birth are not met, then delivery will be by caesarean section. A resistant perineum resulting in significant delay may be an indication for an episiotomy.

 KEY LEARNING POINTS

Management options for delay in the second stage of labour:

- Continued pushing with encouragement.
- Regular reviews of progress and fetal wellbeing.
- Oxytocin to augment contractions.
- Episiotomy for a resistant perineum.
- Instrumental vaginal birth (forceps or ventouse/vacuum).
- Caesarean section.

Fetal compromise in labour

Concern for the wellbeing of the fetus is one of the most common reasons for medical intervention during labour. The fetus may have been compromised before labour, and the reduction in placental blood flow associated with contractions may reveal this and over time lead to fetal hypoxia and eventually acidosis. Fetal compromise may present as fresh meconium staining to the amniotic fluid or an abnormal CTG. However, neither of these findings confirms fetal hypoxia or acidosis. Meconium can be passed for physiological reasons, such as fetal maturity, and it is well recognized that the abnormal CTG carries a very high false-positive rate for the diagnosis of fetal compromise. 'Suspected fetal compromise' is therefore a more accurate term than 'fetal distress'. In many cases, babies delivered by caesarean section or instrumental birth for suspected fetal compromise are found to be in good condition.

Risk factors for fetal compromise in labour

- Placental insufficiency – FGR and pre-eclampsia.
- Prematurity.
- Postmaturity.
- Multiple pregnancy.
- Prolonged labour.
- Augmentation with oxytocin/hyperstimulation.
- Precipitate labour.
- Intrapartum abruption.
- Cord prolapse.
- Uterine rupture/dehiscence.
- Maternal diabetes.
- Cholestasis of pregnancy.
- Maternal pyrexia/chorioamnionitis.
- Oligohydramnios.

Recognition of fetal compromise

Meconium staining of the amniotic fluid is considered significant when it is either thick or tenacious, dark green, bright green or black. Any particulate meconium should also be of concern. Thin and light meconium is more likely to represent fetal gut maturity than fetal compromise. However, when any meconium is seen in the liquor, consideration should be given to starting continuous EFM with the CTG and this is mandatory if the meconium is thick and dark. Another reason for commencing the CTG is if a change in the heart rate is noted with intermittent auscultation, particularly fetal tachycardia, bradycardia or FHR decelerations. The CTG may have already been recorded throughout the labour because of underlying risk factors that predate the labour.

Accurate interpretation of the CTG is a skill that needs to be practised, and there is significant interobserver variability. There are national guidelines, which should be used to classify the CTG as 'normal', 'suspicious' or 'pathological'. Interpretation of the CTG is discussed in more detail in Chapter 4, Assessment of fetal wellbeing.

Management of possible fetal compromise

A number of resuscitative manoeuvres should be considered when a CTG is classified as 'suspicious'. These include repositioning of the mother, intravenous fluids, reducing or stopping the oxytocin infusion and correction of epidural-associated hypotension. It is reasonable to continue observation of the CTG and more complex intervention is not required. If a CTG becomes 'pathological', these reversible factors should also be considered, but it is also important to carry out an immediate vaginal examination to exclude malpresentation and cord prolapse and to assess the progress of the labour. If the cervix is fully dilated, it may be possible to deliver the baby vaginally using the forceps or ventouse. Alternatively, if the cervix is not fully dilated, a fetal blood sampling can be considered. This is usually only possible when the cervix is dilated 3 cm or more. A normal result will permit labour to continue, although it may need to be repeated every 30–60 minutes if the CTG abnormalities persist or worsen. An abnormal result mandates immediate delivery by caesarean section if the cervix is not fully dilated.

Fresh, thick meconium in the presence of a reassuring CTG is still a cause for concern, and although the labour may be allowed to continue, the threshold for intervention will be lowered and a paediatrician should be present at delivery.

Resuscitating the fetus in labour

- Maternal dehydration and ketosis can be corrected with intravenous fluids.
- Maternal hypotension secondary to an epidural can be reversed by a fluid bolus, although a vasoconstrictor such as ephedrine is occasionally necessary.
- Uterine hyperstimulation from excess oxytocin can be treated by turning off the infusion temporarily and using tocolytic drugs, such as terbutaline.
- Venocaval compression and reduced uterine blood flow can be eased by turning the woman into a left lateral position.

Fetal blood sampling procedure

Explanation is given and consent obtained from the woman. She is asked to lie in the left lateral position. An amnioscope is inserted into the vagina and its distal end is applied to the fetal head. The scalp is cleaned and a small cut is made using a blade with a guard. The resulting blood is collected into a microtube. The amount of blood required is approximately 0.25 ml. A normal pH value is above 7.25. A pH below 7.20 is confirmation of fetal compromise. Values between 7.20 and 7.25 are 'borderline'. The base deficit can also be useful in interpretation of the fetal scalp pH. A base excess of more than −12.0 mmol/l demonstrates a significant metabolic acidosis, with increasing risk of fetal neurological injury beyond this level. More than one fetal scalp sample may be necessary over the course of the labour. A downward trend in the fetal scalp pH values is to be expected and should be assessed together with how the labour is progressing.

If an abnormal CTG persists in labour, then, despite normal values, fetal scalp sampling should be repeated every 60 minutes, or sooner if the CTG deteriorates. If the result is borderline, it should be repeated no more than 30 minutes later.

Place of birth

Most births in developed countries take place in hospital. However, depending on the circumstances women may have the opportunity to choose between hospital birth, home birth or birth in a midwifery unit or birth centre. Currently, fewer than 5% of women deliver at home in most areas of the UK. Some midwifery units are based within a hospital environment and some are stand-alone. The published evidence guiding women on the outcomes of birth in the different settings is limited to observational studies, the largest of which is the Birthplace in England Study. The chance of a normal birth at home or in a midwifery unit is higher than in an obstetric unit, and the best outcomes are for women who are multiparous and without complicating factors. There is too little information currently to state conclusively where it is safest to give birth, from a maternal or a fetal perspective. All women should be informed, however, that unexpected emergencies can occur in labour and that the outcome from these may be better in a hospital setting. It should also be made clear that the need for transfer into hospital during labour is possible from home or a midwifery unit. Women with issues that increase the chance of problems occurring during labour should be recommended to deliver in an obstetric unit and guidelines (e.g. NICE) provide a list of obstetric, fetal and medical factors to assist midwives and obstetricians when counselling women. Also, a variety of indications are listed for intrapartum transfer into an obstetric unit, including maternal pyrexia in labour, delayed progress in labour, concerns regarding fetal wellbeing, hypertension, retained placenta and complicated perineal trauma requiring suturing. Use of epidural pain relief is restricted to hospital settings, and is known to increase the chances of delivery by forceps or ventouse. Some women will choose to labour or give birth in water. At present there is insufficient good quality evidence to either support or discourage water birth.

Pain relief in labour

There is a social and cultural dimension to the provision and uptake of analgesia in labour. Some women and their carers believe that there is an advantage in avoiding analgesia, whereas other women will use all methods on offer to limit their pain. Professionals who are knowledgeable about labour and the available options for pain relief should give tailored advice according to the needs and priorities of the individual woman. The method of pain relief is to some extent dependent on the previous obstetric record of the woman, the course of labour and also the anticipated duration of labour. Just as one woman's labour can be made into an unhappy experience by unsolicited and unnecessary analgesia, pain relief that is inadequate or offered too late can ruin another's. Although the final decision rests with the woman, there are certain circumstances in which particular forms of analgesia are contraindicated and should not be offered.

Non-pharmacological methods

One-to-one care in labour from a midwife alongside a supportive birth partner has been shown to reduce the need for analgesia. Relaxation and breathing exercises may help the woman to manage her pain. Prolonged hyperventilation can make the woman dizzy and can cause alkalosis. Homeopathy, acupuncture and hypnosis are sometimes employed, but their use has not been associated with a significant reduction in pain scores or with a reduced need for conventional methods of analgesia.

Relaxation in warm water during the first stage of labour often leads to a sense of wellbeing and allows women to cope much better with pain. The temperature of the water should not exceed 37.5°C. Transcutaneous electrical nerve stimulation (TENS) works on the principle of blocking pain fibres in the posterior ganglia of the spinal cord by stimulation of small afferent fibres (the 'gate' theory). It may be of use in the latent phase of labour and is often used by women at home. It has been shown to be ineffective in reducing pain scores or the need for other forms of analgesia in established labour. It does not have any adverse effects, but is often disappointing.

Pharmacological methods

Opiates, such as pethidine and diamorphine, are still used in most obstetric units and indeed can be administered by midwives without the involvement of medical staff. This may be one of the reasons for their popularity. They should be available in all birth settings but they provide only limited pain relief during labour and furthermore may have significant side-effects.

Side-effects of opioid analgesia

- Nausea and vomiting (they should always been given with an antiemetic).
- Maternal drowsiness and sedation.
- Delayed gastric emptying (increasing the risks of general anaesthesia).
- Short-term respiratory depression of the baby.
- Possible interference with breastfeeding.

Opiates tend to be given as intramuscular injections; however, an alternative is a subcutaneous or intravenous infusion by a patient-controlled analgesic device (PCA). This allows the woman, by pressing a dispenser button, to determine the level of analgesia that she requires. If a very short-acting opiate is used, the opiate doses can be timed with the contractions. This method of pain relief is particularly popular among women who cannot have an epidural and find non-pharmacological options insufficient.

Inhalational analgesia

Nitrous oxide (NO) in the form of Entonox® (an equal mixture of NO and oxygen) is available on most labour wards. It has a quick onset, a short duration of effect and is more effective than pethidine. It may cause light-headedness and nausea. It is not suitable for prolonged use from early labour because hyperventilation may result in hypocapnoea, dizziness and, rarely, tetany and fetal hypoxia. It is most suitable later on in labour or while awaiting epidural analgesia.

Epidural analgesia

Epidural (extradural) analgesia is the most reliable means of providing effective analgesia in labour. Failure to provide an epidural is one of the most frequent causes of upset and disappointment among labouring women. The epidural service must be well organized to be effective, and fortunately resources are now available in most hospital settings so that a significant delay in the placement of an epidural is unusual. The decision to have an epidural sited should be a combined one between the woman, her midwife, the obstetric team and the anaesthetist. The woman must be informed about the benefits and risks and the final decision in most cases rests with the woman unless there is a definite contraindication. It is important to warn the woman that she may lose sensation and movement in her legs temporarily, and that intravenous access and a more intensive level of maternal and fetal monitoring will be necessary, for example with continuous EFM (the CTG).

The effect of epidural analgesia on labour duration and the operative delivery rate has been a controversial issue. The evidence is now clear that epidural analgesia does not increase caesarean section rates. However, the second stage is longer and there is a greater chance of instrumental delivery, which may be lessened by a longer passive second stage awaiting a maternal urge to push. In certain clinical situations, an epidural in the second stage of labour may assist a vaginal delivery by relaxing the woman and allowing time for the head to descend and rotate. The main indication is for effective pain relief. There are other maternal and fetal conditions for which epidural analgesia would be advantageous in labour.

An epidural will limit mobility and for this reason, it is not ideal for women in early labour. However, women in severe pain, even in the latent phase of labour, should not be denied regional anaesthesia. Neither is advanced cervical dilatation necessarily a contraindication to an epidural. It is more important to assess the rate of progress, the anticipated length of time to delivery and the type of delivery expected.

Indications and contraindications for epidural analgesia

Indications
- Prolonged labour/oxytocin augmentation.
- Maternal hypertensive disorders.
- Multiple pregnancy.
- Selected maternal medical conditions.
- A high risk of operative intervention.

Contraindications
- Coagulation disorders (e.g. low platelet count).
- Local or systemic sepsis.
- Hypovolaemia.
- Logistical: insufficient numbers of trained staff (anaesthetic and midwifery).

Complications of epidural analgesia

Accidental dural puncture during the search for the epidural space should occur in no more than 1% of cases. If the subarachnoid space is accidentally reached with an epidural needle, this may allow leakage of cerebrospinal fluid (CSF) and results in a 'spinal headache'. This is characteristically experienced on the top of the head and is relieved by lying flat and exacerbated by sitting upright. If the headache is severe or persistent, a blood patch may be necessary. This involves injecting a small volume of the woman's blood into the epidural space at the level of the accidental dural puncture. The resulting blood clot is thought to block off the leak of CSF.

Bladder dysfunction can occur if the bladder is allowed to overfill because the woman is unaware of the need to micturate, particularly after the birth while the spinal or epidural is wearing off. Overdistension of the detrusor muscle of the bladder can permanently damage it and leave long-term voiding problems. To avoid this, catheterization of the bladder should be carried out during labour if the woman does not void significant volumes of urine spontaneously.

Hypotension can occur with epidural analgesia, although it is more common with spinal anaesthesia. It can usually be rectified with fluid boluses, but may need vasopressors. Occasionally, maternal hypotension will lead to fetal compromise (see below).

Accidental total spinal anaesthesia (injection of epidural doses of local anaesthetic into the subarachnoid space) causes severe hypotension, respiratory failure, unconsciousness and death if not recognized and treated immediately. The mother requires intubation, ventilation and circulatory support. Hypotension must be treated with intravenous fluids, vasopressors and positioning of the woman onto her left side. In some cases, urgent delivery of the baby may be required to overcome aorto-caval compression and so permit maternal resuscitation. Spinal haematomata and neurological complications are rare, and are usually associated with other factors such as bleeding disorders. Drug toxicity can occur with accidental placement of a catheter within a blood vessel. This is normally noticed by aspiration prior to injection.

Short-term respiratory depression of the baby is possible because all modern epidural solutions contain opioids, which reach the maternal circulation and may cross the placenta.

Technique

After detailed discussion, the woman's back is cleansed and local anaesthetic is used to infiltrate the skin. The woman may be in an extreme left lateral position, or sitting upright but leaning over. Flexion at the upper spine and at the hips helps to open up the spaces between the vertebral bodies of the lumbar spine. Aseptic technique is used. The epidural catheter is normally inserted at the L2–L3, L3–L4 or L4–L5 interspace and should come to lie in the epidural space, which contains blood vessels, nerve roots and fat (**Figure 12.30**). The catheter is aspirated to check for position and, if no blood or CSF is obtained, a 'test dose' is given to confirm the catheter

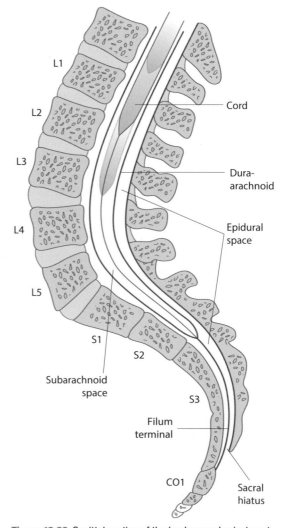

Figure 12.30 Sagittal section of the lumbosacral spinal cord.

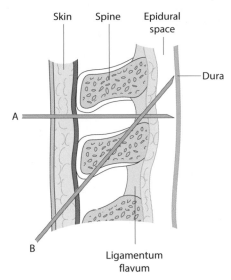

Figure 12.31 Needle positioning for an epidural anaesthetic. Midline (**A**) and paramedian (**B**) approaches.

position (**Figure 12.31**). This test dose is a small volume of dilute local anaesthetic that would not be expected to have any clinical effect. If indeed it has no obvious effect on sensation in the lower limbs, the catheter is correctly sited. If, however, there is a sensory block, leg weakness and peripheral vasodilatation, the catheter has been inserted too far and into the subarachnoid (spinal) space. Inserting the normal dose of local anaesthetic into the spinal space by accident would risk complete motor and respiratory paralysis. If none of these signs is observed 5 minutes after injection of the test dose, a loading dose can be administered. The epidural solution is usually a mixture of low-concentration local anaesthetic (e.g. 0.0625–0.1% bupivacaine) with an opioid such as fentanyl. Combining the opioid with the local anaesthetic reduces the amount of local anaesthetic required and this reduces the motor blockade and peripheral autonomic effects of the epidural (e.g. hypotension).

After the loading dose is given, the mother should be kept in the right or left lateral position, and her blood pressure should be measured every 5 minutes for 15 minutes.

A fall in blood pressure may result from the vasodilatation caused by blocking of the sympathetic tone to peripheral blood vessels. This hypotension is usually short lived, but may cause a fetal bradycardia due to redirection of maternal blood away from the uterus.

It should be treated with intravenous fluids and, if necessary, vasoconstrictors such as ephedrine. The mother should never lie supine, as aorto-caval compression can reduce maternal cardiac output and so compromise placental perfusion. Hourly assessment of the level of the sensory block using a cold spray is critical in the detection of a block that is creeping too high and risking respiratory compromise. Regional analgesia can be maintained throughout labour with either intermittent boluses or continuous infusions. Patient-controlled epidural analgesia is an option. Women should be encouraged to move around and adopt whichever upright position suits them best. Full mobility is unlikely. Reducing the rate of an epidural infusion in the second stage may increase the maternal awareness to push, but care should be taken that the analgesic effect is not compromised. Regional anaesthesia should be continued until after completion of the third stage of labour, including repair of any perineal injury.

Spinal anaesthesia

A spinal block is considered more effective than that obtained by an epidural, and is of faster onset. A fine-gauge atraumatic spinal needle is passed through the epidural space, through the dura and into the subarachnoid space, which contains the CSF. A small volume of local anaesthetic is injected, after which the spinal needle is withdrawn. This may be used as anaesthesia for caesarean sections, trial of instrumental deliveries (in theatre), manual removal of retained placenta and the repair of difficult perineal and vaginal tears. Spinals are not used for routine analgesia in labour.

Combined spinal–epidural (CSE) analgesia has gained in popularity. This technique has the advantage of producing a rapid onset of pain relief and the provision of prolonged analgesia. Because the initiating spinal dose is relatively low, this is a viable option for pain relief in labour.

Labour in special circumstances

Women with an uterine scar

Some women will have a pre-existing uterine scar, usually because of a previous caesarean section. Approximately 20–30% of all deliveries in developed countries are by caesarean section and 99% are performed through the lower segment of the uterus because blood loss is less, healing is better and the risk of subsequent uterine rupture is lower than that following an upper segment or 'classical' caesarean section. There are still a few indications for upper segment caesarean section (e.g. extreme prematurity) and it is important that these women are counselled appropriately. It is estimated that uterine rupture or dehiscence (scar separation) occurs in approximately 1 in 200 women who labour spontaneously with a pre-existing lower segment uterine scar. The risk is 2–3 times higher than this in women with a previous upper segment incision.

Signs of uterine rupture include severe lower abdominal pain, vaginal bleeding, haematuria, cessation of contractions, maternal tachycardia and fetal compromise (often a bradycardia, **Figure 12.32**). Uterine rupture carries serious maternal risks (shock, need for blood transfusion and operative repair, possibly a hysterectomy) and also serious fetal risks (including hypoxia, permanent neurological injury and perinatal death). Rupture of the uterus is more likely to occur late in the first stage of labour, with induced or accelerated labour and in association with a large baby.

Labour after a previous caesarean section is known as 'vaginal birth after caesarean' (VBAC).

Approximately 70–80% of women who attempt a VBAC will give birth successfully and the remainder will need repeat caesarean delivery. The chances of a successful vaginal birth depend on a number of factors, including a previous history of vaginal birth, size of the baby and the original indication for a caesarean section.

If a woman with a previous history of a caesarean section delivery is admitted in labour, close surveillance is required to identify early signs of uterine rupture. Continuous CTG monitoring is strongly recommended and there should be a low threshold for urgent delivery by repeat caesarean section. Some women will have scars on the uterus as a result of a previous myomectomy. In general, there is minimal danger of rupture of a myomectomy scar unless the uterine cavity was opened during the procedure.

Relative contraindications to VBAC

- Two or more previous caesarean section scars.
- Need for induction of labour (IOL).
- Previous labour outcome suggestive of CPD.
- Previous classical caesarean section is an absolute contraindication.

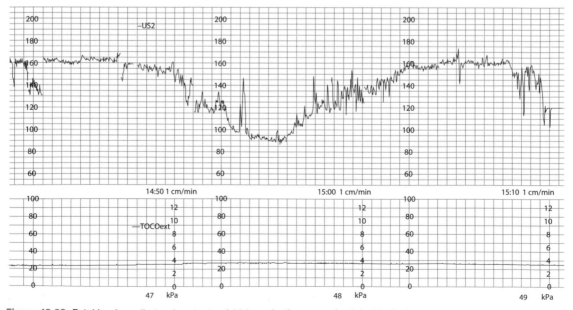

Figure 12.32 Fetal bradycardia to a heart rate of 90 bpm, lasting approximately 11 minutes.

Malpresentation

Breech presentation

The antenatal management of breech presentation and the mechanics of the delivery are discussed in Chapter 6, Antenatal obstetric complications. The majority of breech presentations recognized at term (≥37 weeks) are delivered by caesarean section. Although this is evidence based and it is probably safer for breech babies to be delivered this way, there is still a place for a vaginal breech delivery in certain circumstances. Maternal choice and the failure to detect breech presentation until very late in labour mean that obstetricians need to be expert in the skills of breech vaginal delivery and aware of the potential complications. Poor progress in a breech labour is taken by most to be an indication for caesarean section. However, some obstetricians support the use of augmentation with oxytocin if contractions are infrequent.

Complications of a breech labour and delivery

- Increased risk of cord prolapse: particularly with footling breech.
- Increased risk of CTG abnormalities as cord compression is common.
- Mechanical difficulties with the delivery of the shoulders and/or after-coming head, leading to damage of the visceral organs or the brachial plexus.
- Delay in the delivery of the head may occur with a larger fetus, leading to prolonged compression of the umbilical cord and asphyxia.
- Uncontrolled rapid delivery of the head may occur with a smaller fetus and predisposes to tentorial tears and intracranial bleeding.
- A small or preterm fetus may deliver through an incompletely dilated cervix, resulting in head entrapment.

Face presentation

Face presentation occurs in about 1 in 500 labours and is due to complete extension of the fetal head. In the majority of cases, the cause for the extension is unknown, although it is frequently attributed to excessive tone of the extensor muscles of the fetal neck. Rarely, extension may be due to a fetal anomaly such as a thyroid tumour. The presenting diameter is the submento-bregmatic, which measures 9.5 cm and is approximately the same in dimension as the suboccipito-bregmatic (vertex) presentation. Despite this, engagement of the fetal head is late and progress in labour is frequently slow, possibly because the facial bones do not mould. It is diagnosed in labour by palpating the nose, mouth and eyes on vaginal examination (**Figure 12.25**). If progress in labour is good and the chin remains mento-anterior, vaginal delivery is possible, the head being delivered by flexion (**Figure 12.26**). If the chin is posterior (mento-posterior position), delivery is impossible, as extension over the perineum cannot occur. In this circumstance, caesarean section is performed. Oxytocin should not be used, and if there is any concern about the fetal condition, caesarean section should be carried out. Forceps delivery is acceptable for low mento-anterior face presentations but ventouse is contraindicated.

Brow presentation

Brow presentation arises when there is less extreme extension of the fetal neck than that with a face presentation. It can be considered a midway position between vertex and face. It is the least common malpresentation, occurring in 1 in 2,000 labours. The causes are similar to those of face presentation, although some brow presentations arise as a result of exaggerated extension associated with an OP position. The presenting diameter is the mento-vertical (measuring 13.5 cm) (**Figures 12.14, 12.27**). This is incompatible with a vaginal delivery. It is diagnosed in labour by palpating the anterior fontanelle, supraorbital ridges and nose on vaginal examination (**Figure 12.28**). If this presentation persists, delivery can only be achieved by caesarean section.

Shoulder presentation

This is reported as occurring in 1 in 300 pregnancies at term, but few of these women will go into labour. Shoulder presentation occurs as the result of a transverse or oblique lie of the fetus and the causes of this abnormal presentation include placenta praevia, high parity, pelvic tumour and uterine anomaly (see Chapter 6, Antenatal obstetric complications). Delivery should be by caesarean section. Delay in making the diagnosis risks cord prolapse and uterine rupture.

Multiple pregnancy

About 1 in 80 pregnancies at term are multifetal, although the incidence is rising with increasing maternal age and assisted conception. High-order multiples, such as triplets and quadruplets, are now invariably delivered by caesarean section because of the difficulties in monitoring more than two fetuses and the elevated risks of fetal compromise. For twin pregnancies, the second twin is at greater risk of intrapartum compromise than the presenting twin or a singleton. The published evidence does not support recommending elective caesarean delivery for all twins and this was evaluated in a large multicentre randomized controlled trial (RCT). Nevertheless, caesarean section (elective or emergency) is performed in almost half of all twin pregnancies for a variety of indications.

In 70–80% of twin pregnancies the presenting twin is cephalic, with the majority of the remainder being breech (**Figure 12.33**). Vaginal birth is usually safely achievable where the presenting twin is in a cephalic vertex presentation. However, planned caesarean section will usually be performed if the first twin presents by the breech, and certainly if it is transverse.

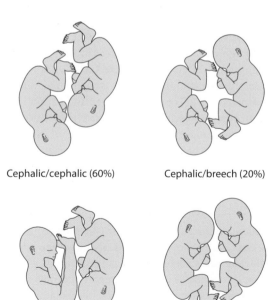

Cephalic/cephalic (60%)   Cephalic/breech (20%)

Breech/cephalic (10%)   Breech/breech (10%)

Figure 12.33 The four most common patterns of fetal presentation in a twin pregnancy.

The mechanics of the delivery of twins is discussed in greater detail in Chapter 7, Multiple pregnancy. Suffice to say that abnormal fetal growth, malpresentation, CTG abnormalities, cord prolapse, need for emergency caesarean section in labour and PPH all occur more commonly in twin than in singleton pregnancies.

🔑 KEY LEARNING POINTS

Normal and abnormal labour management:

- Most labours are uncomplicated and the outcomes are good.
- Labour can be a hazardous journey for the baby and the mother.
- Labour is divided into three stages.
- Progress in the first and second stage of labour is monitored with a partogram.
- Fetal wellbeing is monitored using the FHR, amniotic fluid and, where necessary, FBS.
- The term 'suspected fetal compromise' should be used if there are concerns about fetal wellbeing.
- Abnormalities of the uterine contractions (the 'powers'), the pelvis and lower genital tract (the 'passages') and the fetus (the 'passenger') can cause abnormal labour.
- Augmentation of labour with an oxytocin infusion will often correct inefficient uterine contractions and may help correct a fetal malposition.
- Augmentation of labour with oxytocin can be dangerous in multiparous women with a uterine scar, a malpresentation and where there are concerns about fetal wellbeing.
- Abnormal progress in the first stage of labour can be managed with ARM, oxytocin augmentation or emergency caesarean section.
- Abnormal progress in the second stage of labour can be managed with oxytocin augmentation, episiotomy, instrumental delivery (ventouse or forceps) or caesarean section.
- An abnormal third stage of labour may result in MROP and/or PPH.

Induction of labour

IOL is the planned initiation of labour prior to its spontaneous onset. Approximately 20–25% of deliveries in the UK occur following IOL. The common reasons for IOL are listed below. Broadly speaking, IOL is performed when the risks to the fetus and/or the mother of the pregnancy continuing outweigh those of bringing the pregnancy to an end. It should only be performed if there is a reasonable chance of success and if the risks of the process to the mother and/or fetus are acceptable. If either of these is not the case, the woman should be advised to await spontaneous onset of labour or a planned caesarean section should be performed.

The most common reason for IOL is prolonged pregnancy (previously described as 'post-term' or 'postdates'). There is evidence that pregnancies extending beyond 42 weeks' gestation are associated with a higher risk of stillbirth, fetal compromise in labour, meconium aspiration and mechanical problems at delivery. Because of this, women are usually recommended IOL between 41 and 42 weeks' gestation. Induction for prolonged pregnancy does not increase the rate of caesarean section. The evidence is high quality, and the recommendation a strong one; however, 300–400 pregnancies need to be induced to prevent one perinatal death that would have occurred if the pregnancies had been managed expectantly beyond 42 weeks' gestation. Women who choose not to be induced for this reason are offered more intensive serial fetal monitoring (see Chapter 6, Antenatal obstetric complications).

Prelabour rupture of membranes (PROM) is another common indication for IOL. It is not uncommon for the membranes to rupture and the subsequent onset of labour to be significantly delayed. The longer the delay between membrane rupture and delivery of the baby, the greater the risk of ascending infection (chorioamnionitis) and neonatal and maternal infectious morbidity. At term (beyond 37 weeks), good-quality evidence supports IOL approximately 24 hours following membrane rupture. This policy, endorsed in the NICE guideline on IOL, reduces rates of chorioamnionitis, endometritis and admissions to the neonatal unit. The evidence is less clear at present when PROM occurs preterm (PPROM). Before 34 weeks, some other additional indication is needed to justify IOL if the membranes rupture (e.g. suspected maternal infection, fetal compromise, growth restriction). Between 34 and 37 weeks, in an otherwise straightforward pregnancy, the risks

and benefits of IOL need to be assessed on an individual basis.

Pre-eclampsia and other maternal hypertensive disorders often indicate earlier delivery. Pre-eclampsia at term is normally managed with IOL; however, at very preterm gestations (<34 weeks) or where there is rapid maternal deterioration or significant fetal compromise, caesarean delivery may be a better option (see Chapter 9, Hypertensive disorders of pregnancy).

Maternal diabetes, twin gestation and intrahepatic cholestasis of pregnancy are all common reasons for IOL at 38 weeks' gestation, and sometimes earlier. The published evidence is limited, and a number of RCTs are in progress to address these issues.

Suspected fetal macrosomia (>90th percentile), in the absence of maternal diabetes, is now considered an indication for IOL following publication of a large RCT. The difficulty with this approach is that the estimation of fetal weight by ultrasound has an error margin of 10–20% and some inductions may subsequently prove to have been unnecessary.

'Social' induction of labour is controversial and is performed to satisfy the domestic and organizational needs of the woman and her family. It is mostly discouraged, and there must be careful counselling as to the potential risks involved. These are determined essentially by the parity and the cervical condition. If the situation is favourable for vaginal birth, with higher parity and a favourable cervix (see below, the Bishop score), 'soft' indications are more acceptable. In any circumstance, an induced labour cannot be considered 'normal' and should be carefully supervised.

There are a number of absolute contraindications to IOL, including placenta praevia and severe fetal compromise. Deteriorating maternal condition with major antepartum haemorrhage, pre-eclampsia or cardiac disease may favour caesarean delivery. Breech presentation is a relative contraindication to IOL, and women with a previous history of caesarean birth need to be informed of the greater risk of uterine rupture. Preterm gestation is not an absolute contraindication, but induction at <34 weeks is associated with a much higher risk of failure and the need for subsequent caesarean section.

Indications for induction of labour

- Prolonged pregnancy (usually offered after 41 completed weeks).
- PROM.
- Pre-eclampsia and other maternal hypertensive disorders.
- FGR.
- Diabetes mellitus.
- Fetal macrosomia.
- Deteriorating maternal illness.
- Unexplained antepartum haemorrhage.
- Twin pregnancy continuing beyond 38 weeks.
- Intrahepatic cholestasis of pregnancy.
- Maternal isoimmunization against red cell antigens.
- 'Social' reasons.

The Bishop score

As the time of spontaneous labour approaches, the cervix becomes softer, shortens, moves forward, effaces and starts to dilate. This reflects the natural preparation for labour. If labour is induced before this process has occurred, the induction process will tend to take longer. Bishop produced a scoring system (*Table 12.1*) to quantify how far this process had progressed prior to the IOL. High scores (a 'favourable' cervix) are associated with an easier, shorter induction process that is less likely to fail. Low scores (an 'unfavourable' cervix) point to a longer IOL that is more likely to fail and result in caesarean section.

Methods

IOL was traditionally performed by ARM. In the mid-1950s, synthetic oxytocin (Syntocinon)™ became available and was then used as an intravenous infusion after rupture of the membranes. In unfavourable cases, it was often unsuccessful and sometimes it was impossible to rupture the membranes. In the late 1960s, synthetic prostaglandin became available. Various routes and preparations have been used, but the most common formulation in current use is prostaglandin E2 (PGE2), inserted vaginally into the posterior fornix as a tablet or gel. Two doses are often required, given at least 6 hours apart. A controlled-release pessary is also available and this is left in place for up to 24 hours. Prostaglandins can be used even when the cervix is favourable. Labour may ensue following the administration of prostaglandin, but ARM and oxytocin are often also necessary, particularly in primiparous women. Oxytocin has a short half-life and is given intravenously as a dilute solution. The response to oxytocin is highly variable and a strict protocol exists for its use. The starting infusion rate is low and defined increments follow every 30 minutes until 3–5 contractions are achieved in every 10 minutes. Mifepristone (an antiprogesterone) and misoprostol (another prostaglandin) can be used to induce labour, but complication rates seem higher and this drug combination is currently used in the UK only to induce labour following intrauterine fetal death.

'Membrane sweeping' describes the insertion of a gloved finger through the cervix and its rotation around the inner rim of the cervix. This safe technique strips off the chorionic membrane from the underlying decidua and releases natural prostaglandins. It can be uncomfortable for the woman, and is only possible if the cervix is beginning to dilate and efface. It can be performed more than once and evidence shows that it reduces the need for induction. It is usually only performed at term, and placenta praevia must be excluded before it is offered. It should be considered an adjunct to the normal processes of induction.

Table 12.1 Modified Bishop scoring system

Score	0	1	2	3
Dilatation of cervix (cm)	0	1 or 2	3 or 4	5 or more
Consistency of cervix	Firm	Medium	Soft	–
Length of cervical canal (cm)	>2	2–1	1–0.5	<0.5
Position of cervix	Posterior	Central	Anterior	–
Station of presenting part	−3	−2	−1 or 0	Below spines

Methods of induction

- Membrane sweep (offer weekly from 40 weeks).
- Prostaglandin gel, tablet or pessary to ripen cervix and initiate contractions.
- ARM (cervix must be favourable).
- Oxytocin infusion (membranes ruptured first, spontaneous or artificial).
- Mifepristone and misopostol (for intrauterine fetal death).

Complications of induction of labour

It is generally agreed that a woman is likely to experience more pain with an induced labour and the use of epidural analgesia is more common. The rates of instrumental delivery are higher where epidural analgesia is used, but two recent systematic reviews show no evidence of a higher rate of caesarean section. Long labours augmented with oxytocin predispose to PPH secondary to uterine atony. Fetal compromise may occur during induced labours and this, in part at least, is due to uterine hyperstimulation as a side-effect of use of prostaglandins and oxytocin (**Figure 12.23**). A contraction frequency of >5 per 10 minutes should be treated by stopping the oxytocin and if necessary administration of a tocolytic drug, most commonly a subcutaneous injection of the β2-agonist terbutaline. Uterine hyperstimulation may precipitate a fetal bradycardia and the need for emergency caesarean section if the FHR fails to resolve promptly. If ARM is performed while the fetal head is high, then cord prolapse may occur, again precipitating the need for emergency caesarean section. Women with a previous caesarean section scar are at greater risk of uterine rupture if they are induced. The risk of scar rupture increases from one in 200 in a spontaneous labour to as high as 1 in 70 if IOL is performed using prostaglandins.

IOL may fail and this is said to have occurred if an ARM is still impossible after the maximum number of doses of prostaglandin have been given or if the cervix remains uneffaced and less than 3 cm dilated after an ARM has been performed and oxytocin has been running for 6–8 hours with regular contractions. When an induction fails, the options include a rest period followed by attempting induction again at some point in the future, or performing a caesarean section. Delaying delivery further is only acceptable if there is no major threat to fetal or maternal condition. This may be the case with a failed social induction, for example. Failed induction in the setting of pre-eclampsia or FGR will usually necessitate a caesarean delivery.

Clinical risk management

Risk management is an approach to health care provision that aims to limit harm occurring to patients and also to improve the quality of care. Clinical risk management (CRM) can be applied to all areas of medicine, but the labour ward provides one of the best illustrations of its importance to modern health care.

Labour and delivery carry a serious risk of harm. Maternal trauma (both physical and psychological) and infant neurological injuries are examples of poor outcomes following birth that can potentially be avoided in many cases. Legal action is frequently taken after outcomes such as these, and this is expensive for the National Health Service in litigation payments and distressing for the staff involved. The aim of CRM is to improve standards of care and subsequently reduce the harm occurring to women and their babies. This in turn should reduce the number of complaints made against hospital trusts and the financial costs of litigation.

Shoulder dystocia, for example, can result in brachial plexus injury, intrapartum asphyxia and serious maternal perineal trauma. In many cases, these poor outcomes following shoulder dystocia can be avoided by appropriate management. Regular staff education and the performance of shoulder dystocia 'drills' can limit adverse outcomes. In these drills, the manoeuvres used to safely overcome shoulder dystocia are rehearsed to facilitate timely skilled intervention in the event of a real emergency. The use of guidelines and protocols drawn from evidence-based medicine is another tool of CRM. These help to reduce errors and prevent erratic or incorrect decision-making.

Medical and midwifery staff are encouraged to report when things 'go wrong'. Once a 'near-miss' or an adverse outcome has occurred, careful documentation is vital if claims of negligence are to be defended.

Good communication between the staff and the patient involved may help to clear up misunderstandings and minimize the chances of a formal complaint or legal action. 'Root-cause analysis' is a technique that serves to examine in detail a poor outcome or near-miss, so that every step of the patient-journey is scrutinized to see if the outcome could have been prevented. This approach allows assessment of both systemic (organizational) and individual (doctor/ midwife) contribution to errors. In this way, lessons are learned for the future and Unit policies and guidelines can be adjusted accordingly. It is usually the case that a whole series of failings or errors need to occur together for a poor outcome to result (a cascade effect). Organizational systems as a whole often contribute, and one single individual is rarely solely responsible for a poor outcome.

Audit of labour ward outcomes is an important tool in risk management. If guidelines are not being followed, and certain standards are not being met, this will be detected by audit and steps taken to address the problem. A repeat audit should show that improvements have occurred as a result of the actions taken.

KEY LEARNING POINTS

Important elements of risk management:

- Focus on safety and quality of care.
- Clinical audit.
- Education and training.
- Clinical incident reporting.
- Root cause analysis of adverse events.
- Systems for complaints and claims handling.
- Guidelines and research.
- Service development.

Further reading

Anim-Somuah M, Smyth RMD, Jones L (2011). Epidural versus non-epidural or no analgesia in labour. *Cochrane Database of Systematic Reviews* 12. Art. No.:CD000331.

Birthplace in England Collaborative Group (2011). Perinatal and maternal outcomes by planned place of birth for healthy women with low risk pregnancies in England national prospective cohort study. *BMJ* **343**:d7400.

NICE. Induction of Labour. NICE Clinical Guideline 70. London: NICE, 2008.

NICE. Intrapartum Care; Care of Healthy Women and their Babies during Childbirth. NICE Clinical Guideline 190. London: NICE, 2014.

Self assessment

CASE HISTORY

Ms M, a 28-year-old woman, booked for antenatal care in her first pregnancy. She attended for shared care between her midwife and obstetrician and her pregnancy was uncomplicated. Her membranes ruptured spontaneously at 40 weeks and 4 days. The liquor was clear and her vital signs were normal. She was advised that she could wait for 24 hours to allow spontaneous labour to establish if all was well. Regular contractions started after 4 hours and she presented to the labour ward later that night. On abdominal examination she was assessed to have an average size fetus with one-fifth of the head palpable, confirming engagement. On admission she had strong regular painful contractions at a rate of 3–4 in 10 minutes. The cervix was soft, central, effaced and 5 cm dilated, with the vertex 2 cm above the ischial spines. She was transferred to a labour room in spontaneous labour for ongoing monitoring. She was monitored with intermittent auscultation of the fetal heart rate at 15 minute intervals and her vital signs were checked every 4 hours. She had vaginal examinations at 4-hourly intervals. The contractions spaced out to 2 in every 10 minutes and 8 hours after admission she was found to be 5 cm dilated.

What is the diagnosis and what are the management options?

ANSWER

This is arrest of labour in the first stage, most likely due to inefficient uterine contractions. The membranes have ruptured spontaneously and therefore the next option is to commence a Syntocinon™ infusion to augment labour. In this case, Ms M progressed to full dilatation 4 hours after commencing Syntocinon and progressed to a normal vaginal delivery.

EMQs

1 A Descent.
   B Extension.
   C Engagement.
   D Flexion.

   E External rotation.
   F Restitution.
   G Internal rotation.
   H None of the above.

For each description, choose the SINGLE most appropriate answer from the list of options. Each option may be used once, more than once or not at all.

1 After the head delivers through the vulva, it immediately aligns with the shoulders.
2 The occiput escapes from underneath the symphysis pubis, which acts as a fulcrum.
3 The anterior shoulder lies inferior to the symphysis pubis and delivers first, and then the posterior shoulder delivers subsequently.
4 Terminology for when the widest part of the presenting part has passed successfully through the pelvic inlet

ANSWERS

1F 2B 3H 4C

The mechanism of labour refers to the series of changes that occurs in the position and attitude of the fetus during its passage through the birth canal. The process involves engagement, descent, flexion, internal rotation, extension, restitution, external rotation and delivery of the shoulders and fetal body. Engagement is said to have occurred when the widest part of the presenting part has passed successfully through the inlet.

2 A Latent phase.
   B Third stage.
   C Transition.
   D Passive descent.

   E Braxton Hicks.
   F Effacement.
   G Active second stage of labour.
   H None of the above.

For each description, choose the SINGLE most appropriate answer from the list of options. Each option may be used once, more than once or not at all.

1 Should be considered abnormal if lasting more than 30 minutes.
2 The cervix shortens in length until it becomes included in the lower segment of the uterus.
3 Conventionally should last no longer than 2 hours in a primiparous women.
4 Time between onset of labour and 3–4 cm cervical dilatation.

ANSWERS

1B The third stage of labour is the time from delivery of the fetus until delivery of the placenta and membrane. The time at which the third stage should be considered abnormal may be increased to 60 minutes if the woman has opted for a physiological third stage.
2F The process of effacement may begin during the weeks preceding the onset of labour, but will be complete by the end of the latent phase.
3G The active second stage of labour conventionally lasts no longer than 2 hours in a primiparous women and no longer than 1 hour in a woman who has had a previous vaginal delivery.
4A The duration of labour is highly variable and may be prolonged, especially in primiparous women.

SBA QUESTIONS

Choose the single best answer.

1 A 32-year-old woman is admitted to the labour ward at 39+2 weeks' gestation in her second pregnancy. She is having regular painful contractions and on examination her cervix is 4 cm dilated. Her membranes are intact. She has a birth plan and wishes to birth as naturally as possible. The midwife is intermittently auscultating the fetal heart, which is normal.

Two hours after her initial vaginal examination the cervix is 6 cm on examination. What would your plan of care for this woman be?

A ARM.

B Caesarean section.

C Continue current management.

D Commence CTG.

E Intravenous antibiotics.

ANSWER

C This woman has established labour spontaneously and is making normal progress (usually defined as 1 cm cervical dilatation per hour). The fetal heart is normal and she does not wish for any intervention. There is no indication to perform an artificial rupture of membranes or a caesarean section. The fetal heart is normal on intermittent auscultation and there are no indications for continuous monitoring with CTG.

2 IOL is considered when the maternal or fetal condition suggests that a better outcome will be achieved by intervening in the pregnancy than allowing it to continue. Which of the following is a contraindication to IOL?

A Pre-eclampsia.

B Placenta praevia.

C Intrauterine fetal death.

D Previous caesarean section delivery.

E FGR.

ANSWER

B Normal delivery cannot be achieved in the presence of placenta praevia. IOL is therefore absolutely contraindicated in these circumstances.

LEARNING OBJECTIVES

- To understand the appropriate management of perineal tears.
- To understand the appropriate management of episiotomy.
- To understand the indications, contraindications, procedures and complications of instrumental delivery with ventouse or forceps.

- To understand the indications, procedure, complications and consequences of caesarean section.
- To introduce the concept of risk management in relation to operative delivery.

Introduction

The majority of women aim for a spontaneous vaginal delivery with an intact perineum and fall within the remit of midwifery care. Unfortunately, this outcome is achieved in barely half of all women who labour in the UK. Labour is a physiological process with inherent unpredictability and even the most normal birth can result in complications that require obstetric intervention and some form of operative delivery. The most common form of operative intervention is suturing of a perineal tear or episiotomy. Uncomplicated perineal tears are repaired by a midwife but, if the tear is complex, it will require repair in an operating theatre by an obstetrician. Women who encounter complications in the first stage of labour requiring urgent delivery for either maternal or fetal indications will need to be delivered by emergency caesarean section. Complications that occur in the second stage of labour present a choice between instrumental delivery with a ventouse or forceps and delivery by caesarean section. A further group of women will have a scheduled or elective caesarean section performed before the onset of labour. In all cases, operative intervention should only be performed when the benefits outweigh the potential risks. The needs of the mother and the baby should be balanced with careful consideration of the potential consequences in the short term and for the future. Operative deliveries should only be performed by clinicians who have competency in the procedure or under direct supervision of an experienced trainer.

Perineal repair

Of women who have a vaginal delivery, 85% will have some degree of perineal trauma and 60–70% will require suturing. The first important step following birth of the baby and delivery of the placenta is to examine the woman carefully to classify the perineal tear. Perineal tears should be classified as first, second, third or fourth degree, and when in doubt the operator should classify according to a higher rather than lower grade (*Table 13.1*). This will ensure that the woman receives optimal care.

Some women perform perineal massage in the antenatal period and this may reduce the risk or extent of tearing. Perineal tears occur more commonly with prolonged labour, especially the active second stage, with big babies and in association with instrumental delivery. Third-degree tears are reported in approximately 3% of primigravidae and 0.5% of multiparae. In general terms, external anal sphincter incompetence causes faecal urgency, whereas internal anal sphincter incompetence causes faecal incontinence. Third- and fourth-degree tears are grouped together and termed obstetric anal sphincter injuries (OASI).

Surgical technique

First-degree tears or minor lacerations with minimal or no bleeding may not require surgical repair. A systematic approach should be followed for second-degree perineal repair (**Figure 13.1**). An explanation should be provided to the mother and verbal consent should be documented, or written consent if a complex tear requires repair in an operating theatre. Adequate analgesia should be provided by topping up an epidural or by infiltration with local anaesthetic. The operator should check the extent of grazes and lacerations with a vaginal and rectal examination. Sometimes, the anatomy is not clear and assessment is improved following positioning in lithotomy with effective anaesthesia. If a tear is more complex than initially appreciated, a more experienced operator may be required.

> ▶ **VIDEO 13.1**
>
> Repair of an episiotomy/second-degree perineal tear: http://www.routledgetextbooks.com/textbooks/tenteachers/obstetricsv13.1.php

Table 13.1 Grading of perineal tears

First degree	Injury to perineal skin only
Second degree	Injury to perineum involving muscles but not anal sphincter
Third degree	Injury to perineum involving the anal sphincter complex
IIIa	<50% of EAS torn
IIIb	>50% of EAS torn
IIIc	Both the EAS and IAS torn
Fourth degree	Fourth-degree lacerations involve the perineal fascia and muscles, both the EAS and the IAS, and the rectal mucosa

EAS: external anal sphincter; IAS: internal anal sphincter.

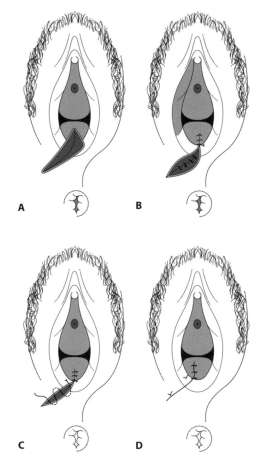

Figure 13.1 Repair of an episiotomy/second-degree perineal tear. **(A)** The perineum prior to the repair; **(B)** continuous repair of the vaginal mucosa; **(C)** subcutaneous suture of the skin; **(D)** completed repair.

It may be helpful to place a pad or tampon high in the vagina to prevent blood loss from the uterus obscuring the view. Care needs to be taken that this is removed at the end of the procedure. The vaginal mucosa is repaired first using rapidly absorbable suture material on a large, round body needle. A knot should be tied above the apex of the cut or tear (as severed vessels retract slightly) and a continuous stitch should be used to close the vaginal mucosa. Interrupted sutures are then placed to close the muscle layer. Closure of the perineal skin follows with either interrupted sutures or a continuous subcuticular stitch, which produces more comfortable results. A gentle vaginal examination should be performed to check for any missed tears and to ensure that good apposition has been achieved. A rectal examination should be performed to confirm that the sphincter feels intact and to ensure that no sutures have been inadvertently placed through the rectal mucosa. If sutures are felt in the rectum they must be removed and replaced. The pad or tampon should be removed and a careful count of swabs, instruments and needles should be completed and documented in the records, alongside the operation note and postoperative instructions. Analgesia should be prescribed.

OASI repair

Repair of third- and fourth-degree tears should be performed or directly supervised by a trained practitioner. There must be adequate analgesia. In practice, this means either a regional or general anaesthetic, as local infiltration does not allow relaxation of the sphincter enough to allow a satisfactory repair. The lighting must be adequate and an assistant is usually needed. Repair of the rectal mucosa should be performed first. The torn external sphincter is then repaired. It is important to ensure that the muscle is correctly approximated with long-acting sutures so that the muscle is given adequate time to heal. Some surgeons opt for an end-to-end repair, while others use an overlap technique; current evidence suggests that the outcome is similar with both methods. The remainder of the perineal repair is as for second-degree trauma. The surgical repair should be documented and a clinical incident form should be completed for risk assessment purposes.

OASI aftercare

Lactulose (laxative) and a bulking agent, such as Fybogel™, are recommended for 5–10 days and the woman should remain in hospital until she has had a first bowel motion. An oral broad-spectrum antibiotic should be prescribed for 5–7 days to reduce the risk of infection. Regular oral analgesia should also be prescribed. All women who have sustained a third- or fourth-degree tear should be offered follow-up in the postnatal period. A team approach is ideal within a specialist clinic; physiotherapy should include augmented biofeedback as this has been shown to improve continence. At 6–12 weeks, a full evaluation of the degree of symptoms should take place. This must include careful questioning with regard to faecal and urinary symptoms and advice in relation to future pregnancy and delivery. Asymptomatic women should be advised that the risk of recurrence in a future pregnancy is 6–8% and that vaginal delivery is safely achievable. Symptomatic women should be offered investigation including endoanal ultrasound and manometry (see Chapter 15, The puerperium). Women with ongoing troublesome symptoms should be offered an elective caesarean section.

Episiotomy

An episiotomy is a surgical incision of the perineum performed during the second stage of labour to enlarge the vulval outlet and assist vaginal birth. Although episiotomies were described in textbooks dating back to the mid-18th century, widespread use of the procedure increased during the early twentieth century. By the 1970s, rates were as high as 90% and it was widely believed that episiotomy was preferable to tearing. A number of randomized controlled trials (RCTs) were conducted comparing restrictive versus routine use of episiotomy. The evidence was collated in a Cochrane systematic review, which demonstrated that a restrictive approach resulted in less posterior perineal trauma and less need for suturing with no difference in pain, urinary incontinence or dyspareunia. A routine episiotomy was not protective of more severe perineal tears (OASI). In the UK, rates now approximate the World Health Organization (WHO) recommendation of 10% of spontaneous vaginal deliveries. However, there remains considerable international variation (rates are 50% in the USA and 99% in Eastern Europe).

Surgical technique

The question of informed consent needs to be addressed as part of antenatal care; when the fetal head is crowning, it is not possible to obtain true informed consent. An episiotomy is performed in the second stage, usually when the perineum is being stretched and it is deemed necessary; for example, when delivery needs to be expedited for a fetal bradycardia. If there is not a good epidural, the perineum should be infiltrated with local anaesthetic. If an effective epidural anaesthetic is in place, and time allows, it should be topped up for delivery with the patient upright to get best coverage of the perineal area.

The incision can be midline or at an angle from the posterior end of the vulva. A mediolateral episiotomy at a 60° angle to the midline is usually recommended; a midline episiotomy is an incision in a comparatively avascular area and results in less bleeding, quicker healing and less pain; however, there is an increased risk of extension to involve the anal sphincter (OASI). A mediolateral episiotomy should start at the posterior part of the fourchette, move backwards and then turn medially well before the border of the anal sphincter, so that any extension will avoid the sphincter (**Figure 13.2**). The episiotomy should be repaired in the same way as a second-degree tear unless there has been involvement of the anal sphincter complex requiring an OASI repair.

Complications

Short-term complications of perineal trauma or episiotomy include pain, infection and haemorrhage. Long-term effects include dyspareunia, incontinence of urine and incontinence of flatus or faeces. The risks are highest with OASI, especially if an anal sphincter injury has been missed. These morbidities can have a profound impact on women's health, relationships and self-esteem.

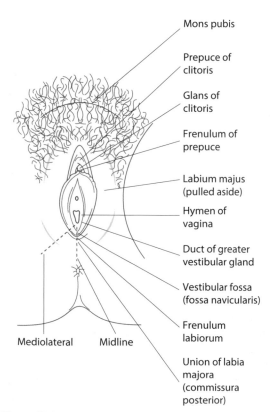

Mons pubis

Prepuce of clitoris

Glans of clitoris

Frenulum of prepuce

Labium majus (pulled aside)

Hymen of vagina

Duct of greater vestibular gland

Vestibular fossa (fossa navicularis)

Frenulum labiorum

Union of labia majora (commissura posterior)

Mediolateral   Midline

Figure 13.2 A right mediolateral episiotomy.

🔑 KEY LEARNING POINTS

- First- or second-degree tearing and uncomplicated episiotomy can be repaired under epidural or local anaesthesia in a labour room by a midwife or obstetrician.
- Assessment of the anal sphincter complex is essential in all cases to ensure that a third- or fourth-degree tear has not been missed.
- Third- or fourth-degree tears require regional anaesthesia and are usually repaired in an operating theatre by an obstetrician with good lighting and an assistant.
- Either 'end-to-end' or overlap repair of the anal sphincter muscle with a long-acting suture material is acceptable.
- Aftercare is important for all women who tear, but women with OASI should receive antibiotics, stool softeners and follow-up specialist review including physiotherapy.
- Women who experience significant pelvic floor symptoms following OASI should be offered an elective caesarean section in a future pregnancy.
- Mediolateral episiotomy should be performed in preference to midline, and it should be used restrictively.

Operative vaginal delivery

Operative vaginal delivery (OVD) refers to a vaginal birth with the use of any type of forceps or vacuum extractor (ventouse). The terms instrumental delivery, assisted vaginal delivery and OVD are used interchangeably. The goal of OVD is to expedite delivery with a minimum of maternal or neonatal morbidity. As with other forms of intrapartum intervention, OVD should only be performed when the safety criteria have been met and when the benefits outweigh the risks. The guidelines of the Royal College of Obstetricians and Gynaecologists (RCOG) advise that obstetricians should achieve experience in spontaneous vaginal delivery prior to commencing training in OVDs. OVDs should be conducted by obstetricians with competency in the chosen procedure or by trainees under direct supervision of an experienced trainer. When these conditions are adhered to, the outcomes of OVD are good.

In the UK, between 10% and 15% of deliveries are assisted with forceps or ventouse. The rate in nulliparous women is as high as 30%. The incidence of OVD varies widely both within and between countries, and this impacts on rates of second-stage caesarean section. Different strategies have been employed to help lower rates of OVD including provision of one-to-one midwifery care in labour, the presence of a birth partner, delayed pushing in the second stage of labour, especially with epidural analgesia, use of oxytocin to enhance expulsive contractions in the second stage of labour and maternal repositioning to enhance the effects of gravity and the maternal urge to push.

The history of forceps delivery is fascinating. Although the use of birth instruments was initially limited to the extraction of dead fetuses via destructive techniques, from as early as 1500 BC there exist reports of successful deliveries of live infants in obstructed labour. In the sixteenth and seventeenth centuries, the male midwife appeared as a new health practitioner and frequently dealt with obstructed labour. The development of the modern obstetric forceps by the Chamberlens, a Huguenot family practising in England, dramatically changed the role of assisted delivery in favour of a live infant. The Chamberlens kept their secret for more than a century; however, it is thought that Peter Chamberlen the Elder was the pioneer in the development of forceps. Hugh Chamberlen, his son, unsuccessfully tried to persuade the great French obstetrician François Mauriceau to adopt obstetric forceps. Chamberlen's visit to Paris failed miserably when Mauriceau mischievously challenged him to deliver a baby in obstructed labour due to a contracted pelvis with maternal rickets; Chamberlen's futile efforts had disastrous effects for both mother and baby. Nonetheless, instrumental delivery became more widely accepted at least in part due to the work of William Smellie, a Scottish doctor working in the poorer parts of London. Smellie was a great teacher of both midwives and physicians, and described the use of forceps in his Treatise on the theory and practice of midwifery, published in 1752. Forceps delivery remains controversial to this day.

Indications

The indications for OVD can be divided into fetal or maternal, although in many cases these factors coexist. The most common fetal factor is suspected fetal compromise, usually based on a pathological cardiotocograph (CTG). The most common maternal factor is a prolonged active second stage of labour. The underlying aetiology for a prolonged second stage should be evaluated in terms of the 3 Ps (see Chapter 12, Labour: normal and abnormal). It may relate to inefficient uterine activity or poor maternal pushing ('powers'), short maternal stature, a less favourable pelvic shape or a tight perineum ('passages') and a macrosomic fetus, malposition or malpresentation ('passenger'). A mismatch between the passages and the passenger may result in cephalopelvic disproportion (CPD). Depending on the overall clinical findings it may be appropriate to use an oxytocin infusion, change the maternal position and offer further encouragement or proceed directly to instrumental delivery. In some cases the findings will be a contraindication to OVD and favour delivery by caesarean section. The indications are summarized in Table 13.2. The complexity of the procedure is reflected in how low the fetal head has descended within the pelvis (station) and whether or not rotation is required. The classification system is described in Table 13.3.

Table 13.2 Indications for OVD

Fetal	Suspected fetal compromise (CTG pathological, abnormal pH or lactate on fetal blood sampling, thick meconium)
Maternal	Nulliparous women – lack of continuing progress for 3 hours (total of active and passive second stage of labour) with regional anaesthesia or 2 hours without regional anaesthesia
	Multiparous women – lack of continuing progress for 2 hours (total of active and passive second stage of labour) with regional anaesthesia or 1 hour without regional anaesthesia
	Maternal exhaustion/vomiting/distress
	Medical indications to avoid prolonged pushing or valsalva (e.g. cardiac disease, hypertensive crisis, cerebral vascular disease, particularly uncorrected cerebral vascular malformations, myasthenia gravis, spinal cord injury)
Combined	Fetal and maternal indications for assisted vaginal delivery often coexist. The threshold to intervene may be lower where several factors coexist

International guidelines (RCOG, ACOG and NICE) largely agree on second stage duration.
Note: No indication is absolute and each case should be considered individually. CTG, cardiotocograph.

Table 13.3 Classification of operative vaginal delivery

Outlet	Fetal scalp visible without separating the labia*
	Fetal skull has reached the pelvic floor
	Sagittal suture is in the antero-posterior diameter or right or left occiput anterior or posterior position (rotation does not exceed 45°)
	Fetal head is at or on the perineum
Low	Leading point of the skull (not caput) is at station plus 2 cm or more but not on the pelvic floor
	Two subdivisions: (a) rotation of 45° or less; (b) rotation more than 45°
Mid	Fetal head is no more than 1/5 palpable per abdomen, usually 0/5
	Leading point of the skull is above station plus 2 cm but not above the ischial spines (station 0 to +1)
	Two subdivisions: (a) rotation of 45° or less; (b) rotation of more than 45°
High	Not appropriate, therefore not included in classification (station –1 or above)

Adapted from RCOG 2011, ACOG 2000.
* Marked caput may give the impression that the vertex is lower than it actually is; systematic abdominal and vaginal examination are required to confirm the classification for assisted vaginal delivery.

Contraindications

A careful assessment should take place to ensure that the safety criteria for OVD have been fulfilled (*Table 13.4*). When the safety criteria are not met, OVD is contraindicated; for example, a high fetal head two-fifths palpable abdominally with station above the ischial spines. The ventouse should not be used in gestations of less than 34 completed weeks because of the risk of cephalhaematoma and intracranial haemorrhage. It is relatively contraindicated at gestational ages 35–36 weeks. It should not be used for a face or breech presentation. There is minimal risk of fetal haemorrhage if the vacuum extractor is employed following fetal blood sampling (FBS) or application of a fetal scalp electrode (FSE). Forceps and vacuum extractor deliveries before full dilatation of the cervix are contraindicated, although possible exceptions occur (e.g. with the vacuum delivery of a second twin where the cervix has contracted somewhat in the interval between delivery of the first and second twins).

Choice of instrument

The guidelines of the RCOG in the UK recommend that obstetricians should be competent and confident in the use of both forceps and the

Table 13.4 Safety criteria for operative vaginal delivery

Full abdominal and vaginal examination	Head is ≤1/5 palpable per abdomen (in most cases 0/5 palpable)
	Cervix is fully dilated and the membranes ruptured
	Station at level of ischial spines or below (0/+1/+2/+3)
	Exact position of the head has been determined so correct placement of the instrument can be achieved
	Caput and moulding is no more than moderate
	Pelvis is deemed adequate
Preparation of mother	Clear explanation given and informed consent obtained
	Trust has been established and woman offers full cooperation
	Appropriate anaesthesia is in place; for midpelvic rotational delivery this will usually be a regional block; a pudendal block may be appropriate in the context of urgency; a perineal block may be sufficient for low-pelvic or outlet delivery
	Maternal bladder has been emptied recently
	In-dwelling catheter has been removed or balloon deflated
	Aseptic technique
Preparation of staff	Operator has the knowledge, experience and skill necessary
	Adequate facilities are available (appropriate equipment, bed, lighting) and access to an operating theatre
	Back-up plan in place in case of failure to deliver:
	• For midpelvic deliveries, theatre staff should be available immediately to allow a caesarean section to be performed without delay (<30 minutes); senior obstetrician should be present if a junior obstetrician is conducting the delivery
	• Anticipation of complications that may arise (e.g. shoulder dystocia, perineal trauma, postpartum haemorrhage)
	• Personnel present that are trained in neonatal resuscitation

Adapted from International Guidelines.

ventouse and that practitioners should choose the most appropriate instrument for the individual circumstances. The choice of instrument should be based on a combination of indication, experience and training. The aim should be to complete the delivery successfully with the lowest possible morbidity and, where appropriate, the preferences of the mother should be taken into account. Ventouse and forceps have been compared in a number of RCTs analysed within a Cochrane systematic review.

The incidence of maternal pelvic floor trauma in deliveries performed with the ventouse is significantly less than with forceps; anal sphincter injury in particular is twice as common with forceps delivery (8% versus 3–4%). There is a paucity of long-term follow-up data; however, one of the largest RCTs showed no difference in pelvic floor symptoms between women delivered by forceps or ventouse when assessed at approximately 5 years after the birth. Ventouse delivery is preferred as a first-line instrument by many obstetricians in terms of reduced maternal trauma, but this needs to be balanced with a failure rate of 10–20% compared to a failure rate with forceps of 5% or less for similar deliveries. The morbidities for the baby differ with a higher incidence of cephalhaematoma and cerebral haemorrhage with ventouse and a higher incidence of lacerations and facial palsy with forceps.

The ventouse compared to forceps is significantly **more** likely to be associated with:

- Failure to achieve a vaginal delivery.
- Cephalohaematoma (subperiosteal bleed).
- Retinal haemorrhage.
- Maternal worries about the baby.

The ventouse compared to forceps is significantly **less** likely to be associated with:

- Use of maternal regional/general anaesthesia.
- Significant maternal perineal and vaginal trauma.
- Severe perineal pain at 24 hours.

The ventouse compared to forceps is **similar** in terms of:

- Delivery by caesarean section (where failed vacuum is completed by forceps).
- Low 5 minute Apgar scores.

Place of delivery

OVDs in the midpelvis are more difficult either because there is a malposition and rotation is required or there is a degree of relative CPD (*Table 13.3*). These deliveries require a higher degree of skill and there is inherent uncertainty whether OVD can be achieved safely. The alternative is to deliver by caesarean section, which can also be a very challenging procedure with the head deep in the pelvis. There have been no RCTs to date comparing these approaches. A prospective cohort study of an entire population of women over 1 year in the UK reported that women who were delivered by caesarean section in the second stage of labour were more likely to have a major haemorrhage and to need a hospital stay of more than 5 days. On the other hand, babies delivered by caesarean section were less likely to have trauma than babies delivered by forceps, but were more likely to require admission for intensive care. It is important to note that the experience of the operator was directly related to the chance of major haemorrhage whatever the mode of delivery. What was striking was the outcome of subsequent pregnancies, where almost 70% of women who had a second stage caesarean went on have a repeat caesarean in the next pregnancy compared to only 10% of women who

had a successful OVD. It should therefore be the aim in the second stage of labour to deliver women vaginally, unless there are contraindications or the woman expresses a clear preference for caesarean section. Although the psychological consequences of transferring a patient to an operating theatre in the second stage of labour should not be underestimated, most midpelvic procedures, which by their nature have a higher rate of complications than outlet or low deliveries, should be performed in an operating theatre with immediate recourse to caesarean delivery should it be required. It is essential that skilled obstetricians supervise complex operative deliveries performed by trainees, whatever the time of day or night they occur.

Procedure

The anatomy of the birth canal and its relationship to the fetal head must be understood as a prerequisite to becoming skilled in the safe use of forceps or ventouse (see Chapter 12, Labour: normal and abnormal).

Evaluation

A thorough abdominal and vaginal examination should take place to confirm the fetal lie, presentation, engagement, station, position, attitude and degree of caput or moulding. This will confirm whether or not the basic safety criteria for OVD have been met. A careful pelvic examination is essential to determine whether there are any 'mechanical' contraindications to performing an OVD. If, for example, a contracted pelvis is the cause of failure to progress in the second stage, then due consideration must be paid to determining the type of instrument to be employed or whether it may be more prudent to perform a caesarean section. The shape of the subpubic arch, the curve of the sacral hollow and the presence of flat or prominent ischial spines all contribute to the decision as to whether a vaginal delivery may be safely performed. Anthropoid (narrow), android (male/funnel-shaped) or platypelloid (elliptical) pelvises all make instrumental deliveries more difficult and may preclude the use of rotational forceps. A trial push is very helpful in determining whether descent is possible and it may also be possible to attempt manual rotation of a fetal malposition at this point.

Analgesia

Analgesic requirements are greater for forceps than for ventouse delivery. Where rotational forceps or midpelvic direct traction forceps are needed, regional analgesia is preferred. For a rigid cup ventouse delivery, a pudendal block with perineal infiltration may be all that is needed and if a soft cup is used, analgesic requirements may be limited to perineal infiltration with local anaesthetic. A requirement for haste should not preclude the use of analgesia. No operator would consider performing a caesarean section without the appropriate anaesthesia and the same should be true for OVD.

Positioning

OVDs are traditionally performed with the patient in the lithotomy position. The angle of traction needed requires that the bottom part of the bed be removed. In patients with limited abduction (such as those with symphysis pubis dysfunction), it may be necessary to limit abduction of the thighs to a minimum. It is the operator's duty to ensure that the bladder is emptied.

Contingency planning

With any OVD there is the potential for failure with the chosen instrument and the operator must have a back-up plan for such an event. It may be possible to complete a failed vacuum delivery with low-pelvic forceps, but failed or abandoned forceps delivery will almost always result in caesarean section. With any difficult instrumental delivery, the risk of shoulder dystocia occurring after successful delivery of the fetal head should be considered, as should the potential for postpartum haemorrhage (PPH). As a consequence, the operator must develop the skills necessary to anticipate such events and to manage the consequences in a logical and calm manner.

Instrument types

Ventouse/vacuum extractors

The basic premise of vacuum extraction is that a suction cup, of a silastic or rigid construction, is connected, via tubing, to a vacuum source (**Figure 13.3**). Either directly through the tubing or via a connecting 'chain', direct traction can then be applied to the presenting part coordinated with maternal pushing to expedite delivery. Recent developments have removed the need for cumbersome external suction generators and have incorporated the vacuum mechanism into 'hand-held' pumps (e.g. OmniCup™). Initial clinical trials suggested that the failure rate is higher with hand-held disposable devices, but this may have been related to the learning curve of adapting to new instruments. More recent large case series have reported success rates similar to that of standard vacuum devices.

Technique

Soft vacuum cups are significantly more likely to fail to achieve vaginal delivery than rigid cups; however, they are associated with less scalp injury. There appears to be no difference in terms of maternal trauma. The soft cups are appropriate for uncomplicated deliveries with an occipito-anterior position (OA); metal cups appear to be more suitable for occipito-posterior (OP), transverse and potentially difficult OA position deliveries where the infant is larger or there is marked caput.

For successful use of the ventouse, determination of the flexion point is vital. This is located at the vertex, which, in an average term infant, is on the saggital suture 3 cm anterior to the posterior fontanelle and thus 6 cm posterior to the anterior fontanelle. The centre of the cup should be positioned directly over this, as failure to do so will lead to a progressive deflexion of the fetal head during traction, and an inability to deliver the baby safely.

The operating vacuum pressure for nearly all types of device is between 0.6 and 0.8 kg/cm². It is prudent to increase the suction to 0.2 kg/cm² first and then to recheck that no maternal tissue is caught under the cup edge. When this is confirmed the suction can then be increased.

Traction must occur in the plane of least resistance along the axis of the pelvis – the traction plane. This will usually be at exactly 90° to the cup and the operator should keep a thumb and forefinger on the cup and fetal scalp to ensure that the traction direction is correct and to feel for slippage. Safe and gentle

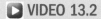

▶ VIDEO 13.2

Operative vacuum delivery:
http://www.routledgetextbooks.com/textbooks/tenteachers/obstetricsv13.2.php

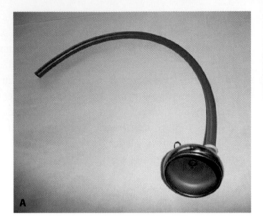

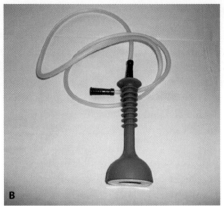

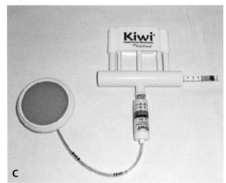

Figure 13.3 Ventouse/vacuum extractor cups. **(A)** Metal ventouse cup; **(B)** silicone rubber cup; **(C)** OmniCup™.

traction is then applied coordinated with uterine contractions and voluntary maternal expulsive efforts. There is a descent phase bringing the head onto the perineum usually achieved in at most three pulls. The crowning phase should occur shortly afterwards, and depending on the resistance of the perineum, may occur with one further pull or some operators prefer to use up to three very small pulls to minimize perineal trauma. With any ventouse, the operator should allow no more than two episodes of breaking the suction 'pop-offs' in a vacuum delivery, and the maximum time from application to delivery should ideally be less than 15 minutes. Rotation is achieved by the natural progression of the head through the pelvis.

It is not acceptable to use a ventouse when:

- The position of the fetal head is unknown.
- There is a significant degree of caput that may either preclude correct placement of the cup or, more sinisterly, indicate a substantial degree of CPD.
- The operator is inexperienced in the use of the instrument.

Forceps

Types of forceps

The basic forceps design has not changed radically over many years; all types in use today consist of two blades with shanks, joined together at a lock, with handles to provide a point for traction. The specific details of construction vary between instruments. The blades may be fenestrated (open), pseudofenestrated (open with a protruding ridge) or solid. Likewise, the length of the shanks, the design of the lock (convergent, divergent or sliding) and the fashioning of the handles are instrument specific.

Non-rotational forceps are used when the head is OA with no more than 45° deviation to the left or right (LOA, ROA). Examples such as Neville Barnes or Simpson forceps (**Figure 13.4**) have a pelvic curve and an English or non-sliding lock. If the head is positioned more than 45° from the vertical, rotation must be accomplished before traction. Forceps designed for rotation, such as Kielland forceps, have minimal pelvic curve to allow rotation around a fixed axis; the sliding lock of the Kielland forceps (**Figure 13.4**) facilitates correction of asynclitism.

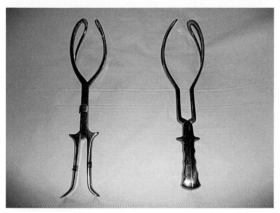

Figure 13.4 Kielland rotational forceps (left) and Simpson non-rotational forceps (right).

Technique

For forceps, all the usual prerequisites for safe delivery apply, but in addition it is essential that the operator checks the pair of forceps to ensure that a matching pair has been provided and that the blades lock with ease (both before and after application). By convention, the left blade is inserted before the right with the operator's hand protecting the vaginal wall from the blades. With proper placement of the forceps blades, they come to lie parallel to the axis of the fetal head and between the fetal head and the pelvic wall. The operator then articulates and locks the blades, checking their application before applying traction (**Figure 13.5**).

Traction should be applied intermittently coordinated with uterine contractions and maternal expulsive efforts. The axis of traction changes during the delivery and is guided along the 'J'-shaped curve of the pelvis. As the head begins to crown, the blades are directed to the vertical and the head is delivered. The majority of forceps deliveries will be completed in no more than three pulls. Specific techniques are required for rotational forceps deliveries and only those who have been properly trained in their use should employ them. Rotation occurs between contractions and the descent phase is similar to non-rotational forceps.

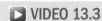

▶ VIDEO 13.3

Operative forceps delivery:
http://www.routledgetextbooks.com/textbooks/tenteachers/obstetricsv13.3.php

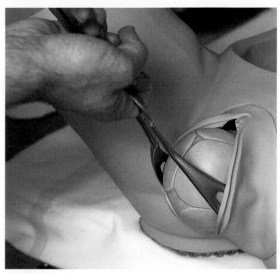

Figure 13.5 Application of forceps.

The role of episiotomy at vacuum and forceps delivery is controversial with conflicting studies reported. A RCT reported that a routine approach to episiotomy was neither protective nor associated with an increased risk of severe perineal tearing. In practice, most obstetricians cut an episiotomy routinely for forceps delivery, especially in nulliparous deliveries where anal sphincter damage is more likely. In parous women, particularly those requiring ventouse delivery, an episiotomy may not be necessary.

Special considerations

Failure of the chosen instrument

Failure to complete delivery vaginally can occur when the choice of instrument is wrong (e.g. a silastic cup ventouse for a rotational delivery), when the application of the instrument is wrong (e.g. ventouse application over the anterior fontanelle) or when the position has been wrongly defined (most commonly OP–OA errors), leading to inappropriately large diameters presenting to the pelvis. Failure is also more common if the fetus is large or maternal effort is poor.

There have been no RCTs assessing the best approach to take following failure to deliver with the first choice of instrument. Observational studies show that outcomes for babies are worse with multiple or sequential use of instruments than if the instrument of first choice is successful. In addition, the rates of third- and fourth-degree tears are higher when a second instrument is used. The operator must choose the approach most likely to result in timely delivery with the least morbidity.

Where the first instrument fails, a number of scenarios may apply. If the reason for failure was cup detachment of a vacuum and the fetal head is OA and on the perineum, a low-pelvic or lift out forceps to complete delivery is acceptable and likely to be less traumatic than a second stage caesarean section. If the instrument failed because there was little or no descent with the first pull of a correctly applied instrument with traction in the correct axis of the pelvis, then delivery must be by caesarean section as the likely diagnosis is CPD. If the instrument failed because the position was incorrectly defined, then the next option will either be a rotational instrumental delivery or a caesarean section. If there is any uncertainty, senior help should be sought immediately and a full re-evaluation should take place, ideally in an operating theatre. In many cases, delivery by caesarean section will be the safer option for the fetus.

Complications

The risk of fetal trauma in relation to forceps delivery, particularly rotational procedures, has been long established. There is now a growing recognition that vacuum delivery can also be associated with significant morbidity. In 1998, the USA Food and Drug Administration (FDA) issued a warning about the potential dangers of delivery with the ventouse; this followed several reports of infant fatality secondary to intracranial haemorrhage. In addition, there has been a growing recognition of the short- and long-term morbidity of maternal pelvic floor injury following OVD. It is not surprising, therefore, that there has been an increase in litigation relating to vacuum and forceps delivery. If we are to offer women the option of safe operative deliveries, we need to improve our approach to clinical care. The goal should be to minimize the risk of morbidity and, where morbidity occurs, to minimize the likelihood of litigation, without limiting maternal choice. It is also important to remember that caesarean section, particularly in the second stage of labour, also carries significant morbidity and implications for future births (see Chapter 14, Obstetric emergencies).

OVDs with both vacuum and forceps can be associated with significant maternal and fetal complications. Maternal deaths have been reported with vacuum deliveries as a result of cervical tearing in women delivered before full dilatation. Traumatic vaginal delivery is considered to be the most important risk factor for faecal incontinence in women and may occur not only after recognized third-degree perineal tears, but also after apparently non-traumatic vaginal delivery. PPH is more common in women needing OVD compared to women who deliver spontaneously, but less common than in women delivered by caesarean section in the second stage. Measures to limit this include early recognition of abnormal bleeding and use of a Syntocinon™ infusion postdelivery, prompt suturing and careful identification of high vaginal wall tears.

Underestimation of blood loss at operative vaginal delivery is common. Where possible, loss should be measured through the weighing of swabs and towels.

Fetal complications are no less important; the incidence of cephalhaematoma is increased with the use of the ventouse, and there are rare reports of severe intracranial injuries and subgaleal haemorrhage. Risks of trauma to the baby correlate with the duration of the operative delivery, the station of the fetal head at the commencement of the delivery and the need for rotation, the difficulty of the delivery and the condition of the fetus immediately prior to OVD. It is important to remember that the risks of traumatic injury significantly increase among babies who are exposed to multiple attempts at both vacuum and forceps delivery.

KEY LEARNING POINTS

- OVD should be classified according to the position and station of the presenting part.
- Clinical assessment and confirmation that the safety criteria have been met are prerequisites for OVD.
- Vacuum or forceps may be suitable depending on the clinical circumstances and operator's preference.
- OVDs with a higher chance of failure should be conducted in an operating theatre.
- Contingency planning is an essential part of any OVD.
- Anticipation and early management of maternal and neonatal complications is essential.

Caesarean section

A caesarean section is a surgical procedure in which incisions are made through a woman's abdomen (laparotomy) and uterus (hysterotomy) to deliver one or more babies. In the UK, between 25% and 30% of all babies are now delivered by caesarean section. The principal aims should be to ensure that women and babies who need delivery by caesarean section receive it and that those who do not are saved from unnecessary intervention. In 1985, concern regarding the increasing frequency of caesarean section led the WHO to hold a consensus conference. This conference concluded that there were no health benefits above a caesarean section rate of 10–15%. More recently it has been suggested that there is maternal and neonatal benefit with caesarean section rates up to 19%. Despite this, rates of caesarean section continue to increase year on year, with marked variation both nationally and internationally.

There are three theories about the origin of the name caesarean. It is said to derive from a Roman legal code called Lex Caesarea, which allegedly contained a law prescribing that the baby be cut out of its mother's womb in the case that she dies before giving birth. The derivation of the name is also attributed to an ancient story, told in the 1st century AD by Pliny the Elder, who claimed that an ancestor of Caesar was delivered in this way. An alternative etymology suggests that the procedure's name derives from the Latin verb *caedere*, to cut, in which case the term 'caesarean section' is redundant. Caesar's mother, Aurelia, lived through childbirth and successfully gave birth to her son, ruling out the possibility that the Roman dictator and general was born by caesarean section. However, the Catalan saint, Raymond Nonnatus (1204–40), received his surname (from the Latin *non natus*, not born) because he was born by caesarean section; his mother died while giving birth to him. The first recorded incidence of a woman surviving a caesarean section was in 1500, in Switzerland: Jakob Nufer, a pig gelder, is supposed to have performed the operation on his wife after a prolonged labour. From the 16th century onwards, the procedure had a high mortality and was performed only when the mother was already dead or considered to be beyond help. In Great Britain and Ireland, the mortality rate in 1865 was 85%. On March 5th, 2000, Inés Ramírez performed a caesarean section on herself and survived, as did her son. She is believed to be the only woman to have performed a successful caesarean section on herself.

Key steps in reducing mortality at caesarean section were:

- Adherence to principles of asepsis.
- Introduction of uterine suturing by Max Sänger in 1882.
- Extraperitoneal caesarean section and then moving to low transverse incision.
- Anaesthetic advances.
- Blood transfusion.
- Antibiotic treatment and prophylaxis.

Classification

Traditionally, caesarean sections have been classified as elective or emergency. Elective caesarean sections are usually booked days or weeks ahead of time and are conducted during daytime hours. There is sometimes confusion between elective caesarean section and non-labour emergency caesarean section. This can be overcome by using the term scheduled caesarean section for procedures that are planned ahead of time. All other caesarean sections can be classified as emergency, irrespective of whether the woman was in labour or not. The degree of urgency should be described clearly using a standard classification to ensure that there is effective communication between the members of the multidisciplinary team, particularly the theatre staff, anaesthetist and obstetrician (*Table 13.5*).

Table 13.5 Classification system for emergency caesarean section

Category 1: Immediate threat to life of woman or fetus
Category 2: No immediate threat to life of woman or fetus
Category 3: Requires early delivery
Category 4: At a time to suit the woman and maternity services

Indications

There are many different reasons for performing a delivery by caesarean section. The four major indications accounting for greater than 70% of operations are:

- Previous caesarean section.
- Malpresentation (mainly breech).
- Failure to progress in labour.
- Suspected fetal compromise in labour.
- Other indications, such as multiple pregnancy, placental abruption, placenta praevia, fetal disease and maternal disease, are less common.

No list can be truly comprehensive and whatever the indication, the overriding principle is that whenever the risk to the mother and/or the fetus from vaginal delivery exceeds that from abdominal delivery, a caesarean section should be undertaken. Absolute indications for recommending delivery by caesarean section are few, almost all indications are relative and there will be circumstances where caesarean section may be best for one woman but not for another. Maternal request caesarean section needs to differentiate between women who request caesarean section because of a previous traumatic birth experience (e.g. emergency caesarean section, difficult OVD or third-degree tear) and women who request caesarean section because they wish to avoid labour. There is also increasing recognition of a condition termed 'tocophobia', which describes an irrational fear of childbirth that can be very incapacitating for the woman. Lack of consent in a woman with capacity to give consent will prohibit caesarean section regardless of the perceived clinical need.

Procedure

Informed consent

Informed consent must always be obtained prior to surgery and ideally the possibility of caesarean section and the potential indications will have been discussed in the antenatal period. The level of information provided in the acute setting must be commensurate with the urgency of the procedure, and a common sense approach is needed. Although it is difficult to impart complete and thorough information when caesarean sections are performed as urgent procedures, women must understand what

> **▶ VIDEO 13.4**
>
> Caesarean section delivery:
> http://www.routledgetextbooks.com/textbooks/tenteachers/obstetricsv13.4.php

is being planned and why. It is important to remember that no other adult may give consent for another (although it is good practice to keep the birth partner fully informed). Where there is incapacity to consent (as may occur with conditions such as eclampsia), the doctor is expected to act in the woman's best interests.

The national consent forms require both the risks and benefits to be discussed with patients and recorded on the consent form. Common medical practice is to highlight risks but not benefits. It is important to remember that the operation is being offered because of perceived benefits, both maternal and fetal in many cases.

Preparation

Most scheduled caesarean sections are performed under spinal anaesthesia with the mother awake and the partner present. If an epidural has been sited during labour, there is usually sufficient time to top-up the anaesthesia in preparation for emergency caesarean section. General anaesthesia is occasionally required where regional anaesthesia is contraindicated or ineffective, or where general anaesthesia is preferred due to the degree of urgency. The bladder should be emptied before the procedure commences and a urinary catheter is usually left *in situ*. A left lateral tilt minimizes aorto-caval compression and reduces the incidence of hypotension (with its consequent reductions in placental perfusion). The anaesthetic block is confirmed and the woman's abdomen is cleaned and draped. Prophylactic antibiotics should be administered intravenously prior to the surgical incision.

Abdominal incision

The skin and subcutaneous tissues are incised using either a transverse curvilinear incision 2 fingerbreadths above the symphysis pubis extending from and to points lateral to the lateral margins of the abdominal rectus muscles (Pfannenstiel incision) or a transverse suprapubic incision with no curve. Subcutaneous tissues are separated by blunt dissection and the rectus sheath is incised transversely along the middle 2 cm. This incision is then extended with scissors before the fascial sheath is separated from the underlying muscle by further blunt dissection. Separation is performed cephalad to permit adequate exposure of the peritoneum in a longitudinal plane. The recti are separated, the peritoneum incised and the abdominal cavity entered. The transverse suprapubic incision has the advantages of improved cosmetic results, decreased analgesic requirements and superior wound strength.

A vertical skin incision is indicated in cases of extreme maternal obesity, suspicion of other intra-abdominal pathology necessitating surgical intervention or where access to the uterine fundus may be required (classical caesarean section). The lower midline incision is made from the lower border of the umbilicus to the symphysis pubis, and may be extended caudally toward the xiphisternum. Sharp dissection to the anterior rectus sheath is performed and is then freed of subcutaneous fat. The rectus sheath is then incised, taking care to avoid damage to any underlying bowel, and extended inferiorly to the vesical peritoneal reflection and superiorly to the upper limit of the abdominal incision. The vertical incision provides greater ease of access to the pelvic and intra-abdominal organs and may be enlarged more easily; however, the incidence of wound dehiscence is increased.

Uterine incision

A lower uterine segment transverse incision is used in over 95% of caesarean deliveries due to ease of repair, reduced blood loss and low incidence of dehiscence or rupture in subsequent pregnancies (**Figure 13.6**). The loose reflection of vesicouterine serosa overlying the uterus is incised and divided laterally, the underlying lower uterine segment is reflected with blunt dissection, the developed bladder flap is retracted and the lower uterine segment is opened in a transverse plane for a distance of 1–2 cm; the incision is extended laterally to allow delivery of the fetus without extension into the broad ligament or uterine vessels. There are relatively few absolute indications for classical caesarean section (which incorporates the upper uterine segment in a vertical incision, **Figure 13.6**). These include a lower uterine segment obscured by fibroids or a lower segment covered with dense adhesions, both of which may make entry difficult. Other indications include placenta praevia, transverse lie with the back down, fetal abnormality (e.g. conjoined twins) or caesarean section in the presence of a carcinoma of

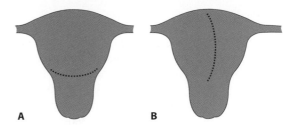

Figure 13.6 Uterine incisions for caesarean section. **(A)** Transverse lower segment incision; **(B)** classical caesarean section incision.

the cervix (so as to avoid damage to the cervix and its vascular and lymphatic supply).

Once the uterus is incised, the membranes are ruptured if still intact, and the operator's hand is positioned below the presenting part. If cephalic, the head is flexed and delivered by elevation through the uterine incision either manually or with forceps. Fundal pressure is applied by the assistant to aid delivery; this should not commence until the presenting part is located within the incision – for fear of converting the lie from longitudinal to transverse. Once the fetus is delivered, an oxytocic agent (5 IU Syntocinon™ IV) is administered to aid uterine contraction and placental separation. The placenta is delivered by controlled cord traction; manual removal significantly increases the intraoperative blood loss and postoperative infectious morbidity.

Closure

Closure of the uterus should be performed in either single or double layers with continuous or interrupted sutures. The initial suture should be placed just lateral to the incision angle, and the closure continued to a point just lateral to the angle on the opposite side. A running stitch is often employed and this may be locked to improve haemostasis. A second layer is commonly used as a means to improve haemostasis and with the aim to improve the integrity of the scar. Once repaired, the incision is assessed for haemostasis and additional 'figure-of-eight' sutures can be employed to control any bleeding points. Peritoneal closure is not routine and depends on the operator's preference. Abdominal closure is performed in the anatomical planes with high strength, low reactivity materials, such as polyglycolic acid or polyglactin. The skin can be closed with either absorbable or non-absorbable suture material or with clips, again depending on operator preference.

Complications

Although caesarean section is relatively safe, the woman needs to be counselled about potential complications. Common complications include haemorrhage, infection of the wound, urinary tract or endometrium, and for the baby transient tachypnoea of the newborn (TTN). Confidential Enquiries into Maternal Deaths have enabled the risks associated with different methods of delivery to be analysed; case fatality rate for all caesarean sections is five times that for vaginal delivery, although for elective caesarean section the difference does not reach statistical significance. Some maternal deaths following caesarean section are not attributable to the procedure itself, but rather to medical or obstetric disorders that lead to the decision to deliver using this approach.

Intraoperative complications

Haemorrhage

Haemorrhage may be a consequence of damage to the uterine vessels or may be incidental as a consequence of uterine atony or placenta praevia. In patients with an anticipated high risk of haemorrhage (e.g. known cases of placenta praevia), blood should be routinely cross-matched. There are many manoeuvres to manage haemorrhage; these range from oxytocin infusion, administration of prostaglandins, bimanual compression and conservative surgical procedures such as uterine compression sutures, to the more radical, but life-saving, hysterectomy.

Caesarean hysterectomy

The most common indication for caesarean hysterectomy is uncontrollable maternal haemorrhage; life-threatening haemorrhage requiring immediate treatment occurs in approximately 1 in 1,000 deliveries. The most important risk factor for emergency postpartum hysterectomy is a previous caesarean section – especially when the placenta overlies the old scar, increasing the risks of placenta accreta (see Chapter 14, Obstetric emergencies). Other indications for hysterectomy are atony, uterine rupture, extension of a transverse uterine incision and fibroids preventing uterine closure and haemostasis. This operation, while a major undertaking, should not be left too late, as the risk of operative complications, maternal morbidity and mortality increases with increasing haemorrhage.

Placenta praevia

The proportion of patients with a placenta praevia increases almost linearly after each previous caesarean section, and as the risk of such a complication increases with increasing parity, future reproductive intentions are very relevant to any individual decision for operative delivery.

Organ damage

Bowel damage may occur during a repeat procedure or if adhesions are present from previous surgery. The risk of bladder injury is increased after prolonged labour where the bladder is displaced caudally, after previous caesarean section where scarring obliterates the vesicouterine space or where a vertical extension to the uterine incision has occurred. If damage is suspected, then transurethral instillation of methylene blue-coloured saline will help to delineate the defect. When such an injury is observed, repair with 2-0 Vicryl™ as a single continuous or interrupted layer is appropriate. The urinary catheter should remain *in situ* for 7–10 days. Damage to the ureters is uncommon as reflection of the bladder displaces them rostrally.

Postoperative complications

Infection

Women undergoing caesarean section have a 5–20-fold greater risk of an infectious complication when compared with a vaginal delivery. Complications include fever, wound infection, endometritis, bacteraemia and urinary tract infection. Other common causes of postoperative fever include haematoma, atelectasis and deep vein thrombosis. Labour, its duration and the presence of ruptured membranes appear to be the most important risk factors, with obesity playing a particularly important role in the occurrence of wound infections. The most important source of microorganisms responsible for post-caesarean section infection is the genital tract, particularly if the membranes are ruptured preoperatively. Even in the presence of intact membranes, microbial invasion of the intrauterine cavity is common, especially with preterm labour. Infections are commonly polymicrobial and pathogens isolated from infected wounds and the endometrium include *Escherichia coli*, other aerobic gram-negative rods and group B streptococcus. General principles for the prevention of any surgical infection include careful surgical technique and skin antisepsis; prophylactic antibiotics should be administered to reduce the incidence of postoperative infection.

Venous thromboembolism

Deaths from pulmonary embolism remain an important direct cause of maternal death, and caesarean section is a major risk factor. The signs and symptoms of pulmonary emboli and deep vein thrombosis are detailed in Chapter 6, Antenatal obstetric complications. The incidence of such complications can be reduced by adequate hydration, early mobilization and administration of prophylactic heparin. Early recognition and prompt initiation of treatment will reduce the consequences of venous thromboembolism.

Psychological

All difficult deliveries carry increased maternal psychological and physical morbidity. The psychological wellbeing of women delivered by emergency caesarean section may be compromised by delayed contact with the baby, a factor that in most cases should be amenable to remedy. The obstetrician who performed the delivery should review the woman prior to hospital discharge to discuss the indication for delivery, the potential for complications, the implications for the future and to answer any questions she or her partner may have.

Subsequent birth following caesarean section

In many units, caesarean section rates for primigravidae are 20–30%. Consequently, the problem of managing a woman with a previous caesarean section in a subsequent pregnancy is common. It is a vital part of antenatal care that women be given a clear understanding of the plan of management from early on in their pregnancy, with the caveat that this may need to be adapted if the pregnancy presents unexpected problems. The management in pregnancy following a caesarean section should be to review the previous delivery, assess the available options and to select the appropriate choice through a shared decision-making process with the woman. The dictum popularized in the USA 'once a caesarean, always a caesarean' is misleading; up to 70% of women with a previous caesarean section who labour achieve a vaginal delivery. It is important, however, to discuss the risks and benefits of elective repeat caesarean section (ERCS) as compared to attempted vaginal birth after caesarean section (VBAC).

From a maternal perspective, ERCS avoids labour with its risk of pelvic floor trauma (urinary and faecal problems), the need to undergo emergency caesarean section and scar dehiscence or rupture with subsequent morbidity and mortality. However, ERCS carries maternal risks: increased bleeding, febrile morbidity, prolonged recovery, thromboembolism, long-term bladder dysfunction and increased risks of placenta praevia in subsequent pregnancies. From a fetal perspective, ERCS reduces the risk of scar rupture, but increases the risk of TTN/respiratory distress syndrome. There is remarkably little robust evidence to inform practice with regard to management of previous caesarean section: there are no RCTs and most of the data relate to observational studies.

Consideration of the risk of scar rupture is probably the most important consideration when determining whether delivery should be by ERCS or by attempted VBAC. Most published studies do not differentiate between scar dehiscence and rupture; however, analysis of observational and comparative studies indicates that the excess risk of uterine rupture following attempted VBAC compared with women undergoing ERCS is between 0.5% and 1%.

Providing the first operation was carried out for a non-recurrent indication, and providing the obstetric situation close to term in the subsequent pregnancy is favourable, then it is appropriate to offer a trial of labour after caesarean (TOLAC) to any woman with a previous uncomplicated lower segment caesarean section and no other adverse obstetric feature. The predominant factors to be weighed when determining the recommended mode of delivery depend on the balance between the preferences of the mother, the risks of a repeat operation, the risks to her child of labour and the risk of labour on the integrity of the uterine scar.

 KEY LEARNING POINTS

- Caesarean section should be recommended only when the benefits outweigh the risks.
- Informed written consent is required.

- Lower uterine segment caesarean section under regional anaesthesia is optimal.
- Common maternal complications include haemorrhage, infection and pain.
- Common neonatal complications include respiratory morbidity.
- Up to 70% of women who labour subsequently achieve a VBAC.
- The risks and benefits of ERCS versus VBAC require counselling on several occasions.
- All adverse outcomes of attempted OVD and caesarean section require a clinical incident form and review.

Clinical risk management

Operative delivery whether by vacuum, forceps or caesarean section has never been free from controversy, and is certainly not without risks. Litigation occurs more frequently following brachial plexus injury, cerebral palsy and maternal pelvic floor damage. Common allegations against practitioners include inadequate indication for operative delivery, excessive use of force with vacuum or forceps, lack of informed consent, delayed delivery by caesarean section and inadequate supervision. The fear of litigation should not dictate good medical practice. It is essential, however, that operators are appropriately trained in decision-making, that they operate within their competencies, have access to senior support and are effective communicators. Clinical incident forms should be completed as part of risk-management procedures when adverse outcomes occur, and both individual and systems-based reviews are important elements of any organization with a learning culture.

Further reading

Caesarean section. NICE guidelines (CG 132), 2011.
Royal College of Obstetricians and Gynaecologists. Operative Vaginal Delivery. Green-top Guideline No. 26. London: RCOG, 2011.
Royal College of Obstetricians and Gynaecologists. Third- and fourth-degree perineal tears, Management. Green-top Guideline No. 29. London: RCOG, 2015.
Royal College of Obstetricians and Gynaecologists. Birth after previous caesarean birth. Green-top Guideline No. 45. London: RCOG, 2015.

Self assessment

CASE HISTORY

Ms A, a 36-year-old nulliparous woman, went into spontaneous labour at 41 weeks' gestation. She had no relevant past medical history and findings on examination were unremarkable; the symphseal fundal height was appropriate for the gestational age. Delay in the first stage of labour led to artificial rupture of the membranes (clear liquor drained) and subsequent use of an oxytocin infusion. When the vaginal examination was repeated, the cervix was fully dilated, with the fetal head at the level of the ischial spines and in a right occipito-transverse position. There was marked caput and moulding. Clear liquor continued to drain and there was a normal, reactive fetal heart rate pattern. The midwife waited 1 hour for passive descent and then commenced active pushing. After 20 minutes there was little sign of progress and there were variable decelerations on the CTG.

A   Were the safety criteria for an operative vaginal delivery met?

B   How should the delivery be effected?

C   What type of forceps should be used?

D   Following traction with another contraction, there was no descent of the fetal head. What is the appropriate management plan?

E   What complications should be anticipated after delivery?

ANSWERS

A The findings on abdominal and vaginal examination are crucial to any consideration of this question. On examination, 0/5th of the fetal head was palpable, the position remained occipito-transverse at the level of the ischial spines with caput and moulding. The pelvic dimensions were average. The prerequisites for a forceps/ventouse delivery were met, but the delivery was classified as midpelvic requiring rotation and was therefore more complex with a higher risk of failure. The appropriate management plan was for transfer to theatre for either a trial of rotational OVD or a caesarean section.

B On the assumption that the delivery was to be performed by an appropriately trained and experienced obstetrician, and that informed consent was obtained, the prerequisites for an operative vaginal delivery were met. Use of either manual rotation and direct traction forceps or rotational forceps, or rotational ventouse would be reasonable. Although the ventouse is associated with less perineal trauma, the obstetrician opted to use manual rotation and forceps as the presence of caput and moulding indicated that the ventouse was more likely to fail.

C The fetal head was rotated manually to the occipito-anterior position prior to application of forceps. Non-rotational forceps (for example, Neville Barnes or Simpsons forceps) with a pelvic curve were applied. The forceps were positioned and 'locked'. Traction was applied with a contraction and with maternal pushing. There was minimal descent of the fetal head. Following traction with another contraction, there was no descent of the fetal head.

D There has been a failed trial of an OVD, with no descent of the fetal head. Delivery must be by caesarean section. The fetal head should be disimpacted manually prior to caesarian section. A lower segment caesarean section was performed, through a Pfannenstiel incision. Although there was difficulty delivering a deeply impacted fetal head, there was no significant extension of the uterine incision. The neonatal birthweight was 4.35 kg. Closure of the uterus and abdomen was unremarkable.

E There was a significant risk of PPH due to uterine atony. In addition to prophylactic antibiotic and anticoagulant therapy (to reduce the likelihood of infective and thrombotic complications), a bolus dose of oxytocin at delivery was followed by an intravenous infusion of oxytocin over 4 hours. No postoperative complications ensued and Ms A was discharged home, with her baby, 4 days after the caesarean section. She was given a hospital follow-up appointment to discuss the events of the labour and delivery and the implications for the future.

EMQ

A Emergency caesarean section in the second stage of labour.

B Emergency caesarean section for failure to progress.

C Emergency caesarean section for fetal distress.

D Caesarean hysterectomy.

E Elective repeat caesarean section.

For each description, choose the SINGLE most appropriate answer from the list of options. Each option may be used once, more than once or not at all.

1 Age 40. Antenatal booking with history of previous pregnancy 4 years ago delivered by emergency caesarean section for fetal distress. Neonatal death from meconium aspiration.

2 Fetal bradycardia after pushing for 40 minutes. Ventouse delivery commenced. Cup came off.

3 Spontaneous labour. Good progress up to 8 cm dilatation. No further progress over next 4 hours.

4 All previous babies delivered by caesarean section. Placenta praevia. Major antepartum haemorrhage followed by uncontrolled massive haemorrhage during delivery.

5 First pregnancy. 42 weeks. Induction of labour. Meconium-stained liquor. Variable decelerations of fetal heart. Cervix 1 cm dilated.

ANSWERS

1E   A woman who has experienced a previous neonatal death related to complications of labour would normally be offered elective delivery at or just before term in any subsequent pregnancy. In this case she was previously delivered by emergency caesarean section and therefore an elective caesarean section would be the most appropriate mode of delivery.

2A   Following failure to achieve an OVD, the normal recourse is an emergency caesarean section in the second stage of labour.

3B   Labour has arrested in the first stage. This is an indication for emergency caesarean section for failure to progress in the first stage of labour.

4D   Life-threatening haemorrhage secondary to a placenta praevia can often only be managed with a caesarean hysterectomy.

5C   The presence of meconium-stained liquor and variable decelerations indicate fetal distress and mandate delivery by emergency caesarean section as the patient is still in the earliest stage of labour.

SBA QUESTIONS

Choose the single best answer.

1   A midwife examines a woman following spontaneous vaginal delivery. She identifies perineal trauma involving the vagina and perineal muscles but not the anal sphincter muscle. How should the tear be classified?

A   First-degree tear.
B   Episiotomy.
C   Third-degree tear.
D   Fourth-degree tear.
E   Second-degree tear.

ANSWER

E   This is a second-degree tear. First-degree tears only involve the perineal skin. Tears that involve the anal sphincter complex are classified as third-degree tears. Fourth-degree tears involve the anal sphincter and the rectal mucosa (see *Table 13.1*). An episiotomy is a deliberate incision in the perineum made to facilitate delivery and reduce the risk of perineal injury.

2   The following are the essential safety criteria that must be fulfilled prior to attempting OVD EXCEPT:

A   The bladder should be empty.
B   The head must be palpable in the abdomen.
C   The cervix must be fully dilated.
D   The position of the fetal head must be known.
E   The fetal head must be at or below the level of the ischial spines.

ANSWER

B   The prerequisites for an OVD are described in *Table 13.4*. A head that is still palpable in the abdomen has not sufficiently engaged and is an absolute contraindication to OVD.

3 A 33-year-old woman, who is known to have a major placenta praevia, has been an inpatient since 34 weeks' gestation. She is now 36 weeks' gestation and complains of a sudden onset of painless heavy vaginal bleeding. Her blood pressure is 90/60, heart rate 110 bpm, respiration rate 16/min and temperature is 36.7°C. Abdominal examination is soft, non-tender. Fetal heart monitoring is normal.

What is the most appropriate management?

A Administer repeat antenatal corticosteroid, as the previous course would not be effective.

B Administer tocolysis as this would help to stop the bleeding and prolong pregnancy.

C Deliver by emergency caesarean section and involve senior obstetric and anaesthetic staff.

D Commence blood transfusion and consider delivery if vital signs do not improve.

E A speculum examination should be performed to help find a cause for the bleeding.

ANSWER

C This patient has a major placenta praevia and is now at an advanced gestation. Heavy vaginal bleeding in this situation that is associated with a maternal tachycardia and falling blood pressure is an indication for immediate delivery. The presence of a major placenta praevia precludes vaginal delivery and is an indication for caesarean section, which can be accompanied by significant intra-operative haemorrhage and should therefore be performed by experienced senior staff.

Obstetric emergencies

FERGUS McCARTHY

LEARNING OBJECTIVES

- To understand the incidence of common obstetric emergencies.
- To understand the risk factors for common obstetric emergencies.
- To be able to understand the early warning signs in obstetric emergencies.
- To be able to provide a stepwise approach in the management of common obstetric emergencies.

Introduction

Obstetric emergencies are common and often result in significant maternal and fetal morbidity and mortality. Regardless of the emergency it is essential they are managed in a methodological stepwise manner to limit morbidity and mortality and maintain safety for the staff and patient. Accurate documentation is also essential. This chapter covers common obstetric emergencies and also rare obstetric emergencies that may result in significant morbidity or mortality. A stepwise approach to managing these obstetric emergencies is suggested.

One maternal death occurs every minute worldwide. In the UK, it is estimated that 1 in every 100 births results in a high dependency unit admission, while 1 in every 1,000 results in an intensive care unit admission. In the 2010 to 2012 triennium, one-third of women died from direct complications of pregnancy such as bleeding. Almost one-quarter of women in the recent Mothers and Babies: Reducing Risk through Audits and Confidential Enquiries across the UK (MBRRACE) report who died had sepsis. Leading causes of maternal mortality include thrombosis and thromboembolism, haemorrhage, sepsis, amniotic fluid embolism and cardiac disease.

An emergency is defined as a serious situation or occurrence that happens unexpectedly and demands immediate action. Prompt recognition and treatment of these emergencies/complications of pregnancy is essential to limit morbidity and mortality. The incidence and outcomes of obstetric emergencies varies hugely country to country (e.g. death from

Table 14.1 Incidence of obstetric emergencies

Obstetric emergency	Estimated rates
Maternal collapse	0.14 and 6/1,000 (14 and 600/100,000) births in the UK
Sepsis	Puerperal sepsis is estimated to complicate at least 75,000 maternal deaths every year The majority are in low-income countries In the USA sepsis is estimated to complicate approximately 1 in 3,000 deliveries
Major obstetric haemorrhage	Estimated incidence in the UK of 3.7/1,000 pregnancies An estimated 125,000 women are thought to die annually worldwide as a consequence of haemorrhage
Amniotic fluid embolism	2.0 per 100,000 deliveries (95% CI 1.5–2.5) with maternal mortality rates of 0.33 per 100,000 pregnancies (UK) and perinatal mortality rates of 135 per 1,000 total births (95% CI 45–288)
Pre-eclampsia and eclampsia	Occurs in 3–5% of first time pregnancies and 2–3% of pregnancies overall Mortality rates of 0.38 per 100,000 maternities (UK) Severe forms of pre-eclampsia and eclampsia estimated to affect up to 18% of pregnant women in parts of Africa with a mortality rate of 10–25%
Thrombosis and thromboembolism	Approximately 50% of maternal venous thromboembolism events occur during pregnancy Overall prevalence of 1 in 1,600 pregnancies; UK incidence of antenatal pulmonary embolism is 1.3/10,000 with case fatality rate of 3.5% Overall mortality rates of 1.08 per 100,000 pregnancies (UK)
Cardiac disease	Prevalence of cardiac disease in pregnancy in the developed world is 0.2–3% Mortality of 2.25 per 100,000 pregnancies (UK)
Shoulder dystocia	Prevalence of 0.58–0.70%

complications such as pre-eclampsia are rare in the UK but prevalent in Africa [*Table 14.1*]). This chapter aims to cover all major obstetric emergencies including the incidence, risk factors, warning signs to recognize at-risk women and suggested management strategies.

Prevention of obstetric emergencies

It is not possible to prevent or predict all obstetric emergencies but it is essential to recognize early warning signs, reduce risk factors and have appropriate support present in anticipation of obstetric emergencies.

The collapsed/ unresponsive patient

The general structured approach to the management of acute illness and trauma is the same for pregnant and non-pregnant patients and is summarized in **Figure 14.1**. Management consists of the following structured approach.

Initial management

Identify life-threatening problems:

A: Airway – with cervical spine control.

B: Breathing – with ventilation. Look for chest movements, listen for breath sounds and feel for movement of air for a maximum of 10 seconds. If breathing is present, give high-flow oxygen. If breathing is absent, start ventilation.

C: Circulation – with haemorrhage control. Minimize aorto-caval compression (**Figure 14.2**). Absence of breathing in the presence of a clear airway is now used as a marker of absence of circulation. If there is no circulation, start cardiopulmonary resuscitation (CPR): 30 chest compressions followed by two ventilations. Manage hypovolaemia/haemorrhage concurrently.

D: Disability – neurological status using the AVPU score (Alert, responds to Voice, responds to Pain, Unresponsive). Following initial

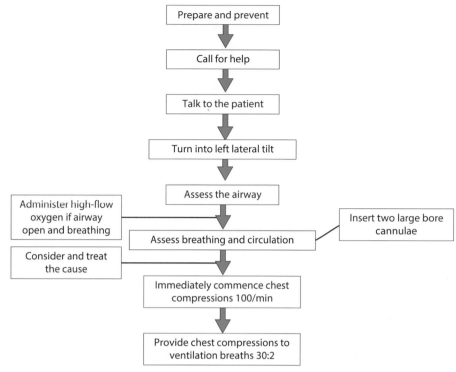

Figure 14.1 The structured approach to managing obstetric emergencies.

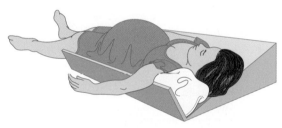

Figure 14.2 Left lateral tilt. The pregnant woman is tilted to the left to move the pregnant uterus off the abdominal vessels, thus improving cardiac output. There are various methods of achieving this; many hospitals have special wedge shaped cushions, but pillows and blankets can be used.

resuscitation perform a Glasgow coma score (GCS). GCS ≤8 indicates a compromised airway and will require intubation.

E: Exposure – depending on environment. Perform full examination of patient remembering risks of hypothermia (use warming blanket if needed) and patient's dignity. Monitoring may include non-invasive blood pressure, pulse oximetry, electrocardiogram (ECG), end tidal CO_2 and respiratory rate. Consider urinary catheter and nasogastric

tube depending on circumstances (e.g. hourly urine output is essential in severe pre-eclampsia).

Resuscitation:

- Deal with any problems as you find them. Consider differential diagnosis (**Figure 14.3**).

- Assess fetal wellbeing and viability: deal with threat to life of fetus. Assess fetal wellbeing using cardiotocography (CTG).

- Notes review: review trends of vital signs/review notes.

- Definitive care: order investigations and plan treatment: specific management depending on underlying cause.

An anaesthetist experienced in obstetric care is critical in the successful management of obstetric emergencies. Difficulties anaesthetists encounter in the resuscitation of the pregnant woman include: increased risk of aspiration of gastric contents; increased metabolic oxygen consumption combined with a decreased functional residual capacity;

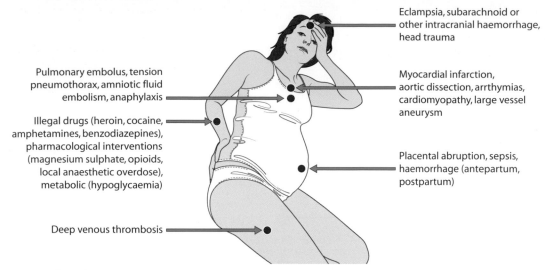

Eclampsia, subarachnoid or other intracranial haemorrhage, head trauma

Myocardial infarction, aortic dissection, arrthymias, cardiomyopathy, large vessel aneurysm

Pulmonary embolus, tension pneumothorax, amniotic fluid embolism, anaphylaxis

Illegal drugs (heroin, cocaine, amphetamines, benzodiazepines), pharmacological interventions (magnesium sulphate, opioids, local anaesthetic overdose), metabolic (hypoglycaemia)

Placental abruption, sepsis, haemorrhage (antepartum, postpartum)

Deep venous thrombosis

Figure 14.3 The differential diagnosis of acute maternal collapse.

pregnancy weight gain and increased breast size makes optimal placement of head and intubation more difficult; and finally aorto-caval compression and the effects of the gravid uterus on venous return.

 KEY LEARNING POINTS

Maternal collapse

- Obtain a left lateral tilt of at least 15–20° at the earliest opportunity to prevent/minimize aorto-caval compression in any patient.
- Resuscitation of a pregnant woman is more difficult due to reduced lung capacity, reduced venous return if supine, greater oxygen demand from the fetus and increased weight.
- The use of Modified Early Obstetric Warning System (MEOWS) scores are key in the early recognition of the clinical deterioration of a patient.

Sepsis

Sepsis in the UK remains an important cause of maternal death. In the 2006–2006 triennium, sepsis was the leading cause of direct maternal death in the UK, with deaths due to group A streptococcal infection contributing significantly. As a result of concerted effort through regulatory bodies, such as the Royal College of Obstetricians and Gynaecologists,

clinical practice guidelines, Confidential Enquiry recommendations and the Surviving Sepsis campaigns, mortality from genital tract sepsis halved between 2006–2008 and 2010–2012.

Sepsis: prevention/risk factors/warning signs

- Prevention: one in 11 of the women in the recent Confidential Enquiry report died from the flu. More than half of these women's deaths could have been prevented by a flu vaccination. All maternal observations should be documented on a MEOWS chart to allow early detection of sepsis and subsequent treatment.
- Risk factors: ruptured membranes, immunocompromised patients, immunosuppressants, obesity, diabetes, minority ethnic group origin, anaemia, urinary tract infections, vaginal discharge, previous pelvic infection, group B streptococcal infection, amniocentesis and other invasive procedures, cervical cerclage, group A streptococcal infection in close contacts.
- Warning signs: pyrexia, hypothermia, tachycardia, increased respiratory rate, hypotension, rise in MEOWS score and oligouria. Patients may rigor, have a rash, have reduced levels of consciousness and not respond to initial treatment.

Management

The Surviving Sepsis Campaign Resuscitation bundles have key points in the timely management of sepsis:

- Obtain blood cultures prior to antibiotic administration.
- Administer broad-spectrum antibiotic within 1 hour of recognition of severe sepsis. Every 1 hour delay in administrating antibiotics increases mortality by approximately 8%.
- Measure serum lactate.
- In the event of hypotension and/or a serum lactate ≥4 mmol/l, deliver an initial minimum 20 ml/kg of crystalloid or an equivalent.
- If there is no response, administer vasopressors for hypotension that is not responding to initial fluid resuscitation to maintain mean arterial pressure (MAP) ≥65 mmHg.
- In the event of persistent hypotension despite fluid resuscitation and/or lactate ≥4 mmol/l, aim to achieve a central venous pressure (CVP) of ≥8 mmHg or a central venous oxygen saturation ≥70% or mixed venous oxygen saturation ≥65%.

Involve a microbiologist or infectious disease physician early, particularly if the woman does not respond to first-choice antibiotics.

Severe sepsis may be defined as:

- Temperature >38°C or <36°C.
- Heart rate >100 beats per minute.
- Respiratory rate >20 respirations per minute.
- White cell count >17 × 10^9/l or <4 × 10^9/l with >10% immature band forms.

Severe sepsis has a higher maternity mortality and requires aggressive prompt treatment and timely involvement of the multidisciplinary team.

Antibiotic use

Each hospital should have its own antibiotic guidelines as the incidence of resistant organisms varies both throughout countries and by country. The selection of antibiotics should be guided by risk factors and potential sources of sepsis. A combination of either piperacillin/tazobactam or a carbapenem plus clindamycin provides very broad coverage for the treatment of severe sepsis. Other antibiotic options include:

- Co-amoxyclav: provides gram-positive and anaerobe cover. Does not cover methicillin-resistant *Staphylococcus aureus* (MRSA), *Pseudomonas* or extended spectrum β-lactamase-(ESBL) producing organisms.
- Metronidazole: provides anaerobic cover.
- Clindamycin: covers streptococci and staphylococci including MRSA. Clindamycin also switches off exotoxin production.
- Gentamicin: provides gram-negative cover against coliforms and *Pesuodomonas*.

KEY LEARNING POINTS

Management of sepsis:

- Blood cultures before antibiotics.
- Culture of other samples should be performed based on clinical suspicion (e.g. high vaginal swab, midstream urine, sputum culture).
- Key organisms involved in puerperal sepsis are Lancefield group A beta-haemolytic streptococcus and *Escherichia coli*.
- Early diagnosis, rapid administration of broad-spectrum antibiotics and review by senior doctors and midwives is essential to reduce mortality and improve outcome.
- Measure lactate and haemoglobin and plan repeat measurements to help assess the response to initial treatment.
- Measure accurate hourly urine output.
- Administer high-flow oxygen

Obstetric haemorrhage

Obstetric haemorrhage is a leading cause of maternal mortality worldwide and is responsible for up to 50% of maternal deaths in some countries. In the UK it is responsible for approximately 10% of all direct maternal deaths.

Antepartum haemorrhage

This is defined as vaginal bleeding after 20 weeks' gestation. It complicates 2–5% of pregnancies and most cases involve relatively small amounts of blood loss. However, significant blood loss poses a risk of mortality and morbidity to both mother and baby. The causes can be classified into placental, fetal and maternal:

- Placental causes:
  - placental abruption;
  - placenta praevia.
- Fetal cause:
  - vasa praevia.
- Maternal causes:
  - vaginal trauma;
  - cervical ectropion;
  - cervical carcinoma;
  - vaginal infection and cervicitis.

Placental causes are the most worrying, as potentially the mother's and/or fetus's life is in danger and often the bleeding may be more severe than with other causes such as cervical ectropion. However, any antepartum haemorrhage must always be taken seriously, and any woman presenting with a history of fresh vaginal bleeding must be investigated promptly and properly. The key question is whether the bleeding is placental and is compromising the mother and/or fetus, or whether it has a less significant cause.

History

- How much bleeding?
- Triggering factors (e.g. postcoital bleed).
- Associated with pain or contractions?
- Is the baby moving?
- Last cervical smear (date/normal or abnormal)?

Examination

- Pulse, blood pressure.
- Is the uterus soft or tender and firm?
- Fetal heart auscultation/CTG.
- Speculum vaginal examination, with particular importance placed on visualizing the cervix (having established that placenta is not a praevia, preferably using a portable ultrasound machine).

Investigations

- Depending on the degree of bleeding, full blood count, clotting and, if suspected praevia/abruption, cross-match 6 units of blood.

- Ultrasound (fetal size, presentation, amniotic fluid, placental position and morphology).

Placental abruption

Placental abruption is the premature separation of the placenta from the uterine wall. The bleeding is maternal and/or fetal and abruption is acutely dangerous for both the mother and fetus (**Figure 14.4**).

Placental abruption: prevention/ risk factors/warning signs

- Prevention: avoidance of precipitating factors such as control of blood pressure, and avoidance of precipitants cocaine and smoking.
- Risk factors: hypertension (including pre-eclampsia), smoking, trauma to the maternal abdomen, cocaine, polyhydramnios, multiple pregnancy, fetal growth restriction (FGR).
- Warning signs: maternal collapse, feeling cold, light-headedness, restlessness, distress and panic, painful abdomen, vaginal bleeding.

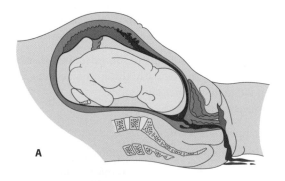

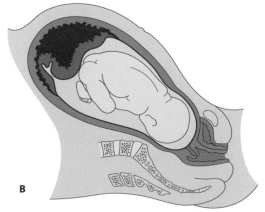

Figure 14.4 (**A**) Placental abruption with revealed haemorrhage; (**B**) placental abruption with concealed haemorrhage.

Clinical presentation

The characteristic presentation of placental abruption is that of painful bleeding associated with a tense rigid abdomen. The absence of a tense abdomen does not rule out a placental abruption. Placental abruption may be diagnosed on ultrasound but the absence of any ultrasound changes does not rule it out and patients should be managed on the basis of their clinical findings. Maternal signs and symptoms may include vaginal bleeding, abdominal pain, sweating, shock, hypotension, tachycardia, absence or reduced fetal movements and tense painful abdomen. CTG may reveal evidence of fetal distress.

The degree of vaginal bleeding does not necessarily correlate with the degree of abruption as abruptions may be concealed (i.e. significant separation between placenta and uterus but blood is concealed between the placenta and uterus so there is little vaginal bleeding seen [**Figure 14.4B**]).

Placenta praevia

A placenta covering or encroaching on the cervical os may be associated with bleeding, either provoked or spontaneous. The bleeding is from the maternal not fetal circulation and is more likely to compromise the mother than the fetus (**Figure 14.5**).

Placenta praevia: prevention/risk factors/warning signs

- Prevention: avoidance of non-clinically indicated caesarean section.
- Risk factors: multiple gestation, previous caesarean section, uterine structural anomaly, assisted conception.
- Warning signs: low-lying placenta at 20 week anomaly scan, maternal collapse, feeling cold, light-headedness, restlessness, distress and panic, painless vaginal bleeding.

Clinical presentation and diagnosis

The characteristic presenting complaint of bleeding associated with a placenta praevia is that of painless vaginal bleeding. The bleeding may trigger preterm labour so often patients with bleeding from placenta praevia will have irregular abdominal pain associated with uterine contractions. A placenta praevia is diagnosed using ultrasound, preferably transvaginal, to allow accurate measurement of the placental edge from the internal os. Often patients will have

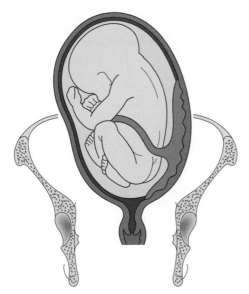

Minor placenta praevia

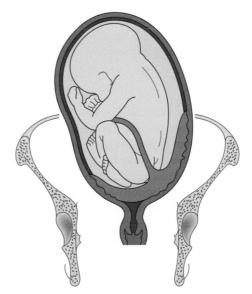

Major placenta praevia

Figure 14.5 Placenta praevia.

been highlighted as having a low-lying placenta at their anomaly scan so there should be a high index of suspicion in any of these patients presenting with vaginal bleeding.

Management

If there is minimal bleeding and the cause is clearly local vaginal bleeding, symptomatic management may be given (for example antifungal preparations for candidiasis) as long as there is reasonable certainty that cervical carcinoma is excluded by smear history and direct visualization of the cervix. Placental causes of bleeding are a major concern. A large-gauge intravenous cannula is sited, blood sent for full blood count, clotting and cross-match, and appropriate fetal and maternal monitoring instituted. If there is major fetal or maternal compromise, decisions may have to be made about immediate delivery irrespective of gestation; an attempt at maternal steroid injection should still be made. If this is the situation, and bleeding is continuing, emergency management is required. If bleeding settles, the woman must be admitted for 48 hours, as the risk of re-bleeding is high within this time frame. Rhesus status is important: if the mother is rhesus negative, send a Kleihauer test (to determine whether any, or how much, fetal blood has leaked into the maternal circulation) and administer anti-D. When there is substantial vaginal bleeding (in excess of 500 ml) antenatal corticosteroids should be considered if gestation is under 35 weeks as the risk of preterm delivery is significant.

Vasa praevia

Vasa previa occurs when fetal vessels traverse the fetal membranes over the internal cervical os. These vessels may be from either a velamentous insertion of the umbilical cord or may be joining an accessory (succenturiate) placental lobe to the main disc of the placenta. The diagnosis is usually suspected when either spontaneous or artificial rupture of the membranes is accompanied by painless fresh vaginal bleeding from rupture of the fetal vessels. This condition is associated with a very high perinatal mortality from fetal exsanguination. If the baby is still alive, once the diagnosis is suspected the immediate course of action is delivery by emergency caesarean section.

KEY LEARNING POINTS

- Placenta praevia is most dangerous for the mother.
- Placental abruption is more dangerous for the fetus than the mother.
- Vasa praevia is not dangerous for the mother but is nearly always fatal for the baby.
- Management involves resuscitation and stabilization of mother and senior input regarding timing of delivery.

Postpartum haemorrhage

Postpartum haemorrhage, defined as blood loss ≥500 ml, affected 13% of all pregnancies in England in 2011 and 2012. In the UK and Ireland there were 17 direct deaths due to obstetric haemorrhage between 2009 and 2012. This gives an overall mortality rate of 0.49 per 100,000 pregnancies (95% CI 0.29–0.78) and a case fatality rate for massive haemorrhage of approximately 1 per 1,200 women. Major obstetric haemorrhage is defined as blood loss ≥2,500 ml, or requiring a blood transfusion ≥5 units red cells or treatment for coagulopathy. Major obstetric haemorrhage affected 0.6% of pregnancies in Scotland in 2011.

Postpartum haemorrhage: prevention/risk factors/ warning signs

- Prevention: haemoglobin levels below the normal range for pregnancy should be investigated and iron supplementation considered if indicated to optimize haemoglobin prior to delivery. Prophylactic use of oxytocin agents for high-risk patients.
- Risk factors for uterine atony (commonest cause of haemorrhage): macrosomia, multiple pregnancy, prolonged labour, oxytocin use, induction of labour, grand multiparity, polyhydramnios, antepartum haemorrhage, placental abruption.

   Other risk factors for obstetric haemorrhage: placenta praevia (**Figure 14.5**) and accreta, previous multiple caesarean sections (risk of placenta accreata is greater than 60% for women who have had 3 or more previous caesarean sections), perineal trauma, full bladder, underlying haemato-logical disorder (e.g. factor VIII deficiency), disseminated intravascular coagulation.

There are three main areas from which haemorrhage occurs: uterus, placenta and cervix/vagina. Uterine causes of haemor-rhage include atony (commonest cause of haemorrhage), uterine inversion and rupture. Remember, haemorrhage may be concealed.

- Warning signs: failure of uterus to contract following delivery of the placenta, maternal collapse.

Signs and symptoms of haemorrhage

- Symptoms: anxiety, thirst, nausea, cold, pain, dizziness.
- Signs: rising fundus, peritonism, reduced urine output, tachypnoea, tachycardia, hypotension, narrow pulse pressure.

KEY LEARNING POINTS
MANAGEMENT OF OBSTETRIC HAEMORRHAGE (FIGURE 14.6)

- Do not delay fluid resuscitation and blood transfusion because of false reassurance from a single haemoglobin result – treat the patient, not the result.

- Be proactive – young fit women compensate extremely well. Therefore, ongoing bleeding should be acted on without delay. Minimal signs of haemor-rhage exist up to 1,000 ml of loss. The commonly used sign of hypotension is a very late sign in blood loss occurring after 2,000 ml of loss.

- Consider the administration of blood components before coagulation indices deteriorate if a woman is bleeding and is likely to develop a coagulopathy.

- Consider early recourse to hysterectomy if simpler medical and surgical interventions prove ineffective.

- In patients where complications are anticipated (e.g. placenta accreata), ideally obtain advanced consent (with partner present if possible) to cover possible interventions including blood transfusion, interventional radiology, leaving placenta *in situ* and hysterectomy.

- Initiate obstetric haemorrhage protocol
- Call for senior help
- Scribe to clearly document timing of events, people present and interventions administered

- Uterine compression/rub up contractions
- Empty uterus and vagina of clot
- Empty bladder
- Uterotonic agents
- Bimanual compression of uterus if atony is the cause
- Intravenous access ×2 large bore cannulae
- Full blood count/group and cross-match/coagulation profile
- Fluid replacement: cross-matched blood or O-negative blood if unavailable
- Rapid infuser with fluid warmer/cell saver set up

A stepwise approach to use of uteronic agents would be:

- 5–10 units IV/IM oxytocin
- 40 units oxytocin in 100 ml normal saline over 4 hours
- 800–1,000 µg rectal misoprostol
- Syntometrine (ergometrine 500 µg and Syntocinon™ 5 units)
- Repeat ergometrine (500 µg) IM or slow IV push
- Carboprost 0.25 mg by IM repeated at intervals of not less than 15 minutes to a maximum of 8 doses (contraindicated in women with asthma)

If ongoing bleeding consider:

- Disseminated intravascular coagulation and replacement of clotting agents
- Senior help – interventional radiology, gynaeoncology
- Transfer to operating theatre for surgical invention (uterine balloon insertion, iliac ligation, uterine artery embolization, hysterectomy)

- Clear documentation of sequence of events and cause of bleeding
- Debrief of staff, family members and patient
- Risk report

Figure 14.6 Algorithm for the management of obstetric haemorrhage.

Eclampsia

Pre-eclampsia is a potentially life-threatening hypertensive disorder of pregnancy characterized by vascular dysfunction and systemic inflammation involving the brain, liver and kidneys of the mother. Eclampsia refers to the occurrence of one or more generalized convulsions and/or coma in the setting of pre-eclampsia and in the absence of other neurological conditions. The UK Obstetric Surveillance System (UKOSS) report gives an estimated incidence of eclampsia of 27.5 cases per 100,000 pregnancies, with a case fatality rate estimated to be 3.1%. Eclampsia is associated with significant maternal morbidity, in particular cerebrovascular events (2.3%). Cerebral haemorrhage has been reported to be the most common cause of death in patients with eclampsia (previously this was pulmonary oedema) and stroke is known to be the most common cause of death (45%) in women with haemolysis, elevated liver enzymes and low platelets (HELLP) syndrome.

Eclampsia: prevention/risk factors/warning signs

- Prevention: low threshold for administration of magnesium sulphate in women with pre-eclampsia who are thought to be unstable or suffering from severe pre-eclampsia. However, remember all patients with pre-eclampsia regardless of perceived severity are at risk of eclampsia.
- Risk factors: difficult to predict, uncontrolled hypertension, two or fewer prenatal care visits, primigravidity, obesity, black ethnicity, history of diabetes and age <20 years.
- Warning signs: epigastric pain and right upper quadrant tenderness, headache, uncontrolled hypertension, agitation, hyper-reflexia and clonus, facial (especially periorbital) oedema, poor urine output, papilloedema.

Management

Call senior help and emergency alert team. Initial approach is similar to the collapsed patient with a focus on airway, breathing and circulation.

Magnesium sulphate is indicated as the first-line anticonvulsant and should be administered as soon as possible either in women at risk of eclampsia or when eclampsia occurs. A loading dose of 4 g is given followed by a maintenance infusion of 1 g/hour generally for 24 hours after delivery. Magnesium sulphate has a narrow therapeutic range and overdose can cause respiratory depression and ultimately cardiac arrest. The antidote is 10 ml 10% calcium gluconate given slowly intravenously.

Amniotic fluid embolism

Amniotic fluid embolism is a rare cause of maternal collapse and is believed to be caused by amniotic fluid entering the maternal circulation. This causes acute cardiorespiratory compromise and severe disseminated intravascular coagulation. In some cases there may be an abnormal maternal reaction to amniotic fluid as the primary event. It is difficult to diagnose when it occurs and is typically diagnosed at postmortem, with the presence of fetal cells (squames or hair) in the maternal pulmonary capillaries.

Amniotic fluid embolism: prevention/risk factors/warning signs

- Prevention: unknown.
- Risk factors: population proportional attributable risks are 35% for induction of labour, 13% for ethnic-minority women 35 years or older and 7% for multiple pregnancy.
- Warning signs: maternal collapse, shortness of breath, chest pain, feeling cold, light-headedness, restlessness, distress and panic, pins and needles in the fingers, nausea and vomiting.

Management

In the case of sudden collapse, management should be the structured ABC approach. The prognosis is poor, with approximately 30% of patients dying in the first hour and only 10% surviving overall. Management is supportive, requiring intensive care, and there are no specific therapies available. Symptoms occurring just before the collapse may be helpful in diagnosis. Perimortem caesarean section should be carried out within 5 minutes or as soon as possible after cardiac arrest. This is for the benefit of the woman to improve the effect of resuscitation.

Umbilical cord prolapse

Umbilical cord prolapse may be defined as the descent of the umbilical cord through the cervix alongside or past the presenting part in the presence of ruptured membranes (**Figure 14.7**). It is estimated to occur in 0.1–0.6% of pregnancies with the perinatal mortality rate estimated at 91 per 1,000.

Umbilical cord prolapse: prevention/ risk factors/warning signs

- Prevention: with transverse, oblique or unstable lie, elective admission to hospital after 37+0 weeks' gestation allows for quick delivery should membranes rupture. Women with non-cephalic prelabour preterm rupture of membranes should be managed as inpatients. Avoid artificial induction of labour when the presenting part is non-stable and/or mobile. When performing vaginal examination avoid upward pressure on the presenting part.

- Risk factors: polyhydramnios, multiparity, multiple pregnancy/ second twin, unstable, transverse and oblique lie, fetal congenital abnormalities, low birthweight (<2.5 kg), internal podalic version, large balloon catheter induction of labour.

- Warning signs: signs of fetal distress on CTG following artificial or spontaneous rupture of membranes.

Management

When suspected, perform speculum or digital examination immediately as early detection is crucial for timely delivery and in the prevention of fetal morbidity and mortality (reported as high as 25–50% of cases). When diagnosed, summon senior help and prepare operating theatre for emergency delivery. If diagnosed, attempt to prevent further cord compression by elevating the presenting part or filling

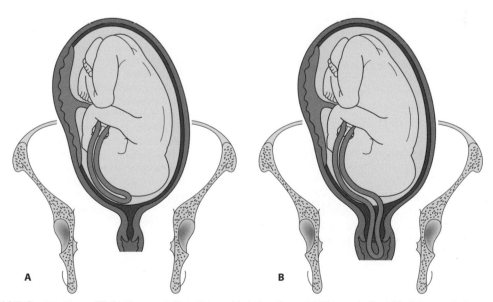

Figure 14.7 Cord prolapse. **(A)** Cord presentation: the cord is below the presenting party (head in this case but commonly a malpresentation) with the membranes intact; **(B)** cord prolapse: the membranes have ruptured and the cord is below the presenting part and has prolapsed into the vagina.

the bladder. Avoid handling the cord as this causes cord spasm. Place mother in knee to chest or left lateral position, ideally with head slightly declined. Confirm fetal viability by auscultation of the fetal heart using CTG. Delivery is generally performed by emergency caesarean section (category 1 if pathological fetal heart pattern or category 2 if normal fetal heart pattern).

Shoulder dystocia

Shoulder dystocia is defined as a vaginal cephalic delivery that requires additional obstetric manoeuvres to deliver the fetus after the head has delivered and gentle traction has been unsuccessful in delivering the shoulders (**Figure 14.8**). It is associated with significant morbidity both for the mother and fetus.

Maternal complications include increased perineal trauma (third- and fourth-degree tear), postpartum haemorrhage and psychological trauma. Fetal complications include brachial plexus injury (2–7% at birth reducing to 1–3% at 12 months of age), fractured clavicle or humerus (1–2%) and hypoxic brain injury.

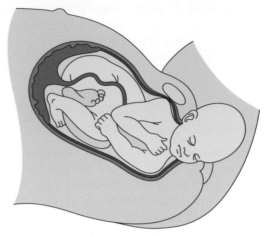

Figure 14.8 Shoulder dystocia. After delivery of the head, shoulder dystocia occurs due to the shoulders being unable to pass under the maternal symphysis pubis.

Shoulder dystocia: prevention/ risk factors/warning signs

- Prevention: diagnosis and optimal control of gestational and insulin-dependent diabetics, reduction of maternal obesity. Careful plan for mode of delivery in women with previous shoulder dystocia delivery (recurrence rate 10–15%).

- Risk factors: macrosomia, poorly controlled gestational and insulin-dependent diabetes, maternal obesity, previous shoulder dystocia, instrumental.

- Warning signs: failure of restitution of head following delivery of the head, retraction of the fetal head against the perineum (analogous to a turtle withdrawing into its shell).

Suggested management algorithm for shoulder dystocia is shown in **Figure 14.9**.

- Call for senior help (neonatology, senior midwife, obstetric consultant)

- Drop the level of the delivery bed as low as it will go and flatten the back of the bed so the woman is completely flat. Remove the foot of the bed to allow access
- McRoberts position – using one assistant on each of the mother's legs, flex and abduct the legs at the hip (thighs to abdomen). This flattens the lumbosacral spine and will facilitate delivery in approximatley 90% of cases
- Suprapubic pressure: apply over the posterior aspect of the anterior fetal shoulder. It can be used in a constant and then rocking motion
- Consider episisiotomy
- Deliver posterior arm and shoulder or consider internal rotational manoeuvres: include Rubin II: insert a hand behind the anterior shoulder and push it towards the chest. This will adduct the shoulders then push them into the diagonal
- Woods' screw: pressure on the anterior aspect of the posterior shoulder to aid rotation. Reverse Woods' screw: rotate the baby in the opposite direction
- Change position to all fours
- Finally consider symphiotomy, cleidotomy or Zavanelli manoeuvres

- Debrief staff, patient and partner
- Write comprehensive notes
- Risk report and risk committe review

Figure 14.9 Algorithm for management of shoulder dystocia.

Thrombosis and thromboembolism

Thrombosis and thromboembolism is once again the leading cause of direct maternal death in the 2009–2012 triennium, resulting in 26 direct maternal deaths (rate of 1.08 per 100,000 pregnancies). Venous thromboembolism (VTE) is 10 times more common in pregnancy compared with non-pregnant women. Women with VTE may be asymptomatic or present with a range of symptoms (specific and non-specific) including calf or groin pain and/or swelling that is often unilateral, low-grade pyrexia to more extreme presentations including haemoptysis, shortness of breath, collapse and death.

Thrombosis and thromboembolism: prevention/risk factors/warning signs

- Prevention: thrombosis assessment should be performed on all patients early in pregnancy as per RCOG guideline, to assess need for antenatal thromboprophylaxis and on each admission to hospital to assess for additional risk factors; managing patients where possible as outpatients and limiting bed rest; thromboembolic stockings; prophylactic low-molecular-weight heparin for at-risk patients.
- Risk factors: immobility, obesity, increased maternal age (≥35), underlying medical conditions, pre-eclampsia, dehydration, multiple pregnancy, raised body mass index (BMI) (≥30 kg/m²), smoker, grand multiparity, thrombophilia.
- Warning signs: immobility, dehydration, calf pain, shortness of breath.

When deep vein thrombosis (DVT) is suspected clinically, compression duplex ultrasound should be undertaken. If this is negative and there is a low level of clinical suspicion, anticoagulant treatment can be discontinued. If clinical suspicion remains high or symptoms fail to resolve, ultrasound may be repeated or magnetic resonance venography may be performed. When pulmonary embolus is suspected, investigative options include chest X-ray (to rule out other respiratory causes of chest symptoms such as pneumonia), low limb Doppler to rule out lower limb VTE and finally a ventilation perfusion (V/Q scan) or computed tomography pulmonary angiography. The measurement of D-dimers is not helpful and should not be performed as they are often elevated secondary to physiological changes in the coagulation system in pregnancy. Treatment of confirmed or suspected VTE is with therapeutic low-molecular-weight heparin given daily in two divided doses according to the patient's weight. In the case of a collapsed patient with pulmonary embolus, management options include intravenous unfractionated heparin, thrombolytic therapy or thoracotomy and surgical embolectomy. This complex management decision is taken by the multidisciplinary resuscitation team including senior physicians, obstetricians and radiologists.

Uterine inversion

Uterine inversion occurs when the uterus is partially or wholly inverted (**Figure 14.10**). Four degrees of inversion have been described: first degree when the inverted fundus extends to but not through the cervix; second degree when the inverted fundus extends through cervix but remains within the vagina; third degree when the inverted fundus extends outside the vagina; finally, total inversion occurs when the vagina and uterus are inverted. Prompt recognition is essential as the longer it is inverted the more difficult it becomes to replace as a retraction ring form forms, preventing eversion.

Uterine inversion: prevention/risk factors/warning signs

- Prevention: senior inhouse supervision and help to deal with this emergency.
- Risk factors: full dilatation sections, malpresentations, prolonged second stage, intravenous Syntocinon™ prior to a decision to deliver by caesarean section, unsuccessful instrumental delivery, prolonged second stage, hyperstimulated uterus.
- Warning signs: see risk factors.

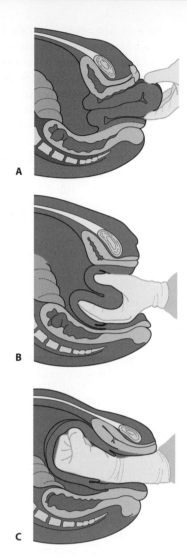

Figure 14.10 Uterine inversion.

Management

Attempt manual replacement as soon as the diagnosis is made. If unsuccessful, transfer to the operating theatre for replacement of the uterus under anaesthetic. If unsuccessful, attempt hydrostatic replacement by running 2–3 litres of warm saline via tubing into the vagina using your hands to create a seal round the vulva. This causes vagina vault and cervical ballooning, which allows the uterus and placenta to gradually reduce thus correcting the inversion. This is then confirmed manually and oxytocin commenced once the uterus contracts in

an attempt to maintain uterine contraction. If this is unsuccessful, surgical procedures including hysterectomy may be necessary.

Uterine rupture

Uterine rupture is a catastrophic event with significant associated maternal and fetal morbidity and mortality. It most commonly occurs in women previously delivered by caesarean section. In the UK between April 2009 and April 2010, the estimated incidence of uterine rupture was 2 per 10,000 pregnancies overall. These rates increased to 21 and 3 per 10,000 pregnancies in women with a previous caesarean delivery planning vaginal or elective caesarean delivery, respectively. Two women with uterine rupture died (case fatality 1.3%, 95% CI 0.2–4.5). There were 18 perinatal deaths associated with uterine rupture among 145 infants (perinatal mortality 124 per 1,000 total births, 95% CI 75–189).

Uterine rupture: prevention/ risk factors/warning signs

- Prevention: reduce rates of primary caesarean section. Avoid vaginal delivery in women with previous myomectomies in which the endometrial cavity has been breached. Act with caution when inducing women with previous caesarean sections.

- Risk factors: previous myomectomies that have breached the endometrial cavity, odds of rupture are increased in women who had two or more previous caesarean deliveries (adjusted odds ratio [aOR] 3.02, 95% CI 1.16–7.85), less than 12 months since the last caesarean delivery (aOR 3.12, 95% CI 1.62–6.02), labour induction and oxytocin use (aOR 3.92, 95% CI 1.00–15.33). The estimated incidence of uterine rupture was 2 per 10,000 pregnancies overall; 21 and 3 per 10,000 pregnancies in women with a previous caesarean delivery planning vaginal or elective caesarean delivery, respectively.

- Warning signs: maternal shock, fetal distress/unable to auscultate fetal heart, unable to palpate any presenting part on vaginal examination; severe sudden abdominal pain.

Management

An urgent laparotomy is required once uterine rupture is diagnosed. Vaginal examination should be performed and the fetus delivered by the quickest route possible. Assisted vaginal delivery is reasonable if the woman is fully dilated and safe vaginal delivery is possible. Regardless, an urgent laparotomy is then required to examine and repair the uterine rupture.

Impacted head at caesarean section

An impacted head at caesarean section can be an extremely stressful situation for the operating clinician and for the parents. Many obstetricians first encounter impaction of the fetal head while in training, often at night without immediate access to senior help. No figures exist for the exact incidence rates but it potentially could affect as many as 20,000 births per year (200,000 caesarean sections in the UK each year with approximately 10% at full dilation).

Impacted head at caesarean section: prevention/risk factors/warning signs

- Prevention: senior in-house supervision and help to deal with this emergency.
- Risk factors: full dilatation sections, malpresentations, prolonged second stage, intravenous Syntocinon™ prior to a decision to deliver by caesarean section, unsuccessful instrumental delivery, prolonged second stage, hyperstimulated uterus.
- Warning signs: see risk factors.

Management

Full dilatation sections should have the obstetric consultant present in anticipation of this complication. Allow the uterus to relax before disimpacting the head. Disengagement of the head requires flexion and rotation of the head into the transverse position prior to delivery by lateral flexion. Forcing the head upwards risks trauma including fractures to the fetal head and extension to the uterine angles, which can result in haemorrhage and damage to the viscera. If you are unable to flex and rotate the head, consider the use of a uterine relaxant such as glyceryl trinitrate (GTN) spray or terbutaline, but beware the risk of postpartum haemorrhage following the use of uterorelaxant agents. Other options include having a senior assistant flex and rotate the head vaginally or the use of newer devices designed to release the vacuum that occurs between the fetal head and pelvis (e.g. C-Snorkel®). However, minimum evidence exists to support their use and extreme care must be taken to avoid iatrogenic trauma.

Further reading

Knight M, Kenyon S, Brocklehurst P, Neilson J, Shakespeare J, Kurinczuk JJ (eds) on behalf of MBRRACE-UK. Saving Lives, Improving Mothers' Care – Lessons learned to inform future maternity care from the UK and Ireland Confidential Enquiries into Maternal Deaths and Morbidity 2009–12. Oxford: National Perinatal. Epidemiology Unit, University of Oxford, 2014.

Managing Obstetric Emergencies and Trauma. The MOET Course Manual, ISBN: 9781107675346.

Royal College of Obstetricians and Gynaecologists. Green-top Guideline No. 56, January 2011. Maternal Collapse in Pregnancy and the Puerperium. Available at https://www.rcog.org.uk/globalassets/documents/guidelines/gtg56.pdf).

Royal College of Obstetricians and Gynaecologists. Green–top Guideline No. 64a April 2012. Bacterial Sepsis in Pregnancy. Available at https://www.rcog.org.uk/globalassets/documents/guidelines/gtg_64a.pdf).

Royal College of Obstetricians and Gynaecologists. Green-top Guideline No. 52 May 2009. Prevention and management of postpartum haemorrhage. Available at https://www.rcog.org.uk/globalassets/documents/guidelines/gt52postpartumhaemorrhage0411.pdf.

Hypertension in pregnancy. The management of hypertensive disorders during pregnancy. NICE clinical guideline 107. Available at http://www.nice.org.uk/guidance/cg107/resources/guidance-hypertension-in-pregnancy-pdf.

RCOG Greentop Guideline Number 50, November 2014. Available at https://www.rcog.org.uk/globalassets/documents/guidelines/gtg-50-umbilicalcordprolapse-2014.pdf.

RCOG Green-top Guideline. No. 37a November 2009. Reducing the risk of thrombosis and embolism during pregnancy and the puerperium. Available at https://www.rcog.org.uk/globalassets/documents/guidelines/gtg37areducingriskthrombosis.pdf.

RCOG Green-top Guideline. No. 37a November 2009. The acute management of thrombosis and embolism during pregnancy and the puerpurium. Available at https://www.rcog.org.uk/globalassets/documents/guidelines/gtg37b_230611.pdf

Self assessment

CASE HISTORY

Ms B is 39 weeks' gestation in her second pregnancy. Her first pregnancy was a term delivery, delivered 11 months previously by caesarean section at 5 cm dilated due to failure to progress. Ms B was induced due to FGR and has been on oxytocin for 4 hours and has made good progress. She is now 9 cm dilated when she develops severe constant lower abdominal pain over the area of her scar. The midwife looking after her labour records the fetal heart rate as 46 beats per minute and calls an emergency alert.

A   What is the likely diagnosis?

B   What risk factors does Ms B have for this complication?

C   How would you manage this situation?

ANSWERS

1   Ms B has likely ruptured her uterus due to the nature and location of pain (constant and severe worse above her scar) and the fetal bradycardia that has now occurred. Differential diagnosis includes fetal distress.

2   Ms B has had a previous caesarean section and has been induced due to FGR. The use of oxytocin also increased the risk of uterine rupture. Ms B has also had a short interpregnancy interval <12 months, which increases the risk of uterine rupture.

3   Management involves calling senior help (senior obstetrician, neonatal team, anaesthetic team), safe delivery of fetus and repair of the rupture. Delivery of the fetus is by safest quickest route. A vaginal examination should be performed and assessment for vaginal delivery made. If vaginal delivery is possible, then this should be performed and assessment made for examination under anaesthetic and/or laparotomy. If vaginal delivery is not possible, the patient should be transferred to the operating theatre for category 1 caesarean section, examination under anaesthetic and laparotomy.

EMQ

A   5–10 units IV/IM oxytocin.

B   Carbaprost 0.25 mg by IM repeated at intervals of not less than 15 minutes to a maximum of 8 doses (contraindicated in women with asthma).

C   Hysterectomy.

D   Repeat ergometrine (500 µg) IM or slow IV push.

E   B-Lynch suture.

F   40 units oxytocin in 100 ml normal saline over 4 hours.

G   Syntometrine (ergometrine 500 µg and Syntocinon™ 5 units).

H   Uterine massage.

I   800–1,000 µg rectal misoprostol.

J   Observe the patient.

K   Indwelling catheter.

For each description, choose the SINGLE most appropriate answer from the list of options. Each option may be used once, more than once or not at all.

1   You are called to review a patient who delivered vaginally 12 minutes previously. She is bleeding moderately vaginally and the midwife has said her uterus is boggy and not well contracted. What is your first step in the management of her uterine atony?

2   Despite uterine compressions the patient continues to bleed. She has already received 5–10 units IV/IM oxytocin. What medication would you next administer?

3   While rubbing up the uterine contraction you notice a palpable bladder. On questioning, the

midwife says urine was last passed 2 hours previously. What is your next management step?

4   At the end of a caesarean section, on swabbing the vagina you express clots and feel the uterus is poorly contracted. The patient is already receiving 40 units oxytocin in 100 ml normal saline over 4 hours and is hypertensive What would your next pharmacological option be?

ANSWERS

1H Uterine massage – uterine atony is the commonest cause of bleeding in obstetrics and generally responds very well to uterine massage. This stimulates the uterus to contract and frequently stops bleeding.

2G Syntometrine (ergometrine 500 µg and Syntocinon™ 5 units) would generally be the second-line pharmacological agent. Preparations containing ergometrine are contraindicated in the presence of hypertension.

3K A full bladder can contribute to atony and should be emptied as soon as possible.

4I   800–1,000 µg rectal misoprostol.

SBA QUESTIONS

Choose the single best answer.

1   What risk factor has the highest association with uterine rupture in a woman with a previous caesarean section?

A   Spontaneous onset of labour.
B   Severe pelvic girdle pain.
C   The use of oxytocin in labour.
D   Prostaglandin E2 induction of labour.
E   Women with systemic lupus erythematosus.

ANSWER

D   The greatest risk factor for uterine rupture in a woman with a previous caesarean section is the use of prostaglandin to induce labour in the presence of an unfavourable cervix. This increases the risk of uterine rupture with an aOR of 3.92 (95% CI 1.00–15.33).

2   Which of the following is NOT a likely finding in a woman with uterine inversion?

A   Lower abdominal pain.
B   Mass in vagina.
C   Well-contracted uterus.
D   Haemorrhage.
E   Unpalpable fundus.

ANSWER

C   Uterine inversion occurs in the presence of a hypotonic uterus that has inverted normally when an attempt has been made to remove the placenta when it is still attached.

CHAPTER

The puerperium | 15

ANDREW D WEEKS

LEARNING OBJECTIVES

- To understand the physiological changes that occur in the normal puerperium.
- To understand the common disorders of the puerperium and how to manage them.
- To understand the process of breastfeeding and common disorders associated with it.
- To be able to recognize and manage common postpartum psychiatric disorders.

Introduction

The puerperium refers to the 6-week period following completion of the third stage of labour, when considerable adjustments occur before return to the prepregnant state. For those with complex medical problems, the early puerperium is especially dangerous and most maternal deaths occur during this time. During this period of physiological change, the mother is also vulnerable to psychological disturbances, which may be aggravated by adverse social circumstances. Adequate understanding and support from her partner and family are crucial. Difficulty in coping with the newborn infant occurs more frequently with the first baby, and vigilant surveillance is therefore necessary by the community midwife, general practitioner (GP) and health visitor.

Physiological changes

Uterine involution

Involution is the process by which the postpartum uterus, weighing about 1 kg, returns to its prepregnancy state of less than 100 g. Immediately after delivery, the uterine fundus lies about 4 cm below the umbilicus or, more accurately, 12 cm above the symphysis pubis. However, by 2 weeks, the uterus becomes no longer palpable above the symphysis (**Figure 15.1**) Involution occurs by a process of autolysis, whereby muscle cells diminish in size as a result of enzymatic digestion of cytoplasm. This has virtually no effect on the number of muscle cells, and the excess protein produced from autolysis is absorbed into the bloodstream and excreted in the urine. Involution appears to be accelerated by the

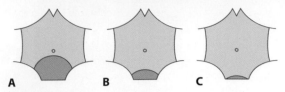

Figure 15.1 Involution of the uterus. (**A**) Day 1, 18 week sized uterus (just below the umbilicus); (**B**) day 7, 14 week sized uterus; (**C**) day 14, 12 week sized uterus. Uterus is larger following caesarean section and in multiparous women.

release of oxytocin in women who are breastfeeding, as the uterus is smaller than in those who are bottlefeeding. A delay in involution in the absence of any other signs or symptoms (e.g. bleeding) is of no clinical significance.

Signs of delayed involution

- Artefact.
- Full bladder.
- Loaded rectum.
- Retained products of conception (or clots).
- Uterine infection.
- Fibroids.
- Broad ligament haematoma.

Genital tract changes

Following delivery of the placenta, the lower segment of the uterus and the cervix appear flabby and there may be small cervical lacerations. In the first few days the cervix can readily admit two fingers; by the end of the first week it should become increasingly difficult to pass more than one finger, and certainly by the end of the second week the internal os should be closed. However, the external os can remain open permanently, giving a characteristic funnel shape to the parous cervix. Assessment of the postnatal cervix is important in diagnosing retained products of conception (see Secondary postpartum haemorrhage below).

Lochia

Lochia is the blood-stained uterine discharge that is comprised of blood and necrotic decidua. Only the superficial layer of decidua becomes necrotic and is sloughed off. The basal layer adjacent to the myometrium is involved in the regeneration of new endometrium and this regeneration is complete by the third week. During the first few days after delivery, the lochia is red (lochia rubra); this gradually changes to pink as the endometrium is formed, serous by the second week (lochia serosa) and then ultimately a scanty yellow-white discharge (lochia alba) that lasts for about 1 month. Persistent red lochia suggests delayed involution that is usually associated with infection or a retained piece of placental tissue (see Secondary postpartum haemorrhage and Puerpural sepsis below).

Recovery after childbirth

Recovery after normal birth

Childbirth is a process of enormous significance in human lives, and with it comes massive physical and emotional changes. Although most parents will describe it as the best, most exciting experience of their lives, others will have bad outcomes and describe it as their worst. But there are very few who are not physically and emotionally drained in the first few weeks after childbirth. The combination of excitement, physical tiredness after labour and dealing with a demanding newborn makes this a time during which mothers (and fathers) often need a lot of support. Around the world, cultures have developed diverse ways of dealing with this. Traditionally, women from China and South India are confined to their homes for the first month postnatally, whereas traditional Sikh women are not allowed to cook for 40 days. Touch between men and women is prohibited while locia is being passed in some Orthodox Jewish couples and those from the Zulu tribe in South Africa. While some of these may seem strange in a modern world, these traditions did recognize the enormity of what the woman had just been through and served to provide new mothers with the chance to recover.

Alongside the psychological changes (covered below), the main physical effects are on the perineum, bladder and bowel.

Perineal pain

Perineal discomfort is a common problem for mothers. About 80% complain of pain in the first

3 days after delivery, with one-quarter continuing to suffer discomfort at day 10. Discomfort is greatest in women who sustain spontaneous tears or have an episiotomy, especially following instrumental delivery. A number of non-pharmacological and pharmacological therapies have been used empirically with varying degrees of success. However, local cooling (with crushed ice, witch hazel or tap water) and topical anaesthetics, such as 5% lignocaine gel, provide short-term symptomatic relief. Effective analgesia following perineal trauma can be achieved with regular paracetamol. If necessary, diclofenac given rectally or orally may also be added. Codeine derivatives are best avoided, as they cause constipation in the mother and drowsiness in some breastfed babies.

The perineum should be kept clean with daily cleaning or showering using tap water only, and with frequent changing of sanitary pads. However, infections of the perineum are surprisingly uncommon considering the risk of bacterial contamination during delivery. Therefore signs of infection (redness, pain, swelling and heat), especially with a raised temperature, must be taken seriously. Swabs for microbiological culture should be taken from the infected perineum and broad-spectrum antibiotics (see below) should be commenced. If there is a collection of pus, drainage should be encouraged by removal of any skin sutures; otherwise, infection would spread, with increasing morbidity and a poor anatomical result.

Spontaneous opening of repaired perineal tears and episiotomies is usually the result of secondary infection. Surgical repair should never be attempted in the presence of infection. The wound should be irrigated twice daily and healing allowed to occur by secondary intention. If there is a large, gaping wound, secondary repair should only be performed when the infection has cleared, there is no cellulitis or exudate present and healthy granulation tissue can be seen.

Bladder function

Voiding difficulty and overdistension of the bladder are not uncommon after childbirth, especially if regional anaesthesia (epidural/spinal) has been used. It is now known that after epidural anaesthesia the bladder may take up to 8 hours to regain normal sensation. During this time, about 1 litre of urine may be produced. Therefore, if urinary retention occurs, considerable damage may be inflicted on the detrusor muscle. Overstretching of the detrusor muscle can dampen bladder sensation and make the bladder hypocontractile, particularly with fibrous replacement of smooth muscle. In this situation, overflow incontinence of small amounts of urine may erroneously be assumed to be normal voiding. Fluid loading prior to epidural analgesia, the antidiuretic effect of high concentrations of oxytocin during labour, increased postpartum diuresis (particularly in the presence of peripheral oedema) and increased fluid intake by breastfeeding mothers all contribute to the increased urine production in the puerperium. Therefore, an intake/output chart alone may not detect incomplete emptying of the bladder.

Women who have undergone a traumatic delivery, such as a difficult instrumental delivery, or who have suffered multiple/extended lacerations or a vulvovaginal haematoma, may find it difficult to void because of pain or periurethral oedema. Other causes of pain, such as prolapsed haemorrhoids, anal fissures, abdominal wound haematoma or even stool impaction of the rectum, may interfere with voiding. The midwife needs to be particularly vigilant after an epidural or spinal anaesthetic to avoid bladder distension. A distended bladder would either be palpable as a suprapubic cystic mass or it may displace the uterus laterally or upwards, thereby increasing the height of the uterine fundus.

A formal assessment of bladder function is best made at 6 hours postnatally, at which time the woman should have passed at least 300 ml of urine. If, after another attempt, she has passed less than that (or none at all), then a small intermittent catheter can be inserted, which should drain less than 150 ml. Those with more than this need close observation, but if there is over 1 litre of urine in the bladder then an indwelling catheter is left in for 48 hours to allow periurethral swelling to settle.

In order to minimize the risk of overdistension of the bladder in women who have had a spinal anaesthetic (for caesarean section or manual removal of placenta), a urinary catheter is left in the bladder for at least 12 hours until the woman is mobile.

Although vaginal delivery is strongly implicated in the long-term development of urinary stress incontinence, it rarely poses a problem in the early puerperium. Therefore, any incontinence should be investigated to exclude a vesicovaginal, urethrovaginal or, rarely, ureterovaginal fistula. Obstetric fistulae are rare in the UK, but are a source of considerable morbidity in developing countries. Pressure necrosis of the bladder or urethra may occur following prolonged obstructed labour, and incontinence usually occurs in the second week when the slough separates. Small fistulae may close spontaneously after a few weeks of free bladder drainage; large fistulae will require surgical repair by a specialist.

Bowel function

Constipation is a common problem in the early puerperium, as a result of an interruption in the normal diet, intrapartum dehydration and opiate use. Advice on adequate fluid intake and increase in fibre intake may be all that is necessary. However, constipation may also be the result of fear of evacuation due to pain from a sutured perineum, prolapsed haemorrhoids or anal fissures. Avoidance of constipation and straining is of utmost importance in women who have sustained a third-degree or fourth-degree tear. A large, hard stool in this situation could disrupt the repaired anal sphincter and cause anal incontinence. It is important to ensure that these women are prescribed lactulose and ispaghula husk or methylcellulose immediately after the repair, for a period of 2 weeks.

The high prevalence of anal incontinence and faecal urgency following childbirth has only recently been recognized. One prospective study using anal endosonography at 6 weeks following vaginal birth identified evidence of occult anal sphincter trauma in one-third of primiparous women (only 13% were symptomatic), and a remarkable 80% of those who had undergone forceps delivery. Larger, retrospective, short-term studies of parous women indicate a symptom prevalence of between 6% and 10%. Long-term anal incontinence following primary repair of a third-degree or fourth-degree tear occurs in 5% of women, and anovaginal/rectovaginal fistulae occur in 2–4% of these women (**Figure 15.2**). It is therefore important to consider a fistula as a cause of anal incontinence in the postpartum period, particularly if the woman complains of passing wind or stool per vagina. Approximately 50% of small anovaginal fistulae will close spontaneously over a period of 6 months, but larger fistulae will require formal repair.

Pelvic floor exercises

It is a widespread belief that pelvic floor exercises tone up the muscles of the pelvic floor and should therefore be advocated in the postpartum period. However, large randomized trials to evaluate their benefit in preventing genital prolapse, urinary incontinence or anal incontinence are lacking. There is also no evidence that antenatal exercises prevent incontinence or prolapse. However, as general

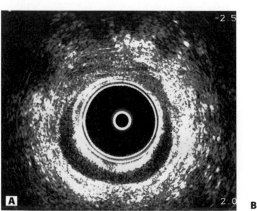
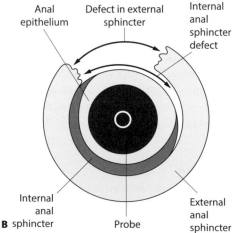

Figure 15.2 (A) Transanal ultrasound showing the anal mucosa and anterior disruption of the internal anal sphincter (dark band) following a third-degree tear at delivery; **(B)** diagrammatic representation of part A.

exercise is known to strengthen striated muscle and pelvic floor exercises are unlikely to be harmful, women are still taught postnatal exercises. This should also serve to cultivate a feeling of pelvic floor awareness, so that women with pelvic floor dysfunction seek medical help sooner.

Recovery from caesarean section

Many women now deliver their baby by caesarean section. Although this reduces the risk of pelvic floor problems, it increases the risk of other complications including infection (wound, urine and chest), anaemia and thromboembolism. The infective risks are discussed in the section below on puerperal sepsis, but are reduced by routine antibiotics at the time of caesarean section and careful wound care. The wound should be covered by a sterile dressing in theatre, which is removed after 24 hours. Women are advised to gently clean and dry the wound daily with tap water. Sutures or staples are removed on the 5th day.

Anaemia is common postoperatively and, given the inaccuracy of blood loss estimation, all women should have their haemoglobin levels measured postoperatively (ideally day 2–3). Asymptomatic women with mild–moderate anaemia (haemoglobin >7 g/dl) can be treated with iron tablets, while the postoperative recovery of those with severe anaemia will be helped greatly from a blood transfusion.

The combination of abdominal surgery, preoperative bed rest and physiological changes in clotting makes women who have had a caesarean section particularly prone to thromboembolism. Other risk factors include obesity, multiple pregnancy, hypertension and postpartum haemorrhage. Early mobilization and good hydration are important for all women, with 1–6 weeks of low-molecular-weight heparin given to those with multiple risk factors. In the UK, early mobilization is now encouraged, with low-risk women being discharged from hospital on day 1–2 following caesarean section. The changes above have contributed to a decrease in thromboembolism deaths in the UK from a peak of 2.2 per 100,000 maternities in 1994–6 to 1.3 per 100,000 in 2009–2011.

After the first few days, women who have undergone caesarean section should not have routine bed rest, but should slowly increase their activity levels aided by oral analgesia as required. They can resume activities such as driving a vehicle, carrying heavy items, formal exercise and sexual intercourse once they have returned to their precaesarean strength with no physical restrictions or distracting effect due to pain.

Postnatal visits

The degree of care provided by the health service varies from country to country. In the UK, a mother who has delivered in hospital may be discharged within 6 hours of an uncomplicated birth, although she may request to stay longer. Traditionally, a midwife would visit the mother and newborn daily for a minimum of 10 days after delivery, with the health visitor taking on continuing care for up to 4 weeks. However, postnatal care is generally now a demand-led service for low-risk women, with only 1–2 routine midwifery visits in the first 10 days and further visits as requested. More frequent visits will be required in high-risk women or if an abnormality has been detected, for example hypertension or maternal pyrexia.

At each visit women should be specifically asked about their recovery, including bowel and bladder function, fatigue, headache and perineum. Further questions will cover the health of the newborn (see Chapter 16, The neonate). During this time, it is crucial that women are also provided with information about danger signs (see *Table 15.1*) and given emotional support. They should also be provided with contact details of where they can get information. Anti-rhesus D immunoglobulin should be given to all rhesus D-negative mothers of rhesus D-positive babies, and mothers who are rubella immune should be offered immunization.

The only routine test to be performed at every postnatal visit in the first week is the maternal blood pressure. Other maternal examinations and observations should be determined by the mother's condition and symptoms (*Table 15.1*). For example, those with offensive vaginal loss or signs of infection will require pulse, temperature, along with an assessment of uterine involution. Those who have had a postpartum haemorrhage (PPH) or who have abnormal vaginal bleeding will require an assessment of uterine involution along with pulse and blood pressure.

Table 15.1 Signs and symptoms of potentially life-threatening postnatal conditions

Signs and symptoms	Condition
Sudden and profuse blood loss or persistent increased blood loss Faintness, shivering, abdominal pain and/or offensive vaginal loss	Postpartum haemorrhage
Fever, shivering, abdominal pain and/or offensive vaginal loss	Infection
Headaches accompanied by one or more of the following symptoms within the first 72 hours after birth: visual disturbances, nausea/vomiting	Pre-eclampsia/eclampsia
Unilateral calf pain, redness or swelling Shortness of breath or chest pain	Thromboembolism

For women with antenatal anaemia, complicated deliveries or PPH, the haemoglobin level should be checked on day 1–3 and iron offered to those who are anaemic. Women who are particularly symptomatic or who have a haemoglobin level of <7 g/dl should be offered a transfusion.

At 2 weeks postnatally, women should be specifically asked about the resolution of the 'baby blues' (see below).

A formal postnatal examination is carried out at about 6 weeks postpartum by the GP, or by the obstetrician if delivery had been complicated. The examination includes an assessment of the woman's mental and physical health, as well as the progress of the baby. In particular, direct questions should be asked about urinary, bowel and sexual function. Incontinence and dyspareunia are embarrassing issues that women do not volunteer to discuss readily. Weight, urine analysis and blood pressure are checked and an examination is performed as required. If a cervical smear is due, it can be taken, although it is preferable to take one after 3 months postpartum. Contraception, pelvic floor exercises and infant immunizations are also discussed.

Puerperal disorders

Hypertension

Women with hypertension in pregnancy are carefully managed with the aim of preventing complications and timing delivery. After childbirth, however, they often receive less attention, even though they remain at significant risk for the first week. Nearly half of all eclamptic fits occur postnatally, and it is the highest risk time for fluid overload. Those

with severe pre-eclampsia should be managed for the first 24 hours on a high-dependency unit until their blood pressure is controlled and they achieve a good diuresis (see Chapter 9, Hypertensive disorders of pregnancy). Those with mild or moderate pre-eclampsia are managed on a postnatal ward until stable. They should continue any antenatally prescribed antihypertensives with the aim of keeping their blood pressure under 150/100 mmHg. Labetolol or slow-release nifedipine are good choices for this, and are commonly needed for 1–2 weeks postnatally. At home the blood pressure is measured every 2 days and the dosage halved when it is <140/90 mmHg. Those who are still on antihypertensives at 6 weeks postnatally should be referred for specialist assessment.

Secondary postpartum haemorrhage

Secondary PPH is defined as fresh bleeding from the genital tract between 24 hours and 6 weeks after delivery (see Chapter 14, Obstetric emergencies). The most common time for secondary PPH is between days 7 and 14. The cause is usually either endometritis or retained placental tissue, and it is often very difficult to distinguish between them. Classically, women with endometritis have constant low abdominal pain and a tender uterus with a closed internal os. In contrast, women with retained products of conception have crampy low abdominal pain, a uterus larger than appropriate (see **Figure 15.1**), with an open internal os, and a history of a prolonged third stage of labour and sometimes passage of bits of placental tissue or tissue. Both endometritis and retained products may have symptoms and signs of infection with low-grade fever, pungent lochia and uterine tenderness. Those bleeding heavily will require circulatory support with fluids or blood along with strong oxytocics (e.g. ergometrine) and uterine evacuation. Antibiotics should be given if placental tissue is found, even without evidence of overt infection. If blood loss is not excessive, the use of pelvic ultrasound to exclude retained products is sometimes used, but is only helpful if the uterus is seen to be empty. Debris, clots and fluid are commonly found even within the normal postpartum uterus and their presence does not mean that there is retained placental tissue. In the absence of a clear diagnosis, expectant management with empirical antibiotics is often used. Other causes of secondary PPH include hormonal contraception, bleeding disorders (e.g. von Willebrand's disease) and occasionally choriocarcinoma.

Obstetric palsy

Obstetric palsy, or traumatic neuritis, is a condition in which one or both lower limbs may develop signs of a motor and/or sensory neuropathy following delivery. Presenting features include sciatic pain, foot-drop, paraesthesia, hypoaesthesia and muscle wasting. The mechanism of injury is proximal nerve damage as the lumbosacral plexus and nerve tracks are stretched and compressed by the fetal head as they cross the pelvic brim. It is almost always associated with prolonged or obstructed labour and is now very rare following modern labour management. If obstetric paralysis develops following a normal labour, then epidural complications and/or herniation of lumbosacral discs should be excluded, particularly if the woman has been in an exaggerated lithotomy position for instrumental delivery. Peroneal nerve palsy can occur when the nerve is compressed between the head of the fibula and the lithotomy pole, resulting in unilateral foot-drop. The development of urinary and faecal incontinence is most likely due to structural damage to the anal sphincter muscle and supporting fascia.

Symphysis pubis diastasis

Spontaneous separation of the symphysis pubis occurs in at least 1 in 800 vaginal deliveries. It is usually noticed after delivery and has been associated with forceps delivery, rapid second stage of labour or severe abduction of the thighs during delivery.

Common signs and symptoms include symphyseal pain aggravated by weight-bearing and walking, a waddling gait, pubic tenderness and a palpable interpubic gap. Treatment includes bed rest, anti-inflammatory agents, physiotherapy and a pelvic corset to provide support and stability.

Thromboembolism

The risk of thromboembolic disease rises fivefold during pregnancy and the puerperium. The majority of fatal thromboembolisms occur in the puerperium and are more common after caesarean section. Those at high risk may be given prophylactic heparin injections. If deep vein thrombosis or pulmonary embolism is suspected, full anticoagulant therapy should be commenced and a lower limb compression ultrasound and/or lung scan should be carried out within 24–48 hours (see Chapter 6, Antenatal obstetric complications, and Chapter 14, Obstetric emergencies).

Puerperal pyrexia

Significant puerperal pyrexia is defined as a temperature of 38°C or higher on any 2 of the first 10 days postpartum, exclusive of the first 24 hours. A mildly elevated temperature is not uncommon in the first 24 hours, but any pyrexia associated with tachycardia merits investigation. In about 80% of women who develop a temperature in the first 24 hours following a vaginal delivery, no obvious evidence of infection can be identified. The reverse holds true for women delivering by caesarean section, when a wound infection should be considered. Common sites associated with puerperal pyrexia include chest, throat, breasts, urinary tract, pelvic organs, caesarean or perineal wounds and legs (*Table 15.2*).

Chest complications

Chest complications are most likely to appear in the first 24 hours after delivery, particularly after general anaesthesia. Atalectasis may be associated with fever and can be prevented by early and regular chest physiotherapy. Aspiration pneumonia (Mendelson's syndrome) must be suspected if there is a spiking temperature associated with wheezing, dyspnoea or evidence of hypoxia following a general anaesthetic.

Table 15.2 Diagnosis and management of puerperal sepsis

Symptoms	Diagnosis	Investigations	Management
Cough Purulent sputum Dyspnoea	Pneumonia	Sputum M, C & S Chest X-ray	Physiotherapy Antibiotics
Sore throat Cervical lymphadenopathy	Tonsillitis	Throat swab	Antibiotics
Headaches Neck stiffness (epidural/ spinal anaesthetic)	Meningitis	Lumbar puncture	Antibiotics
Dysuria Loin pain and tenderness	Pyelonephritis	Urine M, C & S	Antibiotics, Increased fluid intake
Secondary PPH Tender bulky uterus	Endometritis or Retained placental tissue	Clinical diagnosis +/− pelvic ultrasound	Antibiotics and/or Uterine evacuation
Pelvic/calf pain/tenderness	Deep vein thrombosis	Doppler/venogram of legs	Heparin
Chest pain Dyspnoea	Pulmonary embolism	Chest X-ray and blood gases, lung perfusion scan, angiogram	Heparin
Painful engorged breasts	Mastitis or Breast abscess	Clinical examination, M, C & S of expressed milk	Express milk Antibiotics Incision and drainage

M, C & S, microscopy, culture and sensitivity; PPH, postpartum haemorrhage.

Genital tract infection/ puerperal sepsis

Genital tract infection following delivery is referred to as puerperal sepsis and is synonymous with older descriptions of puerperal fever, milk fever and childbed fever. It was not realized until the mid-nineteenth century that the high maternal mortality and morbidity in the UK was due to poor hygiene; the establishment of lying-in hospitals and over-crowding perpetuated the condition to epidemic proportions. Until 1937, puerperal sepsis was the major cause of maternal mortality. The discovery of sulphonamides in 1935 and the simultaneous reduction in the virulence of haemolytic strepto-cocci resulted in a dramatic fall in maternal mortality. The UK Confidential Enquiry into Maternal Deaths reported that in 2010–12 genital tract sepsis accounted for 5% of all maternal deaths. Over 80% of these occurred postnatally. Although some of these cases followed miscarriage or occurred after preterm premature rupture of membranes (PPROM), around one-half occurred following birth at term. Over 50% were due to group A streptococcus.

Aetiology

A mixed flora with low virulence normally colonizes the vagina. Puerperal infection is usually polymicrobial and involves contaminants from the bowel that colonize the perineum and lower genital tract. The organisms most commonly associated with puerperal genital infection are listed in the box below. Following delivery, natural barriers to infection are temporarily removed and therefore organisms with a pathogenic potential can ascend from the lower genital tract into the uterine cavity. Placental separation exposes a large raw area equivalent to an open wound, and retained products of conception and blood clots within the uterus can provide an excellent culture medium for infection. Furthermore, vaginal delivery is almost invariably associated with lacerations of the genital tract (uterus, cervix and vagina). Although these lacerations may not need surgical repair, they can become a focus for infection similar to iatrogenic wounds, such as caesarean section and episiotomy.

Organisms commonly associated with puerperal genital infection

Aerobes

- Gram-positive:
  - beta-haemolytic streptococcus, groups A, B, D;
  - *Staphylococcus epidermidis* and *S. aureus*;
  - Enterococci – *Streptococcus faecalis*.
- Gram-negative:
  - *Escherichia coli*;
  - *Haemophilus influenzae*;
  - *Klebsiella pneumoniae*;
  - *Pseudomonas aeruginosa*;
  - *Proteus mirabilis*.
- Gram-variable.
  - *Gardenella vaginalis*.

Anaerobes

- *Peptococcus* sp.
- *Peptostreptococcus* sp.
- Bacteroides – *B. fragilis, B. bivius, B. disiens.*
- *Fusobacterium* sp.

Miscellaneous

- *Chlamydia trachomatis.*
- *Mycoplasma hominis.*
- *Ureaplasma urealyticum.*

Common risk factors for puerperal infection

- Underlying conditions:
  - obesity;
  - diabetes;
  - human immunodeficiency virus (HIV).
- Antenatal:
  - chorioamnionitis;
  - prolonged rupture of membranes;
  - cervical cerclage for cervical incompetence.
- Intrapartum:
  - prolonged labour;
  - multiple vaginal examinations;
  - instrumental delivery;
  - caesarean section;
  - manual removal of the placenta;
  - retained products of conception.

Prevention

Increased awareness of the principles of general hygiene, a good surgical approach and the use of aseptic techniques have all contributed to the decline in severe puerperal sepsis. Unfortunately, although it is over 150 years since the Hungarian obstetrician Ignaz Semelweiss identified the importance of hand-washing for preventing spread of infection between postnatal women, poor attention to hand-washing remains a significant problem. The arrival of alcohol hand-based hand rubs has facilitated the process: every clinician should use them regularly in clinical areas, at least between every patient contact. The risk of sepsis is higher following caesarean section, particularly when performed after the onset of labour, but can be prevented by routine prophylactic antibiotics. A single intraoperative dose of antibiotics (co-amoxiclav or cephalosporin with metronidazole) is given before the skin incision. The problem with resistant bacteria (e.g. methicillin-resistant *S. aureus* [MRSA]) has led some units to routinely screen all women admitted electively to the hospital so that those carrying the resistant bacteria can be barrier nursed to prevent their spread.

Clinical presentation

Chlamydia trachomatis puerperal parametritis may develop in one-third of women who had a pre-existing infection, but presentation is usually delayed. Investigations for puerperal genital infections are shown in *Table 15.3*.

There are a number of factors that determine the clinical course and severity of the infection, namely the general health and resistance of the woman, the virulence of the offending organism, the presence of haematoma or retained products of conception, the timing of antibiotic therapy and associated risk factors. The common methods of spread of puerperal infection are as follows:

- An ascending infection from the lower genital tract or primary infection of the placental site may spread via the Fallopian tubes to the ovaries, giving rise to a salpingo-oophoritis and pelvic peritonitis. This could progress to a generalized peritonitis and the development of pelvic abscesses.

Table 15.3 Investigations for puerperal genital infections

Investigations	Abnormalities
Full blood count	Anaemia, leukocytosis, thrombocytopaenia
Urea and electrolytes	Fluid and electrolyte imbalance
Culture of blood or swabs from high vagina or infected wound	Bacterial growth
Pelvic ultrasound	Retained products, pelvic abscess
Clotting screen (haemorrhage or shock)	Disseminated intravascular coagulation
Blood lactate	Acidosis
Arterial blood gas	Acidosis and hypoxia (shock)

- Infection may also spread directly into the myometrium and the parametrium, giving rise to an endometritis or parametritis, also referred to as pelvic cellulitis. Pelvic peritonitis and abscesses may also occur.

- Infection may also spread to distant sites via lymphatics and blood vessels. Infection from the uterus can be carried by uterine vessels into the inferior vena cava via the iliac vessels or, directly, via the ovarian vessels. This could give rise to a septic thrombophlebitis, pulmonary infections or a generalized septicaemia and endotoxic shock.

Symptoms of puerperal pelvic infection

- Malaise, headache, fever, rigors.
- Abdominal discomfort, vomiting and diarrhoea.
- Offensive lochia.
- Secondary PPH.

Signs of puerperal pelvic infection

- Pyrexia and tachycardia.
- Uterus – boggy, tender and larger.
- Infected wounds – caesarean/perineal.
- Peritonism.
- Paralytic ileus.
- Indurated adnexae (parametritis).
- Bogginess in pelvis (abscess).

In contrast to pelvic inflammatory disease unrelated to pregnancy, tubal involvement in puerperal sepsis is in the form of perisalpingitis, which, rarely, causes tubal occlusion and consequent infertility. Tubo-ovarian abscesses are also a rare complication of puerperal sepsis.

Management

Mild to moderate infections can be treated with a broad-spectrum antibiotic (e.g. co-amoxiclav or a cephalosporin, such as cefalexin, plus metronidazole). Depending on the severity, the first few doses should be given intravenously.

With severe infections, there is a release of inflammatory and vasoactive mediators in response to the endotoxins produced during bacteriolysis. The resultant local vasodilatation causes circulatory embarrassment and hence poor tissue perfusion. This phenomenon is known as septicaemic, septic or endotoxic shock, and the features are shown in *Table 15.4*. Delay in appropriate management could be fatal and immediate high-dose, broad-spectrum antibiotics and resuscitation with intravenous fluids are provided on a high-dependency unit. Close liaison with microbiologists and internal medicine specialists is vital.

Necrotizing fasciitis is a rare but frequently fatal infection of skin, fascia and muscle. It can originate in perineal tears, episiotomies and caesarean section wounds. Perineal infections can extend rapidly to involve the buttocks, thighs and lower abdominal wall. A variety of bacteria can be involved, but anaerobes predominate and *Clostridium perfringens* is usually identified. In addition to general signs of infection, there is

Table 15.4 Clinical features of sepsis and severe sepsis

Sepsis	Severe sepsis
New onset of confusion or altered mental state	Systolic BP <90 mmHg (or >40 mmHg fall from baseline)
Temperature >38.3°C or <36°C	Oxygen saturations <91%
Heart rate >90 beats per minute	Heart rate >130 beats per minute
Respiratory rate >20 breaths per minute (counted over 60 seconds)	Respiratory rate >25 breaths per minute
Blood glucose >7.7 mmol/l in the absence of known diabetes	Responds only to voice or pain/unresponsive
White cell count >12 or <4 × 10⁹/l	Lactate >2.0 mmol/l (where available)

extensive necrosis, crepitus and inflammation. As well as the measures usually taken to manage septic shock, wide debridement of necrotic tissue under general anaesthesia is absolutely essential to avoid mortality. Split-thickness skin grafts may be necessary at a later date.

Psychiatric disorders

Although the incidence of mild mental health problems is not significantly different during pregnancy, the risk of bipolar or severe depressive illness is greatly increased postpartum and this period represents perhaps the highest risk period in a woman's life for the development of a psychiatric disorder. Furthermore, women with previous serious mental health problems are at high risk of a recurrence during both the antepartum and postpartum periods. A multidisciplinary approach, supervised by specialist perinatal mental health teams, is vital to optimize care, limit morbidity and help prevent the tragic cases of suicide detailed in the maternal mortality reports. The problems of substance and alcohol misuse during pregnancy overlap significantly with mental health issues, and coordination is required between specialist services and providers of maternity care.

The impact of psychiatric disease in pregnancy has been emphasized repeatedly by the UK Confidential Enquiries into Maternal Deaths. The most recent report, 'Saving Lives: Improving Mothers' Care', covers the period 2009–12. It reports on 111 deaths, 95 of which were 'late deaths' occurring between 6 weeks postnatally and 1 year. Suicide during pregnancy is unusually violent (shootings, hangings) in contrast with suicide attempts in younger women, which commonly take the form of overdose and are less frequently successful. This emphasizes the severity of mental health problems occurring after delivery, when most maternal suicides take place. The number of suicides has fallen since the last triennium and it is hoped that recommendations made in these reports are having a positive impact.

The pathophysiology of postpartum affective disorders

The importance of psychosocial factors in the aetiology of non-psychotic mild and moderate postpartum depressive illness is in contrast to the biological factors (e.g. family history) predisposing to puerperal psychosis and severe postpartum depressive illness.

The constancy of incidence across cultures and the temporal relationship with childbirth would tend to suggest a neuroendocrine basis for the more severe conditions. Changes in cortisol, oxytocin, endorphins, thyroxine, progesterone and oestrogen have all been implicated in the causation. Comparable dramatic changes in steroidal hormones outside the postpartum period have a well-known association with affective psychoses and mood disorders. A plausible recent theory is that the sudden fall in oestrogen postpartum triggers a hypersensitivity of certain dopamine receptors in a predisposed group of women and may be responsible for the severe mood disturbance that follows. The occurrence and the severity of the 'postnatal blues' are thought to be related to both the absolute level of progesterone and the relative drop from a prepartum level. However, there is no clear association between the 'postpartum blues' and affective psychoses, and no evidence as yet to implicate progesterone in the aetiology of puerperal psychosis or severe postnatal depression.

Depression is a characteristic feature of hypothyroidism, which may occur as a consequence of postpartum thyroiditis. The other features of hypothyroidism may be missed, and checking thyroid function is important in women with milder depressive symptoms in the first year following childbirth, as correction with thyroid supplements may elevate the mood.

Normal emotional and psychological changes during pregnancy

Diagnosing mental illness in pregnancy is complicated by the wide variety of 'normal' emotional and behavioural changes that may occur.

Postnatal

- The 'pinks': for the first 24–48 hours following delivery, it is very common for women to experience an elevation of mood, a feeling of excitement, some overactivity and difficulty sleeping.
- The 'blues': as many as 80% of women may experience the 'postnatal blues' in the first 2 weeks after delivery. Fatigue, short temper, difficulty sleeping, depressed mood and tearfulness are common but usually mild, and resolve spontaneously in the majority of cases. The following psychological disruptions should not be considered normal and require further assessment:
  - panic attacks;
  - episodes of low mood of prolonged duration (>2 weeks);
  - low self-esteem;
  - guilt or hopelessness;
  - thoughts of self-harm or suicide;
  - any mood changes that disrupt normal social functioning;
  - 'biological' symptoms (e.g. poor appetite, early wakening);
  - change in 'affect'.

Screening for mental health problems during and after pregnancy

The National Institute for Health and Care Excellence (NICE) Clinical Guideline No. 45 'Antenatal and Postnatal Mental Health' sets out screening questions that all postnatal women should be asked (*Table 15.5*). If the answers to these questions raise concerns, then the woman should be referred back to her GP, to her own psychiatrist, if she has one, or to a specialist perinatal mental health team depending on the severity of the symptoms or previous history.

Postpartum (non-psychotic) depressive illness

Between 10% and 15% of women will suffer with some form of depression in the first year after the delivery of their baby. At least 7% will satisfy the criteria for mild major depressive illness (see Symptom box) and many more could be described as having minor depression; 3–5% will suffer a severe major postnatal depressive episode. Without treatment, most women will recover spontaneously within 3–6 months; however, 1 in 10 will remain depressed at 1 year.

Women with a history of severe depression are at even higher risk. Those with a history of depression not related to pregnancy carry between a 1:3 and 1:5 risk of a major postpartum depressive illness, while the recurrence rate of postnatal depression is as high as 50%.

Clinical features

In contrast to puerperal psychosis, non-psychotic postpartum depression usually presents later in

Table 15.5 Screening questions for mental health during and after pregnancy

At booking, and in the postnatal period (at least twice):
During the past month, have you often felt down, depressed or hopeless?
During the past month, have you often been bothered by having little interest or pleasure in doing things?
Are these feelings something you need or want help with?

the postnatal period, most commonly around 6 weeks, with a more gradual onset. The 6-week postnatal check is an ideal opportunity to detect early postpartum non-psychotic depression, but the signs are often missed. The Edinburgh Postnatal Depression Scale is an example of a screening technique, but there are others. NICE recommends that all women are asked about their mood at least twice in the postpartum period by midwives, obstetricians, health visitors or GPs, ideally at 6 weeks and 3–4 months after the birth (*Table 15.5*). Particular attention should be paid to the assessment of women with risk factors for postnatal depressive illness. Indeed, women deemed at highest risk should be under close surveillance by a specialist community psychiatric nurse, with early admission to the local mother-and-baby unit if there are signs of concern.

Severe postnatal affective disorders usually present earlier than milder forms, and in this group, biological risk factors may be more important than psychosocial factors.

Treatment options include:

- Remedy of social factors.
- Non-directive counselling.
- Interpersonal psychotherapy.
- Cognitive–behavioural therapy.
- Drug therapy.

The earlier the onset of the depression and the more severe it becomes, the more likely it is that formal psychiatric intervention will be needed. However, randomized trials have demonstrated the benefits of non-directive counselling from specially trained midwives and health visitors in the management of milder disorders. Even simple encouragement to join a local postnatal group may prevent social isolation and limit depression.

If pharmacotherapy is deemed necessary, tricyclic antidepressants or selective serotonin reuptake inhibitors (SSRIs) are appropriate. There is good evidence to support the safety of the former in breastfeeding, less so for the latter. However, SSRIs in usual doses are probably safe.

There has been a vogue in the past for treating postnatal depression with progestogens in the erroneous belief that the fall in progesterone levels postpartum is the cause of postnatal depression. There is no good evidence to support this, and it may even be harmful if the use of other effective treatments is delayed because of it. This practice should therefore be avoided. High-dose oestrogen regimes have been tried in research trials, but these are not used routinely.

Women with a past history of severe postnatal depressive illness may be candidates for some form of prophylactic treatment, and the help of a specialist in perinatal mental health care should be sought before delivery.

Symptoms of severe postnatal depressive disorder

- Early-morning wakening.
- Poor appetite.
- Diurnal mood variation (worse in the mornings).
- Low energy and libido.
- Loss of enjoyment.
- Lack of interest.
- Impaired concentration.
- Tearfulness.
- Feelings of guilt and failure.
- Anxiety.
- Thoughts of self-harm/suicide.
- Thoughts of harm to the baby.

Adverse sequelae of postnatal depressive illness

Immediate
- Physical morbidity.
- Suicide/infanticide.
- Prolonged psychiatric morbidity.
- Damaged social attachment to infant.
- Disrupted emotional development of infant.

Later
- Social/cognitive effects on the child.
- Psychiatric morbidity in the child.
- Marital breakdown.
- Future mental health problems.

Puerperal psychosis

This very severe disorder affects between 1:500 and 1:1,000 women after delivery. It rarely presents before the 3rd postpartum day (most commonly the 5th), but usually does so before 4 weeks. The onset is characteristically abrupt, with a rapidly changing clinical picture.

Management

The patient should be referred urgently to a psychiatrist and will usually require admission to a psychiatric unit. If possible, this should be a mother-and-baby unit under the supervision of a specialist perinatal mental healthcare team. These units prevent separation of the baby from its mother and this may help with bonding and the future relationship.

Treatments include:

- Acute pharmacotherapy with neuroleptics, such as chlorpromazine or haloperidol.
- Treatment of mania with lithium carbonate.
- Electroconvulsive therapy, particularly for severe depressive psychoses.
- Antidepressants (which will take 10–14 days to be effective) as a second-line treatment.

Recovery usually occurs over 4–6 weeks, although treatment with antidepressants will be needed for at least 6 months. These women remain at high risk of pregnancy-related and non-pregnancy-related recurrences. The risk of recurrence in a future pregnancy is approximately 1 in 2, particularly if the next pregnancy occurs within 2 years of the one complicated by puerperal psychosis. Women with a previous history of puerperal psychosis should be considered for prophylactic lithium, started on the first postpartum day.

Anxiety disorders

Pregnancy, the anticipation of labour and the arrival of a new baby may all exacerbate an existing anxiety disorder. Cognitive–behavioural therapy may limit the need for drug treatment. Neonatal withdrawal effects are evident in the babies born to women who have used regular higher doses of benzodiazepines during pregnancy, and their use should be limited where possible. Breastfeeding may help to reduce the severity of the neonatal withdrawal (neonatal abstinence syndrome), as small amounts do reach breast milk.

The breasts and breastfeeding

Anatomy

The breasts are largely made up of glandular, adipose and connective tissue (**Figure 15.3**). They lie

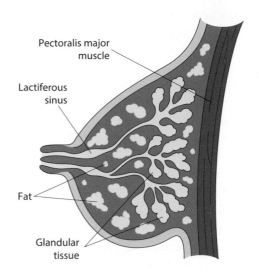

Pectoralis major muscle

Lactiferous sinus

Fat

Glandular tissue

Figure 15.3 The breast during lactation.

superficial to the pectoralis major, external oblique and serratus anterior muscles, extending between the second and sixth rib from the sternum to the axilla. A pigmented area called the areola, which contains sebaceous glands, surrounds the nipple. During pregnancy, the areola becomes darker and the sebaceous glands become prominent (Montgomery's tubercles). The breast is comprised of 15–25 functional units arranged radially from the nipple and each unit is made up of a lactiferous duct, a mammary gland lobule and alveoli. The lactiferous ducts dilate to form a lactiferous sinus before converging to open in the nipple. Contractile myoepithelial cells surround the ducts as well as the alveoli.

Physiology

The human species is unique in that most of the breast development occurs at puberty and is therefore primed to produce milk within 2 weeks of hormonal stimulation. The control of mammary growth and development is not fully understood and many hormones may contribute to this process. In general, oestrogens stimulate proliferation of the lactiferous ducts (possibly with adrenal steroids and growth hormones), while progesterone is responsible for the development of the mammary lobules. During early pregnancy, lactiferous ducts and alveoli proliferate, while in later pregnancy the alveoli hypertrophy in preparation for

secretory activity. The lactogenic hormones prolactin and human placental lactogen probably modulate these changes during pregnancy.

Colostrum

Colostrum is a yellowish fluid secreted by the breast that can be expressed as early as the 16th week of pregnancy, but is replaced by milk during the second postpartum day. Colostrum has a high concentration of proteins but contains less sugar and fat than breast milk, although it contains large fat globules. The proteins are mainly in the form of globulins, particularly immunoglobulin (Ig) A, which plays an important role in protection against infection. Colostrum is also believed to have a laxative effect, which may help empty the baby's bowel of meconium.

Breast milk

The major constituents of breast milk are lactose, protein, fat and water. However, the composition of breast milk is not constant; early lactation differs from late lactation, one feed differs from the next, and the composition can even change during a feed. Compared to cow's milk, breast milk provides slightly more energy, has less protein but more fat and lactose (*Table 15.6*). The major protein fractions are lactalbumin, lactoglobulin and caseinogen. Lactalbumin is the major protein in breast milk, whereas caseinogen forms 90% of the protein in cow's milk. The mineral content (particularly sodium) is much higher in cow's milk, which can therefore be dangerous if given to a baby who is dehydrated from gastroenteritis.

Table 15.6 Comparison between human and cow's milk

	Human breast milk	Cow's milk
Energy (kcal/ml)	75	66
Lactose (g/100 ml)	6.8	4.9
Protein (g/100 ml)	1.1	3.5
Fat (g/100 ml)	4.5	3.7
Sodium (mmol/l)	7	22
Water (ml/100 ml)	87.1	87.3

In addition to IgA, breast milk contains small amounts of IgM and IgG and other factors such as lactoferrin, macrophages, complement and lysozymes. Although breast milk contains a lower concentration of iron, its absorption is better than from cow's milk or iron-supplemented infant formula (75%, 30% and 10%, respectively). The improved bioavailability may be related to lactoferrin, an iron-binding glycoprotein, which also inhibits bacterial growth. With the exception of vitamin K, all other vitamins are found in breast milk and therefore vitamin K is given to the baby to minimize the risk of haemorrhagic disease (see Chapter 16, The neonate).

Prolactin

Prolactin is a long-chain polypeptide produced from the anterior pituitary; levels rise up to 20-fold during pregnancy and lactation. Peak levels of prolactin are reached within 45 minutes of suckling, but return to normal immediately after weaning and in non-breastfeeding mothers. The exact mechanism of action is not fully understood, but prolactin appears to have a direct action on the secretory cells to synthesize milk proteins. Prolactin is essential for lactation and it is hypothesized that nipple stimulation prevents the release of prolactin-inhibiting factor from the hypothalamus, thereby initiating the production of prolactin by the anterior pituitary. This theory is supported by the fact that lactation can be arrested with bromocriptine, a dopamine agonist that inhibits prolactin. A similar phenomenon occurs following pituitary necrosis (Sheehan's syndrome) when prolactin production ceases.

Oxytocin

Once milk has been produced under the influence of prolactin, it has to be delivered to the infant. The milk-ejection or let-down reflex is initiated by suckling, which stimulates the pulsatile release of oxytocin from the posterior pituitary. Oxytocin contracts the myoepithelial cells surrounding the alveoli, as well as the myoepithelial cells lying longitudinally along the lactiferous ducts, thereby aiding the expulsion of milk. Oxytocin release can also be stimulated by visual, olfactory or auditory stimuli (e.g. hearing the baby cry), but can be inhibited by stress. Oxytocin can also stimulate uterine contractions, giving rise to the 'afterpains' of childbirth.

Breastfeeding

Women who opt to breastfeed tend to decide before or very early in their pregnancy. This decision is usually based on previous experience, influence of family or friends, culture and custom. A new mother who is unprepared for breastfeeding may find it a frustrating task and turn to bottlefeeding. There is now evidence to suggest that antenatal classes and literature on breastfeeding given antenatally may be beneficial.

The most common reasons mothers give for abandoning breastfeeding are inadequate milk production and sore and cracked nipples. Both these problems can be overcome by correct positioning of the baby on the breast (**Figure 15.4**). The mouth

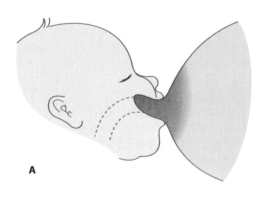

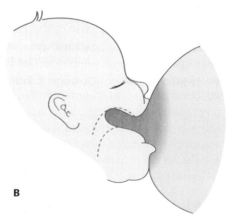

Figure 15.4 **(A)** Poor positioning for breastfeeding; **(B)** good positioning.

should be placed over the nipple and areola so that suction created within the baby's mouth draws the breast tissue into a teat that extends as far back as the junction of the soft and hard palate. The tongue applies peristaltic force to the underside of the teat against the support of the hard palate. In this way, there should be no to-and-fro movement of the teat in and out of the baby's mouth, thus minimizing friction. The mother should also be taught how to implement the rooting reflex. When the skin around the baby's mouth is touched, the mouth begins to gape. At this point, the mother should reposition the baby so that the lower rim of the baby's mouth fits well below the nipple, allowing a liberal mouthful of breast tissue. When the baby is properly attached, breastfeeding should be pain free. The use of creams and ointments for cracked nipples has not been shown to be beneficial and the use of a nipple shield merely reduces milk production.

Although no study has identified the threshold of the critical time limit for successful breastfeeding, early suckling appears to be beneficial. However, this should not be rushed, and perhaps should be done initially under supervision when the mother is comfortable and in privacy.

There is no scientific evidence to justify a rigid breastfeeding schedule. Babies should be fed on demand and left on the breast until feeding finishes spontaneously. An imposed time limit on feeding can have a deleterious effect on calorie intake.

Supplementary feeds of formula, glucose or water are sometimes given to breastfed infants in the mistaken belief that the baby is still hungry or thirsty. This should be discouraged as it increases the risk of total abandonment of breastfeeding.

Test-weighing infants before and after a feed to establish the quantity of milk intake has no role in healthy babies but is sometimes used by specialists to explore the reasons for poor weight gain.

When treating a breastfeeding woman, care needs to be taken to avoid drugs that can be passed onto the baby through the breast milk (*Table 15.7*).

Table 15.7 The use of common drugs in breastfeeding mothers

Breastfeeding contraindicated	Aspirin (at doses of 300 mg or more) Amiodarone Lithium Anticancer drugs (antimetabolites) Radioactive substances (stop breastfeeding temporarily)
Continue breastfeeding	
Neonatal side-effects possible (monitor baby closely)	Benzodiazepines (e.g. diazepam), psychiatric drugs and anticonvulsants Carbimazole
Use alternative drug if possible	Chloramphenicol, tetracyclines, metronidazole quinolone antibiotics (e.g. ciprofloxacin)
Monitor baby for jaundice	Sulfonamides, dapsone, sulfamethoxazole/trimethoprim (cotrimoxazole), sulfadoxine/pyrimethamine
Use alternative drug (may inhibit lactation)	Oestrogens, including oestrogen-containing contraceptives, thiazide diuretics, ergometrine
Safe in usual dosage (monitor baby)	Most commonly used drugs: analgesics and antipyretics: short courses of paracetamol, low-dose aspirin, ibuprofen; occasional doses of morphine and pethidine Antibiotics: ampicillin, amoxicillin, cloxacillin and other penicillins, erythromycin Antituberculosis drugs, antileprosy drugs (see dapsone above) Antimalarials (except mefloquine, sulfadoxine/pyrimethamine), anthelminthics, antifungals Bronchodilators (e.g. salbutamol), corticosteroids, antihistamines, antacids, drugs for diabetes, most antihypertensives, digoxin Nutritional supplements of iodine, iron, vitamins

Advantages of breastfeeding

- Readily available at the right temperature and ideal nutritional value.
- Cheaper than formula feed.
- Has a contraceptive effect with associated amenorrhoea.
- In the longer term it is associated with:
  - reduced necrotizing enterocolitis in preterm babies;
  - reduced childhood infective illnesses, especially gastroenteritis;
  - reduced atopic illnesses (e.g. eczema and asthma);
  - reduced juvenile diabetes;
  - reduced childhood cancer, especially lymphoma;
  - reduced premenopausal breast cancer.

Non-breastfeeding mothers

There are various reasons why a woman may not breastfeed, ranging from a choice based on personal preference to the tragedy of a stillbirth. Previously, all women infected with HIV were discouraged from breastfeeding due to the presence of the HIV virus in breast milk. However, it is now clear that the highest risk of mother to child transmission is from mixed breast and bottle feeding. Furthermore, in resource-poor settings, child mortality is increased by not breastfeeding. Therefore, while HIV-positive women in resource-rich settings are advised not to breastfeed, the World Health Organization recommends that women in low-resource settings take antiretroviral medication and exclusively breastfeed.

Non-breastfeeding mothers may suffer considerable engorgement and breast pain. Dopamine receptor stimulants, such as bromocriptine and cabergoline, inhibit prolactin and thus suppress lactation. However, both commonly cause drowsiness, hypotension, headache and gastrointestinal side-effects. Furthermore, fluid restriction and a tight brassiere have been shown to be as effective as bromocriptine usage by the second week and therefore this is the method of choice for the suppression of lactation.

Breast disorders

Blood-stained nipple discharge

Blood-stained nipple discharge of pregnancy ('rusty pipe syndrome') is typically bilateral and believed to be due to epithelial proliferation. It usually occurs in late pregnancy or early breastfeeding and lasts for up to 1 week. As the condition is self-limiting, no investigation or treatment is necessary, and the woman should be reassured.

Painful nipples

Nipples become very sensitive during late pregnancy and in the first week of breastfeeding. 'Sensitive nipples' can cause marked discomfort during the first minute of breastfeeding, but it settles spontaneously. 'Painful nipples', however, occur after the first week of feeding and worsen during feeds. A common cause of this is cracked nipples (small fissures in the nipple) and this is associated with an increased risk of breast abscess. The cause is usually poor positioning of the baby on the breast, although thrush (candidiasis) may also cause soreness. The treatment is to correct the underlying problem, but may also require local antibiotic ointment, analgesics, or even resting the affected nipple. The milk can be expressed during this time and the breastfeeding restarted once the nipples have healed.

Galactocele

A galactocele (or lactocele) is a sterile, milk-filled retention cyst of the mammary ducts following blockage by thickened secretions. It is identified as a fluctuant swelling with minimal pain and inflammation. It usually resolves spontaneously assisted by massage of the breast towards the nipple, but may also be aspirated; with increasing discomfort, surgical excision may become necessary.

Breast engorgement

Engorgement of the breasts usually begins by the second or third postpartum day and if breastfeeding has not been effectively established, the overdistended and engorged breasts can be very uncomfortable. Breast engorgement results in a puerperal fever of up to 39°C in around 15% of women. Although the fever rarely lasts more than 16 hours, other infective causes must be excluded. A number of remedies for the treatment of breast engorgement, such as manual expression, firm support, cabbage leaves, ice bags and electric breast pumps, have all been recommended in the past, but allowing the baby easy access to the breast is the most effective method of treatment and prevention.

Mastitis

Inflammation of the breast is not always due to an infective process. Mastitis is commonly related to breastfeeding problems, and occurs when a blocked duct obstructs the flow of milk and distends the alveoli. If this pressure persists, the milk extravasates into the perilobular tissue, initiating an inflammatory process. The affected segment of the breast is painful and appears red and oedematous. The woman also experiences flu-like symptoms with a tachycardia and pyrexia. In contrast to breast engorgement, the pyrexia with infective mastitis develops later (typically third to fourth postpartum week) and persists for longer. The most common infecting organism is *S. aureus*, which is found in 40% of women with mastitis.

Other bacteria include coagulase-negative staphylococci and *Streptococcus viridans*. Early localized mastitis can be managed with massage of the breast (towards the nipple) and analgesia. If the mastitis worsens, then a sample of the milk should be taken for microbiological culture and flucloxacillin commenced while awaiting sensitivity results. Breastfeeding should be continued during this process. About 10% of women with mastitis develop a breast abscess (diagnosed using ultrasound). Treatment is by a radial surgical incision and drainage under general anaesthesia.

Contraception

The exact mechanism of lactational amenorrhoea is poorly understood, but the most plausible hypothesis is that during lactation there is inhibition of the normal pulsatile release of luteinizing hormone from the anterior pituitary. Breastfeeding therefore provides a contraceptive effect, but it is not totally reliable, as up to 10% of women conceive while breastfeeding. However, it has recently been shown that a mother who is still in the phase of postpartum amenorrhoea while fully breastfeeding her baby has a less than 2% chance of conceiving in the first 6 months. Although this is comparable to some other forms of contraception (see *Gynaecology by 10 Teachers*, 20th edition, Chapter 6), most women in developed countries use some sort of additional contraception, such as barrier methods. If an intrauterine contraceptive device is preferred, it is best to wait for 4–8 weeks to allow for involution. Care needs to be exercised during insertion as there have been reports of increased rates of uterine perforation in breastfeeding mothers. The combined oral contraceptive pill enhances the risk of thrombosis in the early puerperium and can have an adverse effect on the quality and constituents of breast milk. The progesterone-only pill (the minipill) is therefore preferable and should be commenced about day 21 following delivery. If done before this, there may be puerperal breakthrough bleeding. Injectable contraception, such as depot medroxyprogesterone acetate (Depo-Provera™) given 3-monthly or norethisterone enantate (Noristerat™) given 2-monthly, is also very effective. Injectable contraception can be given within 48 hours of delivery for convenience, but it can cause breakthrough bleeding and therefore should preferably be given 5–6 weeks postpartum.

Sterilization can be offered to mothers who are certain that they have completed their family. Tubal ligation can be performed during caesarean section or by the open method (mini-laparotomy) in the first few postpartum days. However, it is better delayed until after 6 weeks postpartum, when it can be done by laparoscopy. This allows the mother to spend more time in comfort with her newborn baby and, furthermore, laparoscopic clip sterilization is less traumatic and associated with a lower failure rate.

Women who are not breastfeeding should commence the pill 3 weeks after delivery, as ovulation can occur by 4–6 weeks postpartum.

Perinatal death

- Stillbirth: a baby born with no signs of life.
- Perinatal death: stillbirth >24 weeks gestation or death within 7 days of birth.
- Live birth: any baby that shows signs of life irrespective of gestation.

Bereavement counselling following perinatal death requires special expertise and is best left to a senior clinician and a trained bereavement counsellor. Inappropriate management of this traumatic period can have a devastating effect on the woman's emotional and marital life. Effective communication and support are crucial and women should be encouraged to make

Table 15.8 Investigation into perinatal death

Investigations	Reason
Full blood count	Anaemia, leukocytosis
Clotting screen	Disseminated intravascular coagulation
Liver function tests and bile acids	Obstetric cholestasis
Kleihauer test	Fetomaternal transfusion
Virology, infection screen	Cytomegalovirus, parvovirus
Autoantibody screen (anticardiolipin and lupus anticoagulant)	Antiphospholipid syndrome, systemic lupus erythematosus
Placental swab for culture	Infections such as *Listeria monocytogenes*
Blood group antibodies	Haemolytic disease
Toxoplasma antibodies	Toxoplasmosis
HBA1c	Undiagnosed diabetes
Placental pathology	Evidence of infection or vasculopathy
Cytology of placenta	Fetal chromosomal abnormality
Skin biopsy/cardiac blood/placental biopsy	Fetal chromosome abnormalities
Full-body X-ray or MRI	To identify congenital defects

HBA1c, glycosated haemoglobin; MRI, magnetic resonance imaging.

contact with organizations, such as SANDS (Stillbirth and Neonatal Death Society).

The grieving process can be facilitated by practices such as seeing and holding the dead baby, naming the baby and taking hand/foot prints and photographs. Coming to terms with the perinatal death of a twin is even more difficult because the mother has to mourn one baby and celebrate the arrival of the other.

A postmortem is the most important diagnostic test, even though there may be no positive findings. Couples who decline a postmortem may do so because of religious reasons or because they fear mutilation. In this situation, a partial postmortem should be discussed whereby an autopsy of a single organ or a tissue biopsy can be performed. A full-body X-ray or, preferably, magnetic resonance imaging may be useful in some cases (*Table 15.8*).

If the baby was stillborn, a stillbirth certificate should be completed by the attending doctor; otherwise, the paediatrician should complete the certificate. The certificate should be given to the parents to register the death with the Registrar of Births and Deaths. Funeral arrangements can be made privately or by the hospital.

Every mother who has lost a baby should have the 6-week postnatal visit at hospital to discuss the underlying cause and to plan for the future.

 KEY LEARNING POINTS

- The puerperium refers to the 6-week period following childbirth.
- Care during this transition period is crucial as the woman returns to her prepregnant state.
- Perineal discomfort is a major complaint following vaginal delivery and therefore adequate analgesia should be prescribed.
- All women should be screened for depression at least twice in the postpartum period.
- Common disorders include puerperal sepsis, thromboembolism, bowel and bladder dysfunction.

Further reading

Knight M, Kenyon S, Brocklehurst P, Neilson J, Shakespeare J, Kurinczuk JJ (eds.) on behalf of MBRRACE- UK. Saving Lives, Improving Mothers' Care - Lessons learned to inform future ma-ternity care from the UK and Ireland Confidential Enquiries into Maternal Deaths and Morbidity 2009–12. Oxford: National Perinatal Epidemiology Unit, University of Oxford 2014.

National Institute for Health and Care Excellence. NICE Guideline CG37: Postnatal Care. NICE 2014.

World Health Organization. WHO recommendations on postnatal care of the mother and new-born. WHO Press, WHO, Geneva 2014.

Self assessment

CASE HISTORY 1

An 18-year-old woman with a body mass index of 35 who had a forceps delivery after a prolonged second stage of labour 10 days previously presented with heavy, fresh vaginal bleeding and clots. She felt unwell and complained of abdominal cramps. On examination she had a temperature of 38.2°C and there was mild suprapubic tenderness. Vaginal examination revealed blood clots, but no products of conception. The cervix admitted one finger and the uterus was tender and measured 16 weeks in size. A review of the delivery notes revealed that the placenta was delivered complete, but the membranes were noted to be ragged.

A What is the most likely diagnosis?
B What are the key features that suggest retained products of conception?
C How should the patient be managed?

ANSWER

A Secondary PPH due to infected retained products of conception.
B Secondary postpartum haemorrhage. Enlarged uterus. Open cervical os.
C Blood cultures. Intravenous broad-spectrum antibiotics (e.g. cephalosporin and metronidazole). Surgical evacuation of the retained products.

CASE HISTORY 2

A recent Eastern European immigrant to the UK, with minimal English, was seen by her GP at 12 weeks' gestation. The only history of note was that her father had suffered a long-standing psychiatric illness that the woman believed to be 'schizophrenia'. He had died when she was young in a road traffic accident. Her pregnancy proceeded without complication, and she went home on the second postnatal day following a normal delivery at term.

Within a couple of weeks, her partner reported to the community midwife that he had concerns about her mood. She seemed agitated, fearful and unduly concerned about the wellbeing of the baby and refused any help offered by him. The GP saw her, without an interpreter, and diagnosed 'postnatal depression'. He commenced tricyclic antidepressants. However, 1 week later she became frankly delusional and believed that her partner was trying to kill the baby. She was hardly sleeping and eating very little, but was continuing to breastfeed her baby.

A What is the most likely diagnosis?
B How should this be managed?
C How should her breastfeeding be managed?
D In retrospect, how should the pregnancy have been managed?

ANSWER

A The most likely diagnosis is puerperal psychosis.
B She should be admitted to a regional mother-and-baby unit with her newborn where she can receive multidisciplinary care from the specialist medical, nursing and midwifery staff. The antidepressants should be stopped and she should be treated with antipsychotics (e.g. trifluoperazine).
C She should be encouraged to continue breastfeeding but the baby should be monitored for side-effects.
D Ideally, the woman should have been asked to explore the nature of her family history. This would have revealed that her father suffered from schizophrenia. If this had been known, then it could have prompted review by a specialist in perinatal mental health, leading to regular postnatal review by a community psychiatric nurse being organized. This might have led to earlier intervention and prevented her deterioration to such a severe state.

EMQ

A Tonsillitis.
B Chronic bronchitis.
C Atelectasis.
D Pneumonia.
E Cholecystitis.
F Pancreatitis.
G Tubo-ovarian abscess.

H Appendicitis.
I Chorioamnionitis.
J Endometritis.
K Infected retained products of conception.
L Pelvic abscess.
M Wound infection.
N Deep vein thrombosis.

For each description, choose the SINGLE most appropriate answer for the cause of the pyrexia from the list of options. Each option may be used once, more than once or not at all.

1 A 38-year-old woman had ruptured membranes at 28 weeks' gestation. She was given a 10-day course of prophylactic antibiotics, and monitored as an inpatient. At 32 weeks' gestation her white cell count and C-reactive protein levels rose, and she went into spontaneous labour. When 6 cm dilated in active labour, she spikes a temperature of 39°C and has a soft, tender uterus.

2 A severely overweight 18-year-old is induced for pre-eclampsia at 36 weeks, but ends up with an emergency caesarean section for 'failure to progress'. She is given prophylactic antibiotics at the time of the caesarean, and is discharged home 2 days later feeling well. 10 days later her midwife admits her from home with a grumbling low-grade pyrexia of 37–37.5°C. She has no chest symptoms and her uterus is palpable just above the pelvic brim. Both legs remain markedly swollen, but the left calf is also tender.

3 A 24-year-old smoker with no medical history of note is 5 days after the normal delivery of her third child. She develops central abdominal pain, anorexia, nausea and a pyrexia of 38°C.

On admission to hospital for observation she remains intermittently pyrexial, but the pain has localized to the right iliac fossa. The uterus is firm and equivalent to a 14-week gestation size, and the lochia is normal. On palpation of the lower abdomen there is rebound tenderness in the right iliac fossa.

4 A 28-year-old smoker has a history of asthma for which she takes regular inhaled steroids. She labours spontaneously in her first pregnancy at term, but delivers by emergency caesarean section due to marked cardiotocograph abnormalities. A spinal anaesthetic is tried initially but is unsuccessful and she eventually has a general anaesthetic. She is admitted to the high dependency unit for postoperative care, and at 4 hours postoperatively you are called to see her. She has a pyrexia of 37.5°C and is noticeably short of breath. Her respiratory rate is 28 per minute and her oxygen saturation is low at 93%. On auscultation of her chest there are no wheezes, but fine inspiratory crepitations at both lung bases.

ANSWER

1I This is a classic case of chorioamnionitis. The prolonged rupture of membranes allows ascending infection into the uterus causing markers of infection and premature labour.

2N Deep vein thrombosis does not commonly present with a low-grade pyrexia, but 10 days postnatal is the classic time for development of thrombosis and this woman has multiple risk factors for it. Having swollen legs is common in the first few postnatal days but usually settles quickly with the physiological postpartum diuresis and would not usually still be present at 10 days postpartum. In overweight women who have undergone emergency caesarean, a high index of suspicion is needed for thrombosis as it is common and the signs may be masked by obesity.

3H Just because a woman is postnatal does not mean that she cannot get common non-obstetric surgical problems. The case describes the classic symptoms and signs of appendicitis. Postpartum genital tract infection is a differential diagnosis, but is usually bilateral and presents initially with offensive lochia.

4C This woman is at high risk of postoperative chest complications. Chest infections, however, tend to occur at day 1–2 rather than immediately postoperatively, and the lack of wheezes makes an exacerbation of asthma unlikely as a cause of her respiratory problems. This is a classic case of atelectasis and should respond to deep breathing exercises and vigorous physiotherapy of her lungs, aided by good analgesia.

SBA QUESTIONS

Choose the single best answer.

1 You are asked by a midwife to review an overweight 42-year-old woman 6 weeks after the birth of her third child. Her booking blood pressure was 145/85 mmHg, but it reduced during pregnancy and she went on to have a spontaneous labour and normal birth at term. Her blood pressure was again raised during labour with proteinuria (+), and she was treated with labetalol. Despite continuing this therapy postnatally, her blood pressure has continued to be raised, averaging 150/95 mmHg. What is the most likely cause of her raised blood pressure?

A   Pre-eclampsia.

B   Essential hypertension.

C   Cushing's disease.

D   Coarctation of the aorta.

E   Pregnancy-induced hypertension.

ANSWER

B   Blood pressure typically reduces during pregnancy and returns to its prepregnancy level at term. Those with essential hypertension therefore often have normal blood pressure in pregnancy, but are hypertensive postnatally. The risk of essential hypertension increases with age and weight. Pre-eclampsia does cause proteinuria, but classically occurs in the first pregnancy and, like pregnancy-induced hypertension, rarely persists more than 1 week postnatally. Cushings and coarctation can both cause hypertension, but are very rare.

2 A 24-year-old 'primip' is due to have a caesarean section because of placenta praevia and is planning to breastfeed. Prior to her operation, she asks your advice on effective contraception. Which of the following is appropriate advice?

A   She could start the combined oral contraceptive at 3 weeks postnatal.

B   An intrauterine device could be inserted at the time of the caesarian section.

C   No contraception is needed until she stops breastfeeding.

D   No contraception is needed until her periods return.

E   She could start the progesterone-only pill at 3 weeks postnatal.

ANSWER

E   Oral contraceptives should only be started at 6 weeks postnatal due to the thromboembolism risk and because they can affect breastfeeding. Breastfeeding is contraceptive, but is not a reliable method. Intrauterine devices are normally inserted at 6 weeks postnatal once the uterus has returned to its usual size.

LEARNING OBJECTIVES

- To understand and be able to describe the unique features of newborn babies and the transition to extrauterine life.
- For common neonatal problems be able to describe:
  - key features from an obstetric point of view;

  - urgent action in the delivery room or soon afterwards;
  - important messages for parents.
- To describe key points relevant to postnatal management that need to be communicated by professionals involved in antenatal care.

Introduction

Neonatology is the continuation of antenatal care. Many of the outcomes on neonatal units are determined or influenced by events before birth and it is important for obstetricians to know what happens to babies after they are born. More importantly, the transition from fetus to neonate occurs as a continuum for babies and their parents. Accordingly, postnatal care needs to be based on continuity and a shared understanding between professionals involved in the care of mother and baby.

This chapter is about babies and how they are looked after in hospital during the 7 days after birth. It will tell you what you need to know as an obstetrician to support families and colleagues on the neonatal unit. This chapter mainly focuses on neonatal conditions that are related to obstetric management or which benefit from close collaboration between maternity and neonatal teams. There is some information relevant to antenatal counselling about postnatal outcomes. This chapter does not cover routine care for healthy babies in detail.

Communication between antenatal and post-natal teams is very important. This communication occurs in several ways: between individual care-givers, through clinical records and through systems. Senior medical staff have an important role in ensuring that clinical notes and systems are fit for purpose, even if they are not directly involved in the care of every mother and baby. Each of these approaches to communication can fail, so all professionals have a duty to ensure that information that will influence the care of an individual baby is shared.

Neonatal anatomy and physiology

Newborn babies are not small adults, or even small children. After babies are born they go through a number of unique processes. Firstly, there is the physical transition to the extrauterine environment. This involves processes that change how the baby's body works before significant anatomical and physiological changes take effect. The main transition is the replacement of lung fluid with air. The next phase is anatomical and physiological adaptation of the baby's body to extrauterine life. Examples of anatomical/physiological adaptation include reduction in the pressure in the pulmonary arteries that allows increased blood flow in the lungs so that blood can become oxygenated and closure of the ductus arteriosus; and altering renal blood flow so that glomerular filtration increases. Then there is an adjustment phase during which the baby overcomes any problems that arose during transition and adaptation and resumes the developmental pathways that were present before birth. Finally, the babies grow. Each of these stages varies in duration according to gestational age. Some of these stages will be delayed or prolonged by inter-current illness, as described below.

Airway

Immediately after birth the airways can be blocked by mucus, by the position of the head and neck and by poor muscle tone. Simple manoeuvres can overcome these problems. The head is relatively large, the neck is short and the occiput is prominent. The larynx is anterior and high. The combination of these features means that the airway can be maintained using a neutral position (neonates do not need the 'sniffing the morning air position' used in airway management in older age groups).

Respiratory system

At birth the lungs are very stiff because they are filled with fluid. It is important to establish a functional residual capacity (FRC) (i.e. make sure that some air is left in the lungs after maximal expiration). Once that has been done it is important to maintain an end-expiratory pressure. Healthy babies do this by crying and deploying surfactant. Fetal lung fluid is usually cleared via lymphatics in the hours after birth.

Cardiovascular

The absence of placental blood flow leads to closure of the ductus venosus. There is an increase in blood flow to the lungs. During the week after birth there is a reduction in pulmonary vascular resistance. The ductus arteriosus gradually closes during the first week. In healthy term babies these processes are not apparent.

Some newborn babies become sick. This can be associated with delayed reduction of pulmonary vascular resistance, which can cause profound hypoxia. Persistent pulmonary hypertension is more likely if the baby is cold, acidotic, infected or suffering from meconium aspiration but it can happen for no apparent reason.

Metabolic

Glucose

The newborn baby needs to adapt from a continuous infusion of maternal glucose via the placenta to intermittent feeds. Healthy term babies can cope with gaps between feeds because they have enough stores and the endocrine milieu will mobilize the stores. Therefore, glucose concentrations are not measured in healthy babies born at term.

Things can go wrong for a number of reasons. If babies are at risk of not being able to cope with intermittent feeds they are screened by measuring blood glucose before feeds. This means that there is a need for clear communication about risk factors from the antenatal team to the postnatal team.

Prolonged neonatal hypoglycaemia damages the brain and is largely avoidable.

> **Reasons why babies are at risk of hypoglycaemia and the antenatal problems that are associated with these reasons**
>
> - Low stores of glycogen/fats: seen in fetal growth restriction (FGR), prematurity, perinatal asphyxia.
> - Inadequate hormonal responses to birth: seen in prematurity and FGR, and can be important if the baby's catecholamine response is suppressed by, for example, maternal consumption of beta-blockers.
> - Hyperinsulinism (infant of diabetic mother).
> - Feeding difficulties (preterm, FGR, asphyxia, infection).

Bilirubin

In the days after birth the production of bilirubin is more than the liver enzymes that render bilirubin water soluble and ready to eliminate can handle. This leads to an increase in the circulating concentrations of unconjugated bilirubin. This can show as jaundice and is a concern because very high concentrations of unconjugated bilirubin are neurotoxic. The liver enzymes are induced over the first 3–4 days after birth. Breastfed babies take longer to induce their enzymes but this does not cause harm.

Pathological jaundice is a sign of a departure from the expected adaptation. Visible jaundice within 24 hours of birth is pathological and is usually due to infection or haemolysis.

Conjugated bilirubin is not neurotoxic. High circulating concentrations of conjugated bilirubin reflect problems excreting bile. This can be due to an obstruction. In term babies this can relate to the rare but important condition of biliary atresia. In preterm babies, obstructive jaundice is often related to parenteral nutrition. In all age groups conjugated or prolonged jaundice has an extensive differential diagnosis that requires detailed evaluation.

Renal

Before birth there is low glomerular filtration and poor tubular function because the placenta eliminates the products of metabolism. Renal adaptation is similar to the lung in that there are shifts in renal blood flow during the week after birth that lead to increased renal function. This means that the dosage of drugs needs to be adjusted after the first few days as renal clearance increases. Occasionally, babies have high creatinine levels that may be related to maternal renal function. Preterm babies often have high creatinine levels in the first week after birth and this does not appear to increase their risk of long-term renal damage.

Infection

Infection is a major source of neonatal mortality and morbidity. Neonates are exposed to infective agents antenatally, during labour and postnatally. Neonates have different immune function when compared to older children and adults, including relatively lower effective bacterial killing due to immature function of neutrophils and complement.

Endocrine

The most common neonatal endocrine problem is maternal hypothyroidism, which can cause symptomatic neonatal hypothyroidism. Maternal hyperthyroidism (active or latent) due to Graves's disease can lead to neonatal hyperthyroidism. In most babies with a maternal history of abnormal thyroid function it is safe to observe for symptoms and check the baby's thyroid function several days after birth. Babies with symptoms of thyroid disorders are rare and need urgent attention from an experienced paediatric endocrinologist.

Weight loss

Newborn babies lose weight in the days after they are born. This reflects a loss of extracellular fluid. A rule of thumb is that healthy term babies can lose 10% of their birthweight and get back to their birthweight within 1 week. Deviations from these limits may indicate a pathology but exceeding these limits is not in itself diagnostic of a disease. Weight loss may be greater during the establishment of breastfeeding. This may rarely be associated with hypernatraemia. In the UK, this complication is rare and does not lead to long-term harm if babies who appear unwell or dehydrated during the establishment of breastfeeding are promptly admitted to hospital and treated.

Neonatal care

Principles of neonatal care

1 Keep families together whenever possible.
2 If separation is required to deliver care then optimize contact between mother (and father) and baby. Move to skin-to-skin care as quickly as possible.
3 Breast is best – all neonatal care must promote breastfeeding unless there is a contraindication to breastfeeding.
4 Keep babies at the right temperature. Preterm babies also need to be kept at the optimal humidity.
5 Communication is central:
   • from maternity team to neonatal team (we need good systems including documentation and sharing of risk factors for neonatal disease, daily meetings between Consultants/shift Leaders to coordinate work, regular contact between individuals);
   • between neonatal team and parents.
6 Good neonatal care is guideline-driven and based on the application of standardized principles. This allows optimization of care while taking account of individual circumstances. Even when the best pattern of care has not been defined rigorously, consistent care improves outcomes.
7 Support transition and adaptation to extrauterine life followed by growth and development while treating any intercurrent illnesses.

Neonatal care is carried out by a range of professionals. Much routine care is supervised by midwives. With the relevant training and support midwives are often responsible for the routine examination of the newborn (EON or baby check). On the neonatal unit nurses provide care, working with families. Some nurses have extended roles including intubation and prescribing. In many countries advanced neonatal nurse practitioners (ANNPs) play an important role. ANNPs diagnose, prescribe, conduct all clinical procedures and contribute to audit and research. You will also find doctors on a neonatal unit; many of them have less experience than nurses and ANNPs. Accordingly, it is important to treat all neonatal professionals with respect.

Common problems: term babies

In most term babies the process of transition, adaptation, adjustment and growth is clinically seamless, although it is often a stormy time for the parents. The process can go wrong if transition is interrupted (usually breathing problems) or adaptation is delayed (often due to cardiovascular problems). Adjustment can be complicated by delayed metabolic shifts (jaundice or hypoglycaemia) or by consequences of antenatal events (meconium aspiration/encephalopathy). Intercurrent illnesses include infection.

Management at birth

• Stabilize the baby using a well-defined approach, such as Neonatal Life Support (Further reading).
• Use age-specific oxygen saturation targets bearing in mind that too much oxygen may be harmful.
• Keep the baby warm by keeping the birth room at a suitable temperature. Premature babies should not be dried but need to be placed in a plastic bag immediately after birth in order to avoid loss of heat and water.

Poor condition at birth

Poor condition at birth can be caused by a number of processes. Most of the time these are self-limiting or benefit from simple interventions. Condition at birth is conventionally assessed using the Apgar score. This is a mnemonic for assessment that has minimal predictive value.

The approach to a baby in poor condition at birth is consistent: follow standardized procedures for neonatal life support. It is important to keep skills up to date. Newborn life support cannot be taught in a book. Go on a course.

Breathing difficulties

Most initial problems with breathing are caused by obstruction of the airway that can be corrected by good positioning. In a newborn baby the airway needs a 'neutral' position (i.e. no flexion and no extension of the neck). This is different from the position advised in adults. Secretions may be a problem but be aware that excessive suctioning can cause bradycardia. Breathing difficulties that persist despite initial supportive care may be due to surfactant deficiency, transient tachypnoea of the newborn, meconium aspiration or infection.

Surfactant deficient lung disease (SDLD) is rare in term babies, but can occur. It is more common in the infants of insulin-dependent diabetic mothers. As discussed below, SDLD is managed with supplementary oxygen, ventilatory support and the administration of surfactant. The chest X-ray shows evidence of alveolar fluid with a ground-glass appearance or air bronchograms.

Transient tachypnoea of the newborn (TTN) is found in 5/1,000 live births and is characterized by a high respiratory rate and requirement for some supplementary oxygen (usually less than 40%). The condition gradually resolves over 1–3 days. This condition is thought to be caused by the persistence of fetal lung fluid. TTN is more common after caesarean section in the absence of labour. TTN is treated conservatively with supplementary oxygen as required. Oral or enteral feeds may need to be suspended because increased work of breathing makes feeding more difficult. If breastfeeding is ever suspended because of neonatal problems it is essential to support the mother to express her breast milk. In TTN the chest X-ray is relatively clear and can show perihilar shadowing and fluid in the lateral fissure.

Meconium aspiration syndrome is a chemical pneumonitis. Clinically significant meconium aspiration occurs before birth. The condition gets worse over 24–48 hours and then gradually improves. Clinically relevant meconium aspiration requires mechanical ventilation. Babies with meconium aspiration may benefit from surfactant. Extracorporeal membrane oxygenation is an option if babies are not responding to optimal medical care, including supplementary surfactant, high frequency oscillation and treatment for pulmonary hypertension. Suction on the perineum is no help. The damage is done before the first breath. Babies only require inspection of the vocal cords if they have respiratory difficulties.

None of these conditions can be reliably differentiated from infection. All babies with significant respiratory distress at birth need to be treated with antibiotics until infection can be ruled out.

Suspected bacterial infection

In newborn babies a number of risk factors and signs of infection can be seen. The problem is that these signs are common and are not specific while proven infection is devastating but rare.

The solution to this problem is to treat suspected infection promptly with a low index of suspicion. Aggressive treatment is continued if there is an infection or if clinical condition is poor. Treatment is stopped promptly if there is no evidence of infection. For example, treatment for suspected infection can be stopped after 36 hours if the baby is well, blood cultures are negative and two measurements of C-reactive protein (CRP) are less than 10 mg/l.

Early

The incidence of proven early onset neonatal infection is 2–4 per 1,000 live births. Around 1 in 10 neonates are treated with antibiotics for suspected early-onset neonatal infection. Most of these courses of antibiotics are stopped within 48 hours. Early-onset neonatal infection is caused by a limited range of bacteria. A baby may be well at birth and gradually deteriorate in the hours after birth. Sometimes the baby is acutely unwell at birth and the course is fulminant, requiring multiorgan support in intensive care.

The most common gram-positive cause of early-onset neonatal infection in the UK is group B streptococcus (GBS, *Streptococcus agalactiae*). Invasive GBS illness is severe. As described in Chapter 11, Perinatal infections, this bacteria is part of the intestinal flora for many people. About 20% of the population carry GBS in their stool at any one time, including pregnant women. Women colonized with GBS are at increased risk of having a baby with invasive GBS. For this reason, women are screened for GBS carriage, either universally or in a targeted manner. Evidence of GBS colonization triggers intrapartum antibiotic prophylaxis (IAP), which reduces the incidence of invasive GBS disease. GBS is susceptible to benzyl penicillin, therefore benzyl penicillin is a useful agent for IAP and treatment. A treatment course for proven GBS infection is at least 7 days.

Other gram-positive causes of early-onset neonatal infection are *Staphylococcus aureus* and group A streptococcus.

A common cause of gram-negative early-onset neonatal infection is *Escherichia coli*. As in other age groups, *E. coli* can cause a life-threatening systemic infection requiring full intensive care. Antimicrobial susceptibility varies with the local prevalence of antimicrobial resistance. Given the vertical pattern of infection, resistance patterns will vary with patterns of community resistance. In the UK, gentamicin is used for the initial treatment of *E. coli* (and other gram-negative bacteria).

Haemophilus influenzae is an occasional cause of early-onset neonatal infection due to vertical transmission. This is due to non-capsulate, non-serotypable forms that are not covered by the routine immunization against *H. influenza b*. This is treated with cefotaxime.

Late

Some late-onset neonatal infection occurs at home, in which case the babies will have community acquired bacteria rather than hospital ones.

Neonatal meningitis

Early or late neonatal infection can be associated with meningitis, which is often associated with a poor outcome in childhood. Meningitis may not have clinical signs so neonatologists have a low threshold for performing a lumbar puncture.

Syphilis

Babies born to women with positive treponemal serology need clinical evaluation and syphilis serology testing unless there is definitive proof of maternal biological false-positive serology or cure.

In the UK congenital syphilis is rare. It affects around 10 babies a year, usually among women presenting to maternity services in the third trimester with backgrounds of socioeconomic deprivation and chaotic lifestyles. The diagnosis of congenital syphilis is difficult so maternity staff need to work closely with paediatricians, genitourinary medicine specialists and paediatric infectious disease specialists.

Babies are treated if congenital syphilis is suspected or maternal treatment is within 4 weeks of birth or incomplete. The usual treatment is intravenous benzyl penicillin for 2 weeks or more.

Viral infections

Herpes simplex

Neonatal herpes simplex virus (HSV) infection is often fatal (20%) and leads to significant disability among survivors (>60%). Neonatal HSV is usually vertically transmitted. If an active, maternal primary infection is underway at the time of birth the baby has a 50% risk of developing systemic herpes. If a recurrence of genital herpes is underway at the time of birth the risk of neonatal herpes is much lower (<5%). Thus it is very important to notify the neonatal team if a mother has evidence of genital herpes and to provide as much information as possible about the clinical history and diagnosis. Caesarean section is an effective way to reduce the incidence of infection among women known to have primary genital herpes.

Neonatal HSV infection presents in three ways: localized, central nervous system (CNS) and disseminated. The localized form is relatively benign but the neurological and disseminated manifestations of neonatal HSV are severe illnesses often requiring extensive intensive care. The treatment is intravenous aciclovir.

Varicella zoster

Neonatal varicella occurs in the babies of mothers who develop chicken pox. If the baby is born more than 5 days after the mother develops the rash, then transplacental antibodies provide some protection and the illness is not severe. If the baby is born fewer than 5 days after the mother develops the rash, then the baby is not protected and can develop a severe infection complicated by pneumonitis.

The severity of neonatal varicella can be reduced if the baby receives zoster immunoglobulin (ZIG) as soon after birth as possible.

Babies of women who develop chicken pox 7 days before or 7 days after birth should receive ZIG. If a woman has shingles, then the baby is protected from infection with varicella zoster virus by maternal antibodies; mother and baby can stay together.

Human immunodeficiency virus

The management of babies born to mothers with human immunodeficiency virus (HIV) is well described in national guidelines. The principles are that each woman needs an individualized care plan that reflects her risk status and is drawn up by a multidisciplinary team.

UK guidance is that babies born to women with a low viral load (<50 HIV ribonucleic acid [RNA] copies/ml plasma) should receive monotherapy with zidovudine for 4 weeks.

If a woman has >50 HIV RNA copies/ml plasma or maternal HIV is diagnosed within 3 days of birth, combination postexposure prophylaxis with three agents should be started under expert supervision.

With appropriate postexposure prophylaxis less than 1% of babies born to HIV-positive mothers will be infected. In the absence of postexposure prophylaxis, 15% of babies born to HIV-positive mothers became infected in a UK cohort study.

Cytomegalovirus

Symptomatic congenital cytomegalovirus (CMV) causes learning disabilities or sensorineural hearing loss. Congenital CMV can be treated with ganciclovir intravenously for 6 weeks. This reduces the severity of CNS damage and hearing loss.

Jaundice

The management of neonatal jaundice involves strong overlap between maternity and neonatal services. Antenatal information about conditions that lead to jaundice is invaluable for starting treatment promptly. Postnatal management can usually be conducted on the postnatal wards, keeping mother with baby.

The management of neonatal jaundice involves well-established pathways that include escalations of therapy guided by bilirubin measurements. Treatment of jaundice is based on phototherapy, which uses light in the visible spectrum to conduct a photoisomerization of toxic bilirubin to safe isomers, some of which are excreted rapidly. The key to successful phototherapy is to expose the baby to the phototherapy. If overhead lights are used, then the eyes should be protected. Phototherapy can be interrupted for breastfeeding unless there is a high likelihood of exchange transfusion.

If phototherapy does not prevent the concentrations of bilirubin from climbing to levels associated with brain injury, then exchange transfusion is performed. Exchange transfusion involves withdrawing a small aliquot of blood from the baby and replacing it with a small aliquot of cross-matched blood. This is repeated every 5 minutes over 4 hours. The aim is to replace twice the baby's circulating volume (130 ml/kg). If there is evidence of active alloimmune disease (e.g. rhesus or ABO incompatibility) on direct antiglobulin testing (DAT), then

immunoglobulin (Ig) during phototherapy can reduce the need for exchange transfusion.

Causes of neonatal jaundice include abnormalities of red cell enzymes or morphology, extravasated blood (e.g. cephalohaematoma), increased enterohepatic circulation and endocrine conditions such as hypothyroidism. Appropriate investigations are undertaken if the clinical course suggests they are needed.

Hypoglycaemia

As noted above some babies become hypoglycaemic and some of them become symptomatic. Most of these have risk factors. The solution is to monitor blood glucose in babies with risk factors. Prefeed glucose is the important measurement. Postfeed measurements have limited value because of inconsistencies in absorption. Severe or symptomatic hypoglycaemia can cause brain damage so is an emergency requiring intravenous glucose.

It is standard practice in neonates to check the blood sugar in any unwell baby.

Seizures

Seizures are relatively common in the newborn period, affecting 1–2 per 1,000 livebirths. Hypoxic-ischaemic encephalopathy is the most common cause of neonatal seizures, causing about half of neonatal seizures. However, there is a broad differential. Other causes of neonatal seizures include: cerebral infarction (stroke); intracranial haemorrhage (intraventricular haemorrhage and subdurals); meningitis; electrolyte disturbances (hypocalcaemia, hypomagnesemia); and hypoglycaemia.

The assessment of neonatal seizures is based on description followed by interpretation. Neonates have specific patterns of seizures, including tonic, clonic, subtle and myoclonic. Tonic–clonic seizures are rare in neonates. Clinical observation is not reliable. Ideally electroencephalography (EEG) or cerebral function monitoring (CFM) is used. Other features such as autonomic changes (respiratory rate, blood pressure, oxygen saturations) are also important features of seizures. Jitters are not seizures. Jitters affect up to half of babies. Jitters involve repeated movements at 1–3 Hz, typically on stimulation. Jitters can be restrained in contrast to seizures.

Investigations are directed towards finding the cause of the seizures and looking for prognosis. Brain magnetic resonance imaging (MRI) is the first-line imaging modality.

The evidence base for the treatment of neonatal seizures is minimal. Conventional therapy involves phenobarbital. Supplementary agents include midazolam, levetiracetam, phenytoin and sodium valproate.

The prognosis of neonatal seizures depends on the cause. Overall, about one-half of children with neonatal seizures will have neurodevelopmental abnormalities. The proportion is much higher if there is cerebral dysgenesis. Ten to 20% of children with neonatal seizures have seizures in later life (this proportion will be higher if there is a brain malformation).

The rate of neonatal seizures is sometimes suggested as a marker of the quality of perinatal care. This suggestion may have some value when examining large differences in quality. When high-quality perinatal care is in place the differences in diagnosis and the underlying contribution of factors such as brain malformation, infection and stroke mean that the signal about quality from seizure frequency is unreliable.

Feeding difficulty

Feeding difficulties are common in the days after birth. The healthy, well-grown neonate is equipped for a few days of semi-starvation while feeding is established. Healthy well-fed babies usually need a bit of practice before they establish feeds and they respond to patient support. It usually takes three people to support feeding: the baby, the mother and a skilled helper. Staff who support feeding are essential, particularly if the community does not have a strong tradition of breastfeeding. If formula milk is needed, then the marketed infant feeds are indistinguishable from a medical perspective and the mother's choice should be supported.

When breastfeeding is interrupted because the baby is unwell, it is essential to support the mother to express her milk. This can be frozen until it can be used. This is particularly important for premature babies because expressed breast milk protects them from necrotizing enterocolitis (NEC).

If feeding difficulties persist, then a systematic approach is needed to exclude medical causes for poor feeding. The baby should be examined to rule out problems with infection, neurology (brain, nerve, muscle, coordination) or anatomy (cleft palate etc).

Tongue-tie

Many cases of tongue-tie do not cause any problems: asymptomatic tongue-tie does not need treatment. Some cases of difficulty with breastfeeding are associated with tongue-tie. If routine support for breastfeeding is unsuccessful, then surgical division of tongue-tie can be performed.

Congenital anomalies

Dysmorphic features

Dysmorphic features are common in the general population. One or two dysmorphic features may not lead to a diagnosis or have any effect on the child. If in doubt look at the parents and wait 24 hours for swelling to subside.

Trisomy 21 in neonates

The most common syndrome in the neonate is trisomy 21, Down's syndrome. This can be expected on the basis of sonographic or genetic analyses conducted during pregnancy or can be unexpected. Unexpected cases occur in people who decline antenatal screening for this condition and in people who have been screened as low risk. A risk of 1:2,000 does mean that 1 in 2,000 women will have a baby with Down's syndrome.

Honesty and transparency is important when dealing with a case of suspected Down's syndrome. The ideal is to share suspicions with both parents in a calm, private setting. However, this is not always possible. If a parent raises concerns about Down's syndrome those concerns should be acknowledged and a paediatric opinion sought as soon as possible.

A paediatric assessment of suspected Down's syndrome will usually take the form of a shared examination of the baby with the parents. All features of the baby are described and positives are shared. Features that are different from many children are pointed out (not abnormal features).

A genetic test is always done, even if an experienced clinician is able to make a definitive diagnosis on the basis of the examination alone. If there is even the slightest clinical suspicion of trisomy 21, it is usually worth doing the genetic test even if the likelihood is low. If one set of clinicians raise the concern, other groups are likely to raise the same concern. The genetic test is usually a fluorescent *in situ* hybridization (FISH) test that can give a result within 24–48 hours. A definitive karyotype is needed to report the type of trisomy and advise about the value of genetic testing in parents and future risk. Disjunction does not need testing of family members and is associated with a low risk of recurrence (1%).

The days after diagnosis are traumatic for the family. The dominant clinical problem is establishing feeds. Some babies with trisomy 21 can learn to feed on the postnatal wards with their mother, but most are admitted to the neonatal unit for a period to tube feeding. A cardiac defect is seen in about one-third of cases of trisomy 21 and is sought using echocardiography. The parents are given information about the condition and the possibility of peer support from other families is raised. Babies go home when they are able to feed.

Cleft lip/palate

In the UK the care of babies with cleft lip or palate is centralized into 11 networks (nine in England and Wales, one each in Scotland and Northern Ireland). The immediate management is based on individualized assessment of the baby's feeding abilities. Many children with cleft lip or palate need adaptations to the feeding process; for example, by giving expressed breast milk using a flexible teat. Corrective surgery is not urgent and is usually done several months after birth.

Heart murmur

In the neonatal period the management of antenatal diagnosed congenital heart disease is stratified according to the need for treatment.

Urgent intervention (within 6–12 hours of birth) is needed for a small number of conditions in which a functional anatomy cannot be maintained with medical treatments; for example, transposition of the great arteries without interatrial or intraventricular communication. In these cases, an urgent septostomy is required.

Urgent medical treatment is instituted for conditions that are likely to be duct-dependent. These include pulmonary (cyanotic) conditions, where the duct is needed to oxygenate blood, and systemic conditions, where the duct is needed to allow oxygenated blood to reach the majority of the body. Fetal cardiology assessment usually identifies these babies and prompts the initiation of a postnatal care pathway. The duct is kept open using an intravenous infusion of prostaglandin E2.

Some causes of congenital heart disease lead to cardiac failure. In the acute phase these are treated with inotropes and possibly with diuretics.

Congenital heart disease can present in the newborn period unexpectedly. Babies with congenital heart disease present with cyanosis, heart failure (manifest as respiratory distress) and cardiovascular collapse or are asymptomatic. This often happens a few days or a week after birth when the duct closes.

Cyanosis can indicate respiratory failure or a structural heart condition that prevents blood getting into the lungs to be oxygenated. In respiratory failure there is usually a failure in ventilation as well as in oxygenation, in which case there is respiratory acidosis that requires significant support with a ventilator. Giving extra oxygen will usually change the oxygen saturation in respiratory failure. In contrast, cyanotic heart disease will have a much greater deficit in oxygenation and increasing inspired oxygen does not make a difference to oxygen saturation. Causes of early cyanotic heart disease include transposition of the great arteries, atresia or stenosis of the pulmonary valve (including tetralogy of Fallot and double outlet right ventricle with severe pulmonary stenosis) and totally anomalous pulmonary venous drainage.

Heart failure in the newborn usually presents with respiratory failure without evidence of lung disease. Structural causes of early heart failure include hypoplastic left heart, coarctation of the aorta, interrupted aortic arch and critical aortic stenosis. Other causes of early heart failure include arrhythmias, myocardial ischaemia, myocarditis, dilated cardiomyopathy, endocardial elastofibrosis and hypertrophic cardiomyopathy.

Cardiovascular collapse can be due to hypoplastic left heart, aortic valve atresia or critical stenosis, coarctation of the aorta and interrupted arch.

All these distinctions are easy to make *post hoc* but clinical presentations overlap so that the neonatal assessment is complicated.

Hypospadias

Hypospadias occurs in 1 in 300 boys. It involves an abnormally placed urinary meatus, chordee of the penis and a limited foreskin. Surgical correction takes place between 6 months and 1 year after birth. It is important to advise the parents to avoid circumcision because the foreskin is used during the operation.

Hypospadias may be part of ambiguous genitalia. Consider ambiguous genitalia if both testes cannot be palpated.

If a baby has ambiguous genitalia it is important to share concerns with the family, to avoid assigning a sex and to arrange urgent review by a skilled multidisciplinary team (including paediatric endocrinologists, surgeons and radiologists).

Encephalopathy

Neonatal encephalopathy is a clinical condition suggesting that brain injury has occurred. There is a broad differential diagnosis. Neonatal encephalopathy is often, but not always, associated with events during and after labour. Thus the neonatal approach is to evaluate with an open mind about the diagnosis and assess the baby systematically before making a diagnosis and offering a prognosis. It may take 1 week or more to come to a conclusion. In the meantime, the baby is treated aggressively for a number of conditions.

Causes of neonatal encephalopathy include hypoxic-ischaemic encephalopathy (HIE), infection (bacterial and viral, e.g. HSV), drugs (maternal therapeutic, maternal abuse, neonatal therapeutic), CNS malformations, metabolic conditions (hypoglycaemia, aminoacidaemias, organic acidaemias, pyridoxine dependency, mitochondrial disorders, urea cycle disorders, etc). The assessment is based on the questions in the Box. Answering these questions requires collaboration between antenatal and postnatal teams.

Questions to answer during the evaluation of neonatal encephalopathy

- Is there positive evidence of HIE?
  - during labour: evidence of fetal distress on history, on cardiotocograph (CTG), on cord gas analysis, with passage of meconium;
  - after birth: poor condition at birth and prolonged resuscitation.
- Is there positive evidence of other conditions?
  - look for infection: blood cultures for bacterial infection; serology or viral detection for HSV and electron microscopy of any vesicle fluid.
- Look for abnormal brain structure: MRI scan is useful, cranial ultrasound is usually not informative during the assessment of neonatal encephalopathy.
- Look for hypoglycaemia.
- Can other conditions be ruled out?
  - metabolic conditions are unlikely if the blood gases, glucose and lactate can be normalized and if serum ammonia is normal.

It is important to consider these diagnoses because some of these conditions need specific management and some of these conditions can exacerbate HIE or make the baby more vulnerable during labour.

Encephalopathy represents altered brain function. This leads to changes in the conscious level and the tone. The level of consciousness can be increased or reduced. Tone can be increased or reduced. It is important to describe the baby and then offer an interpretation. One way to summarize the observations is to use the Sarnat grading (*Table 16.1*). This is designed to structure the assessment of a baby with one type of encephalopathy: HIE. The clinical characteristic of HIE is that it evolves.

Treatment continues while the diagnostic questions are answered. It can take several days to rule

Table 16.1 Sarnat scoring

	Grade I mild	Grade II moderate	Grade III severe
Alertness	Hyperalert	Lethargy	Coma
Muscle tone	Normal or increased	Hypotonic	Flaccid
Seizures	None	Frequent	Uncommon
Pupils	Dilated, reactive	Small, reactive	Variable, fixed
Respiration	Regular	Periodic	Apnoea
Duration	<24 hours	2–14 days	Weeks

out infection and other causes. Treatment is based on supportive care that includes:

- Airway: severe encephalopathy involves loss of tone in the pharynx so an endotracheal tube may be required.
- Breathing: encephalopathy reduces respiratory drive so artificial ventilation is usually required. This continues until respiratory drive is restored and the airway is secure.
- Circulation: a severe hypoxic-ischaemic insult affects the heart leading to poor myocardial function that is treated with inotropes.
- Renal failure: a severe hypoxic-ischaemic insult affects the kidneys leading to a condition similar to acute tubular necrosis. This initially leads to poor urine output followed by high urine output.

Specific care includes antibiotics in line with local policy. If there is any uncertainty about the diagnosis or any evidence of HSV infection, aciclovir is started to treat HSV.

Therapeutic hypothermia improves the outcome of HIE. A series of trials in several countries has shown that cooling reduces mortality and improves neurodevelopmental outcomes at the age of 18 months. In the Cochrane review of 11 trials, among babies allocated to care without cooling, death or major disability in survivors was seen in 409/666 (61%) while among babies allocated to cooling death or major disability in survivors was seen in 312/678 (46%). This gives a risk ratio of 0.75 in favour

of cooling (95% confidence interval 0.68–0.83). Therapeutic hypothermia is now the standard of care for treatment of HIE.

Therapeutic hypothermia should be started as soon as possible after birth if the clinical picture suggests HIE. Hypothermia can be administered through whole body cooling or selective head cooling. 'Passive' cooling can also be used before the child has access to formal equipment for cooling. Debate continues about whether to use hypothermia for conditions not included in the inclusion criteria for the trials that identified the value of cooling; for example, in babies born between 34 and 37 weeks' gestation.

The residual morbidity from HIE even with cooling is prompting research into adjuncts to hypothermia. Agents under investigation include xenon, melatonin and caspase inhibitors. It has been argued that phenotypic variation in cases of HIE may mean that more than one adjunct is needed or that there is a residue of injury that cannot be easily treated.

The progress of the encephalopathy can be followed clinically or with amplitude integrated electroencephalography (aEEG, otherwise known as cerebral function monitoring, CFM). aEEG allows a partial assessment of brain activity by measuring two EEG leads and summarizing the signals in ways that are analogous with the CTG. aEEG can show evidence of normal brain activity and changes in behavioural states; or profound abnormality: burst suppression patterns or a 'flat line' isoelectric signal. There are intermediate patterns such as loss of continuity.

Brain imaging is central to the diagnosis of neonatal encephalopathy and the prognostication of HIE. Cranial ultrasound will show some gross structural defects of the brain. Computed tomography (CT) scanning can be very helpful if traumatic brain damage is suspected (e.g. subdural haematoma). MRI is the key investigation. MRI results can be informative between days 2 and 14 after birth so that the timing of the scan is down to local circumstances and preferences. Altered signals in the basal ganglia suggest a rapid onset of hypoxia that is short-lived (<20–30 minutes) while altered signals in the cerebral cortex suggest a more chronic period of hypoxia. The basal ganglia are the most metabolically active part of the neonatal brain and are hit by a rapid insult. The cerebral cortex is less metabolically active so is less susceptible to damage during acute hypoxia, but is vulnerable to chronic hypoxia if blood is redirected to the metabolically active parts of the brain.

An integrated view of clinical progress and the results of investigations lead to an individualized prognosis. It can take more than 1 week to define a baby's prognosis since behaviour after cooling and the brain MRI are of central importance to establishing the prognosis. Some diagnostic features are not very informative about prognosis. These include: cord pH or base excess; the CTG; and Apgar scores in the 10 minutes after birth.

Features that suggest a good outcome include: rapid return to normal behaviour; rapid return to normal CFM; normal brain MRI. It is said that if a baby can take an oral feed within 7 days of birth they are very unlikely to have a bad outcome.

Features that suggest a poor outcome include: prolonged resuscitation; seizures within 6 hours of birth; unresponsive to stimulation; no gag response when off all medication; multiorgan failure; burst suppression pattern on the CFM when off all medication; prolonged return of CFM baseline to normal; abnormal signal on the internal capsule on brain MRI; extensive abnormality on the brain MRI. A baby with these features is highly likely to have extensive disability.

Other features are intermediate and it can be difficult to provide a firm prognosis. CFM or advanced brain imaging techniques such as MR spectroscopy may bring clarity in the future, but at present babies need neurodevelopmental follow-up.

Brain MRI findings are associated with specific outcomes: basal ganglia injury is associated with dyskinetic cerebral palsy (CP); internal capsule injury is associated with upper motor lesions (e.g. spastic hemiplegia); cerebral cortex injury is associated with learning difficulties.

Sometimes it is clear within 24 or 48 hours of birth that a baby has sustained a catastrophic brain injury. In other cases the features of a poor prognosis are not apparent for several days, until the baby is breathing spontaneously.

One outcome of HIE

A baby boy is born by emergency caesarean section after a clear history of placental abruption. The cord pH is 6.7 and he is given full resuscitation, requiring cardiac massage for 30 minutes at birth. 36 hours later the baby is completely unresponsive and ventilator-dependent with profound hypotonia, no respiratory effort and no seizures. Creatinine and liver enzymes are markedly elevated. He is not on anticonvulsants, sedatives or analgesia so the neurological assessment is unclouded.

Discussion with parents

In this case the parents would be told that the child has very little or no prospect of survival and any survivors would have no prospect of meaningful quality of life. A joint decision-making process would follow. In most cases care would be redirected toward palliation and the child would be taken off the ventilator. In such a case the decisions would be made without waiting for imaging.

This is an extreme case. Most babies with HIE do not have such a clear-cut clinical story and a decision toward palliation is often not indicated.

Other problems

Localized neurology

Upper limb

Brachial plexus palsies are often noted after birth. These may be associated with difficult births but this does not explain all the cases. Erb's palsy affects the C5 and C6 nerve roots, giving rise to a distinctive posture with the arm held at the baby's side, internally rotated and pronated. Klumpke's palsy affects C8 and T1 but is rare.

Total recovery occurs in 75% of babies over a few weeks to months. Referrals to physiotherapy and orthopaedics are essential to minimize complications such as contracture and assess for surgical intervention if there is no improvement.

Back

Small 'dimples' at the bottom of the back are common, affecting around 5% of babies. They can be associated with spinal lesions if the bottom of the dimple is not visible or if there is a change to the skin nearby. Ultrasound of the lower spine is indicated if there is any suspicion of a worrying feature.

Face

Facial palsy is seen in neonates and is likely to be due to pressure from the mother's sacral promontory during labour. The use of forceps may exacerbate this in some cases. Recovery is usually complete within 3 weeks.

Neonatal fractures

The most common sites of neonatal fracture are clavicle, humeral shaft and femoral shaft. Less common sites are at epiphyses of humerus or femur. Some fractures are sustained during birth. Almost all neonatal fractures heal without sequelae. Immobilization is difficult in this age group and may not help. Analgesia is important (e.g. with paracetamol).

Vitamin K deficiency bleeding

Vitamin K deficiency is a preventable cause of death and disability among the newborn; therefore, give vitamin K. There is no evidence for or against either oral or intramuscular preparations of vitamin K except that IM is a one-off treatment.

Neonatal abstinence syndrome

Neonatal abstinence is a common complication of maternal substance misuse. A wide range of substances is misused during pregnancy. Neonatal management is similar for all cases. The principles are structured observation, most commonly using a dedicated scoring system, and then treat according to the severity of the withdrawal. The medicine is then weaned according to a structured process. This can take weeks or months. A range of medications is in use. There is no evidence to choose between them. Neonatal treatment does not change the outcome but aims to make life less miserable for the baby and their carers. Extensive multidisciplinary team working is needed.

Routine management on postnatal wards

Similar to antenatal care, postnatal care is based on a risk assessment and stratification into groups that are used to guide management, with movement between groups very important if the baby's needs change.

Routine care is conducted by mothers with contact by maternity staff members to support feeding, advise mothers (e.g. if it is their first baby), anticipate social problems and detect jaundice.

Targeted care is aimed at babies at risk of conditions such as infection or hypoglycaemia. Neonates who have risk factors for infection may be safely observed rather than given antibiotics. Babies at risk of hypoglycaemia because of FGR or maternal diabetes have prefeed estimations of glucose.

Advice about how to avoid sudden infant death syndrome (SIDS, otherwise known as cot death) should be given to parents and reinforced frequently. In the UK advice about how to reduce the risk of SIDS is based on a series of detailed epidemiological studies.

Advice to parents on how to minimize the risk of sudden infant death

- Place the baby on their back to sleep in a cot in the same room as the parents.
- Don't smoke during pregnancy and don't let anyone smoke in the same room as a baby.
- Parents who smoke or take drugs need to avoid sharing a bed with a baby and parents who have been drinking alcohol need to avoid sharing a bed with a baby.
- Parents must avoid sleeping with a baby on a sofa or armchair.
- Don't allow babies to get too hot or too cold.
- Keep a baby's head uncovered.
- Tuck blankets in at shoulder level.
- Place a baby with their feet touching the surface of the cot or pram.

Neonatal screening

It is important to screen babies for conditions that are difficult to diagnose antenatally. There are three components of neonatal screening: physical examination, hearing check and blood tests.

Physical examination

A top to toe examination is traditional, done flexibly to adapt to the baby's behaviour. A few components of the neonatal physical examination are useful screening tests. Neonatal examination can detect congenital cataracts that need treatment in themselves, but are often the presenting feature of a metabolic condition that needs treatment to avoid more general problems.

Most neonatal heart murmurs are not associated with cardiac lesions and reflect the transition to postnatal circulation. Auscultation of the heart can detect murmurs arising from conditions that are difficult to diagnose antenatally. In some areas this is supplemented with pulse oximetry. Pulse oximetry can detect postductal hypoxia. This can be due to cardiac lesions that are difficult to detect on antenatal ultrasound. The head circumference is measured. In boys the testes are examined.

Hips

The neonatal examination includes examination of the hips to exclude developmental dysplasia of the hips. The hips are abducted and adducted in order to elicit dislocated or dislocatable hips. If the hips are dislocated or dislocatable, the baby is referred for orthopaedic management.

Developmental dysplasia of the hip (DDH) occurs in 1–2 per 1,000 live births with up to 20 per 1,000 live births having unstable hips. Untreated DDH leads to abnormal gait, limp and early onset of hip osteoarthrosis, causing early hip replacement. Treatment of DDH is effective. Neonatal screening for DDH is well established.

When the neonatal screen for DDH is positive the baby is referred for ultrasound and orthopaedic assessment. If DDH is confirmed the initial treatment is with a Pavlik harness that holds the legs in the best position to support the growth of the acetabulum. The harness is used for several weeks or months. If the harness does not solve the problem, surgical approaches are likely.

Many babies have stable joints but are found to have a 'clicky hip'. This is not abnormal but can be associated with an unstable joint, so babies with clicky hips are referred for a hip ultrasound and orthopaedic review.

Hearing

Some cases of permanent hearing loss can be detected in the newborn period and this allows early provision for the child and family. In high-income settings screening should be done with objective tests. In the UK newborn hearing screening is conducted with otoacoustic emissions. This procedure involves playing clicks to the baby. A healthy cochlea responds by making noises that can be detected. Screen failure or an uncertain response leads to an automated auditory brainstem response (AABR) test. In income-constrained settings questionnaires or behavioural testing can be used in a targeted or unselected way, but need to be piloted and linked to educational and other support.

Blood spot testing

In the UK the newborn blood test is done about 5 days after birth. The diseases screened for are: sickle cell disease, cystic fibrosis, congenital hypothyroidism and six metabolic conditions: phenylketonuria (PKU), medium-chain acyl-CoA dehydrogenase deficiency (MCADD); maple syrup urine disease (MSUD); isovaleric acidaemia (IVA); glutaric aciduria type 1 (GA1); homocystinuria (pyridoxine unresponsive) (HCU).

Immunizations

Immunizations are central to public health. National immunization schedules cover a range of diseases depending on the assessments made in each country. In the UK the national immunization schedule is updated regularly (http://www.nhs.uk/conditions/vaccinations/pages/vaccination-schedule-age-checklist.aspx).

Two vaccines are often administered in the neonatal period and both of them depend on good communication between maternity and neonatal services. Hepatitis B immunization is given to all babies whose mothers have serological evidence of hepatitis B (HBV). HBV immunization should start within 24 hours of birth. Women who present in labour without having had their booking bloods done should have hepatitis serology sent urgently so that the results can prompt immunization within 24 hours of birth, if appropriate. In addition, HBV Ig is given to all mothers with serological evidence of hepatitis B unless the mother has anti-Hep e antibodies. Thus, the only babies of HBV-positive mothers who do not get HBV Ig are babies whose mothers have serological evidence that they are not infective.

Tuberculosis (TB) continues to be a major cause of morbidity and mortality in many parts of the world. Neonatal bacillus Calmette-Guérin (BCG) is an effective way to reduce the incidence of TB infection, particularly TB meningitis. Neonatal BCG may be offered on the postnatal wards or elsewhere. In the UK BCG is offered to all infants aged 0–12 months in areas where the annual incidence of TB is 40/100,000 or greater, and to infants who have a parent or grandparent who was born in a country where the annual incidence of TB is 40/100,000 or greater.

Baby check

All babies should have a comprehensive examination within 48 hours of birth by someone trained to do this. This can be midwife, doctor, neonatal nurse or ANNP. This can be done at home.

Preterm babies

The burden of prematurity takes two forms: low numbers of babies with high-impact complications of extreme prematurity (<29 weeks), and high numbers of babies with moderate- or low-impact conditions born between 29 weeks and term. While neonatal services seem preoccupied with extremely premature babies, we all need to remember that the consequences of moderate or late prematurity are significant.

Outcomes of preterm birth

The outcomes of preterm birth are summarized below in *Table 16.2*. The information shown provides indicative information. Up to date figures should be used in the light of local experience and adapted to the circumstances of the family.

Events following preterm birth

In preterm babies adaptation can take several days because of surfactant deficiency, immature systemic haemodynamics and pulmonary haemodynamics. The adjustment and growth phases of postnatal life can be deranged due to alterations in the developmental pathway, mainly in the lungs.

Table 16.2 Outcomes for babies born at less than 28 weeks

1 Survival and early morbidity					
Condition	Gestational age at birth (weeks)				
	22	23	24	25	26
Intrapartum stillbirths as percentage of those alive at the start of labour	44	19	11	5	2
Survival to discharge as percentage of all live births	16	30	47	70	78
Bronchopulmonary dysplasia (supplementary oxygen at 36 weeks PMA) as percentage of survivors	100	86	80	67	61
Survival without disability at 3 years as a percentage of all births	50	53	65	72	79
Survival with severe disability as a percentage of all births	10	30	19	16	10
Survival with moderate disability as a percentage of all births	40	17	16	12	10

These data are drawn from the EPICure2 study that examined all births between 22 and 26 weeks in England. See Further reading for the papers that include definitions of the terms.

EPICure2 data provide an overview but all information must be tailored to the local situation and the circumstances of an individual pregnancy.

Pay attention to the denominator for each statistic (e.g. alive at start of labour vs. live birth). Percentages refer to each gestational age category.

PMA, postmenstrual age.

(continued)

Table 16.2 (continued) Outcomes for babies born at less than 28 weeks

2 Non-neurological					
System	**Age (years)**				
	First year	**1–5**	**5–10**	**10–17**	**18+**
Respiratory (worse if the baby had bronchopulmonary dyplasia)	Increased hospital admissions			Reduced lung volumes and exercise capacity but asymptomatic	
Growth	Some differences in length at discharge			Difference narrows but is persistent	
General health			5–10% increase in prevalence of general ill-health (c. 20% in term controls)		
Blindness or severe visual impairment			4–8% if born at 24–25 weeks 1–2% if born at 26–27 weeks		
Hearing impairment			1–4%		
Support for language development		30–50% (2% for term controls)			
Completion of secondary education/high school					23–27 weeks: 68% (term controls: 75%)

These values are 'ballpark' figures drawn from a range of reviews. The information is indicative rather than definitive.

Table 16.3 Patient pathway for a very premature baby

Gestational age	Stage			% of live births in England
	Immediate transition	**Adaptation/adjustment**	**Growth**	
22	Not successful			
23	Often not successful	Needs careful attention to environment (temperature/humidity) Often needs support with inotropes Development of lungs is often deranged leading to prolonged requirement for respiratory support (weeks or months)	Initially dependent on technology Dependent on avoiding intercurrent illnesses Needs support with oral feeding until 34 weeks PMA or later	0.1
24–26	Usually needs supplementary oxygen and active support (positive airway pressure and surfactant)			0.5
27–30	May need active support (positive airway pressure and surfactant)	Needs careful attention to environment (temperature/humidity) Often needs supplementary oxygen May need support with other organs Development of lungs may be deranged leading to requirement for respiratory support for weeks	Initially dependent on technology Dependent on avoiding intercurrent illnesses Needs support with oral feeding until 34 weeks PMA or later	1.3
31–33	Sometimes needs active support	Takes 10–14 days Can need extra support with feeding and warmth May need supplementary oxygen	Needs support with oral feeding until 34 weeks PMA	1.2
34–36	Rarely needs support	Takes 5–10 days Can need extra support with warmth	May need support to establish oral feeding	4.6
37+	Rarely needs support	Takes 2–3 days Rarely needs support beyond routine care	Dependent on nutrient supply	92.3

PMA: postmenstrual age.

Intercurrent illnesses include infection (bacterial and fungal), NEC and complications of intensive care (lung secretions, infections, parenteral nutrition). Establishing growth can be a problem because enteral feeds may not be easy to establish or because parenteral nutrition does not meet all the requirements of the babies. The pattern of brain injury in preterm babies is different from that seen in term babies. Premature neonates can often withstand lower oxygen levels because they have a lower metabolic requirement because of the stage of development.

Immaturity at birth gives rise to other vulnerabilities. These can result in haemodynamic-related brain injury: intraventricular haemorrhage or parenchymal brain injury related to infection, inflammation or hypoxia; periventricular leucomalacia. Prediction of long-term outcomes remains a challenge.

General points

Antenatal management is an important way to optimize outcomes of preterm birth (*Table 16.3*). There is a key role for antenatal steroids and strategies that optimize the delivery of antenatal steroids are very useful (e.g. tocolytics). There is a role for antenatal magnesium in neuroprotection but the absolute effect is not large.

The universal elements of neonatal care are: optimal environment (warmth and humidity); minimal handling; developmental care; optimizing nutrition; and scrupulous efforts to minimize infection (*Table 16.4*). The culture of neonatal units is based round the need for routines to reduce risks while allowing flexibility for parents.

The economics of care for premature babies are favourable. Inpatient hospital care during the initial admission for a baby born at 24 weeks' gestation costs around £100,000. When averaged over the 20-year-span commonly used for health technology assessment, this works out about £5,000 a year. Since many survivors have a reasonable quality of life, intensive care for neonates represents good value for money when compared to treatments such as renal dialysis.

Care for babies who are born before extrauterine life is viable

Neonatal care extends to babies born before they are viable, although the gestational age cut-off for formal neonatal involvement varies between hospitals. Babies born between 20 and 24 weeks' gestation frequently show signs of life. The median duration of signs of life among these babies is 1 hour, but 10% of babies born between 20 and 24 weeks' gestation will have signs of life for more than 6 hours. This requires careful preparation of the families and sensitive support by professionals.

In the UK a useful framework is provided by the Nuffield Council on Bioethics Report on Critical Care Decisions in fetal and neonatal medicine: ethical issues (See Further reading). This suggests that babies born at 20 or 21 weeks' gestation are offered comfort care only. Babies born at 22 weeks' gestation are offered comfort care unless a research-driven effort to support them is available (such efforts have not been conducted in the UK). The management of babies born at 23 weeks can be driven by parental preference or, if the parents do not express a preference during careful discussion, by team preference. Babies born at 24 weeks and above are usually offered full intensive care from birth unless there is a reason not to offer that care.

Initial care of a viable premature baby

The initial care of a premature baby is centred around the environment, assessment of the baby's condition, supporting transition to extrauterine life, stabilizing the baby prior to transfer to the neonatal unit and keeping the family informed about progress.

Ensuring the birth room is warm and free from draughts is essential for the environmental care of an extremely premature baby. The baby is placed into a clear plastic bag immediately after birth. This avoids evaporation and consequent hypothermia (which is associated with poor outcome).

Initial care of a premature baby should not be treated as a 'resuscitation' but as 'stabilization'. Many premature babies will gradually adapt to breathing as long as age-specific oxygen saturation targets are respected.

On the intensive care unit a thermoneutral environment is maintained (i.e. the baby is maintained at a temperature that results in minimal energy expenditure and stress to the infant). Vascular access is obtained, preferably both arterial and venous. The umbilical vessels are a convenient site for vascular

Table 16.4 Pattern of care at different gestational ages

Mary R is a 32-year-old married teacher with a healthy 2-year-old daughter					
		PMA	Event	Impact on John	Impact on parents
January	2nd	22	Mary is admitted at 22 weeks' gestation with threatened preterm labour	Settles, discharged the next day	Upsetting discussion with obstetricians and neonatologists about the lack of benefit for neonatal intensive care at this gestational age
	16th	24	Mary is admitted at 24 weeks' gestation with threatened preterm labour	Tightenings continue, Mary is admitted	Separation from 2-year-old daughter
	17th	24	Mary is transferred to a tertiaty neonatal unit 40 miles from home (two nearer units are full)		Separation from daughter Travel costs Time off work
	20th	25	John is born at 4:30 am	Placed in a plastic bag Intubated Given surfactant Transferred to Neonatal Unit	Very worried because they only catch glimpses of their newborn son who is hidden by a plastic bag
			John arrives on Neonatal Unit at 4:46 am	Umbilical venous and arterial catheters are sited Parenteral nutrition is started Antibiotics are started ECG leads are placed on John's chest and a saturation probe is placed on his left hand	Very worried until 2 hours after John's birth when they are taken to the neonatal unit and shown him. Initially elated to see him alive and pleased to hear about all the care he will receive from the nurses. However, they are upset after a discussion with the senior doctor on the Neonatal Unit. John may not survive. If he survives he is likely to be disabled. He will be in hospital until Mary's due date or later
			Second dose of surfactant	Improvement in lung function but becomes hypotensive 3 hours later (unrelated to surfactant)	
	23rd		Fresh blood appears in the endotracheal tube	Pulmonary haemorrhage	Shocked by sight of blood in his tubes and on his face Terrified that he will die

| John's treatment | | | | | Other medication | Other possible events | Worst case scenario (these are rare but plausible outcomes) |
Respiratory support	Nutrition	Analgesia	Inotropes	Antibiotics			
							Fetal death *in utero*
40%; 18/4							John does not survive birth
40%; 18/4	Total PN	Morphine		Benzyl penicillin Gentamicin	Caffeine Vitamin K		John develops pulmonary hypertension, is treated with high-frequency oscillatory ventilation and inhaled nitric oxide but dies
60%; 22/4	Total PN	Morphine	Dopamine	Benzyl penicillin Gentamicin	Caffeine		John dies from hypotension that does not respond to treatment
100%; 24/3	Total PN	Morphine	Dopamine Dobutamine	Benzyl penicillin Gentamicin	Caffeine		John dies from pulmonary haemorrhage

(continued)

Table 16.4 (continued) Pattern of care at different gestational ages

Mary R is a 32-year-old married teacher with a healthy 2-year-old daughter

		PMA	Event	Impact on John	Impact on parents
	24th		Cranial ultrasound scan	Intraventricular haemorrhage	Upset to hear that there is a 'bruise in John's brain' and that he may be disabled when he grows up
	26th	26	Abdominal distension and blood in orogastric tube Intestinal perforation noted on abdominal X-ray	NEC Started on three antibiotics	Terrified to see that his tummy is large and shiny
	27th	26	Operation	20 cm of ileum removed Ileostomy sited	Very scared to hear that he needs an operation and that he may die during the operation
February		26	Recovery	Continues on antibiotics and nil by mouth for 10 days	Relieved that he tolerated the operation well and is gradually getting better
		27	Extubated on post op day 5	Put on nasal CPAP	First cuddle
		27	Cranial ultrasound scan	Cystic periventricular leucomalacia	Devastated by news that John may be disabled with difficulty walking by himself (cerebral palsy) and possible learning difficulties
March		28	Started on expressed milk on post op day 10		Enjoying doing most of his cares and having cuddles every day

John's treatment					Other medication	Other possible events	Worst case scenario (these are rare but plausible outcomes)
Respiratory support	Nutrition	Analgesia	Inotropes	Antibiotics			
	Total PN	Morphine			Caffeine		The cranial ultrasound shows bilateral damage to the brain tissue (IVH Grade 4). John develops seizures. Family and staff recognize that John will not have a meaningful quality of life if he survives and care is realigned away from intensive care. John dies in his mother's arms
70%; 22/5	Total PN	Morphine		Amoxycillin Gentamicin Metronidazole	Caffeine		John dies from fulminant NEC
50%; 20/4	Total PN	Morphine			Caffeine		John is found to have pan-intestinal NEC. Family and staff recognize that further treatment is futile. Care is realigned away from intensive care. John dies in his mother's arms after compassionate extubation
40%; 16/4	Total PN				Caffeine	"Stuck" on ventilator. Given diuretics for 5 days followed by a course of steroid	
70%	Total PN				Caffeine		
						Family ask for care to be discontinued but this is not possible since John is breathing for himself	
70%	Partial PN and some expressed breast milk				Caffeine		

(continued)

Table 16.4 (continued) Pattern of care at different gestational ages

	PMA	Event	Impact on John	Impact on parents
	29	Develops episodes of low heart rate (bradycardia) and low oxygen levels on pulse oximetry (desaturations)	Diagnosed with infection Started on antibiotics that are continued for 5 days	Very worried to hear he is sick again and upset that he may go back on the ventilator, but glad when he carries on breathing without a ventilator
	30	Moved to high-dependency area		Very pleased that he is strong enough to leave the Intensive Care Unit
	31	Time in high-dependency area		Getting into a routine as he goes for days and days without a setback
April	32	Moved to Mary's booking hospital		Relieved that they don't have to travel back and forth to the hospital with the Intensive Care Unit
	33, 34	Time in high-dependency area		Very frustrated because the hospitals do things differently
May	35	Starts to breastfeed		
	35	Time in special care		Practising being at home!!
	36	Cranial ultrasound scan	Cystic periventricular leucomalacia	Devastated again by repeat scan that reminds everybody that John may be disabled
June	38	Fully breastfed		
	39	Home		Hooray!

CPAP: continuous positive airways pressure; ECG: electrocardiogram; IVH: intraventricular haemorrhage; NEC: necrotizing enterocolitis; PMA: postmenstrual age; PN: parenteral nutrition.

access in the newborn baby. Parents are reunited with the baby as soon as possible. A long process of education about prematurity and how to look after premature babies is started, emphasizing that parents are at the centre of the baby's care.

Premature babies are cared for in an environment that supports their development. Noise and light are avoided whenever possible. The clinical team adopt a policy of minimal handling. This is done so that the baby can devote their energy to growth and development. Family-centred care is becoming increasingly prominent in neonatal units. Parents are encouraged to spend as much time as they can with their baby, taking account of other family commitments. Skin-to-skin (or kangaroo) care is an important part of neonatal care as soon as the baby is stable enough. It provides reassurance to the parents and is associated with improved physiological stability in the baby (**Figure 16.1**).

| John's treatment | | | | | Other medication | Other possible events | Worst case scenario (these are rare but plausible outcomes) |
Respiratory support	Nutrition	Analgesia	Inotropes	Antibiotics			
70%	Partial PN and some expressed breast milk			Amoxycillin Gentamicin	Caffeine		John dies from fulminant gram-negative infection
60%	Fully enterally fed				Caffeine		
					Caffeine		
50%	Fully enterally fed				Caffeine		
40%	Fully enterally fed						
40%	Fully enterally fed				Caffeine		
0.5 l/min	Fully enterally fed						
0.3 l/min	Fully enterally fed						
0.1 l/min	Fully enterally fed						
Air	Breast fed						

Breathing

Preterm babies are prone to atelectasis because the chest is less stiff than it is in other age groups. This is most marked immediately after birth when low levels of surfactant mean that surface tension also is very high. These problems are overcome by applying a positive end expiratory pressure. This can be done using continuous positive airway pressure (CPAP) or intermittent mandatory ventilation (IMV). CPAP is administered nasally: a variety of delivery devices is available. IMV is administered with an endotracheal tube (ETT) (i.e. by intubation). If a baby is not breathing well then surfactant is administered. This can be done through an ETT or during CPAP by visualizing the vocal cords and placing a tube into the trachea while surfactant is administered. The choice

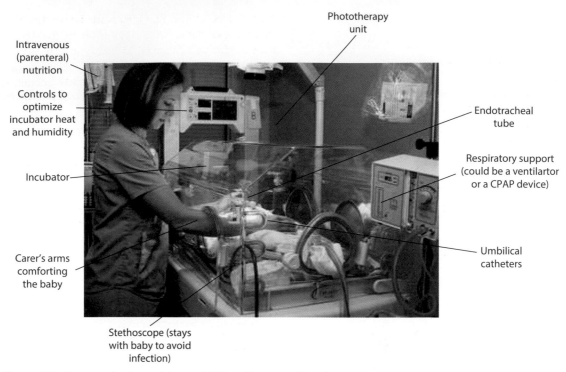

Figure 16.1 Components of neonatal care. CPAP, continuous positive airways pressure.

between these methods depends on local preference and practice. Commercially available surfactants are carefully prepared extracts of pig or cow lung or are completely synthetic.

Many preterm babies will have an uncomplicated course once they make their own surfactant within 12–24 hours of birth. Complications include pneumothorax but this is rare if antenatal steroids and postnatal surfactant have been administered.

Preterm birth before 30 weeks disrupts the developmental programme of the lungs. This shows as bronchopulmonary dyplasia, otherwise known as chronic lung disease of prematurity (CLD). Babies with bronchopulmonary dyplasia have abnormal lung architecture and reduced gas exchange. This is managed by administering oxygen and positive pressure. There are a number of ways of delivering positive pressure, some of which are invasive (ETT and continuous mandatory ventilation) and others are non-invasive (CPAP, biphasic positive airway pressure and variations on this). Over a number of weeks the development programme modifies lung architecture changes and gas exchange improves.

This improvement is manifest as a reduced oxygen requirement and reduction in the extent of positive pressure. Once the need for invasive ventilation is over, further ventilation aid can be given using nasal CPAP, high-flow oxygen, nasal cannula or ambient oxygen, among other methods. During the recovery from bronchopulmonary dyplasia supplemental oxygen and positive pressure are gradually reduced. Recovery may take weeks or months and can be interrupted by intercurrent infection. Diuretics and/or corticosteroids may be used to accelerate the clinical features of improvement.

A few babies have extensive derangement of lung architecture a week after birth that is described as pulmonary interstitial emphysema (PIE). This manifests as very poor gas exchange and a requirement for high ventilator settings.

Babies with respiratory insufficiency in the days and weeks after premature birth often have a patent ductus arteriosus (PDA). It is unclear whether the PDA is a cause or effect of severe bronchopulmonary dyplasia. Accordingly, the management of bronchopulmonary dyplasia varies considerably.

Circulation

In the days after premature birth the heart may not be able to meet the needs of the body. This is partly because the fetal heart is working close to capacity (high rate, high filling volume) and partly because the myocardium and catecholamine-mediated regulation of the heart are immature. This manifests as poor circulation, most commonly seen as hypotension. Inotropes are frequently used to overcome this transient problem. The most commonly used inotropes are dopamine and dobutamine. Hydrocortisone and adrenaline are also used frequently. Among survivors the need for inotropes resolves during the first week after birth.

Extreme prematurity is associated with specific cardiovascular problem during transition and adaptation. A PDA that does not start to close can increase the work required from the heart and increase blood flow into lungs. Rapid shifts of blood into the lungs sometimes cause pulmonary haemorrhage, which can be fatal. Poor ventricular contractility is a common problem among extremely preterm neonates due to weaker myocardium and receptors.

Antenatal conditions do not appear to have specific effects on neonatal haemodynamics. Babies with severe FGR or infection/inflammation (e.g. babies born to women with chorioamnionitis) tend to have severe circulatory problems but clinically these follow a common final pathway.

Nutrition

As always, breast is best. Ideally, expressed maternal breast milk is gradually introduced in the 2 weeks after birth. However, this is unpredictable because of variation in the establishment of peristalsis. If maternal milk is not available, donor breast milk is very useful.

In the smallest babies parenteral nutrition is used to bridge the gap between placental nutrition and expressed breast milk. Enteral tube feeding is continued until the baby is able to take oral feeds. Babies can start to feed orally by breast, cup or bottle around 34 weeks' gestation if they are not receiving respiratory support.

Necrotizing enterocolitis

NEC is a condition of unknown aetiology that occurs in 5–10% of babies born weighing <1,500 g.

NEC is a condition that affects the bowel mucosa. Factors associated with disruption to the bowel mucosa include hypoxia, infection and nutrition (particularly high osmotic load). The clinical features of NEC are feed intolerance (the stomach does not empty between feeds), bile-stained gastric fluid, abdominal distension and blood-stained stool. Abdominal X-ray shows distended bowel loops and, in confirmed cases, air in the bowel wall (pneumoatosis intestinalis). Intestinal perforation is seen commonly. The clinical challenge is that feed intolerance, bile-stained gastric fluid and abdominal distension are seen commonly in neonates who do not have NEC.

NEC is often associated with a systemic inflammatory response and infection that needs aggressive multiorgan support. Antibiotics are used to provide 'triple coverage' for gram-positive, gram-negative and anaerobic bacteria.

The definitive treatment is surgery but this may not be possible if the baby is very unstable. An abdominal drain may be useful as a bridge to surgery.

The intestinal outcomes of NEC vary from loss of 5–10 cm of small bowel to panintestinal NEC, which is not compatible with survival. Many babies end up with short bowel syndrome and long-term dependence on parenteral nutrition, which is frequently complicated by cholestatic jaundice. Babies with short bowel syndrome due to NEC can spend many months in hospital and end up requiring a liver transplant. Bowel transplant or bowel lengthening procedures may be suitable in some cases. The risk of long-term neurodevelopmental sequelae is increased substantially in babies who develop NEC.

Suspected infection

Early-onset bacterial infection is suspected in many preterm babies. Bacteria are isolated rarely and are similar to the bacteria isolated from term babies with early-onset infection. The features of late-onset neonatal infection among preterm babies include bradycardia, apnoea, desaturations and feed intolerance, but are not specific. More than 80% of babies with suspected late-onset neonatal infection are treated for fewer than a couple of days because symptoms resolve, there is no laboratory evidence of infection and blood cultures are negative. In high-resource settings the most common bacteria isolated from babies suspected of late-onset infection are coagulate-negative staphylococci species. Gram-negative bacteria are also found. The importance of late-onset neonatal infection among preterm neonates is twofold. Firstly, these babies are unwell and need increased care, which disrupts the family and has resource implications. Secondly, the systemic inflammation may damage the brain and increase the risk of neurodevelopmental sequelae. For these reasons it is essential to prevent late-onset neonatal infection as much as possible. Accordingly, it is essential to follow scrupulous hand hygiene when visiting a neonatal unit. On arrival on the unit you need to wash your hands thoroughly. Every time you enter a nursery or move between patients you must apply alcohol-based hand wash thoroughly. If you make contact with body fluids you must wash your hands thoroughly.

Fungal infection is a serious complication of neonatal intensive care. The incidence varies between 1% and 10%. The onset of fungal infection is often insidious and it may take 7–10 days to manifest after birth.

Eyes

Babies born before 32 weeks' gestation or weighing less than 1,500 g are at risk of retinopathy of prematurity (ROP). Untreated this condition leads to vascular proliferation in the retina and potentially retinal detachment and blindness. Treatment is effective and a screening programme is well established. The first successful treatment was cryotherapy, which has been superseded by laser treatment. Laser treatment may be superseded by other treatments such as intraocular injection with antibodies that block the actions of vascular endothelial growth factor (VEGF). In the past ROP was thought to be due to administration of excessive amounts of oxygen. More recently, it has become clear that oxygen is only part of the problem. Other factors such as low birthweight, poor growth, low levels of insulin-like growth factor and excessive activity of VEGF are now thought to contribute to the development of ROP.

Premature babies with no, or successfully treated, ROP may have visual problems because of cortical blindness or squints.

Antenatal counselling

Antenatal counselling about birth at extreme prematurity should be a joint effort between experienced obstetric and neonatal staff. The neonatal team will make a number of points that are shown below.

Neonatal aspects of antenatal counselling about birth at extreme prematurity

- The pattern of care is tailored to the individual.
- Survival ranges from 20% following birth at 23 weeks and 50% following birth at 24 weeks to 95% following birth at 30 weeks.
- If the baby survives then she/he will probably go home around the expected date of delivery, give or take a month or two.
- A number of other problems may arise including infection, NEC and ROP.
- There is a very wide range of outcomes among survivors. Some attend mainstream school (although all babies born at 23 or 24 weeks will need help in the classroom). Some have obvious disability. Some are profoundly disabled.
- Even if a baby responds to initial treatment after birth there is no way to predict how each baby will progess. Cranial ultrasound scans can predict some outcomes in some babies but are not always accurate. Even a baby with a normal set of ultrasound scans can develop a disability.

Families often have a different perspective after birth compared to before birth. Some families who would discontinue a pregnancy for a poor fetal prognosis would not agree to discontinue intensive care when offered the same prognosis postnatally (and *vice versa*). This means that decisions made by families and the neonatal team may appear strange from the obstetric perspective.

Outcomes of conditions seen in fetal medicine units

- *Hydrops*: affected babies usually need repeated chest or peritoneal drains. Pleural effusions and ascites can recur. Mortality among babies born alive with severe hydrops is around 50%.

- *Twin-to-twin transfusion syndrome* (TTTS): in established TTTS both twins are at risk after birth. Donor twins have chronic hypoxia that leaves them with haemodynamic insufficiency and a risk of NEC. Recipient twins have high-output cardiac failure. Neither donor nor twin in severe TTTS has a clear survival advantage over the other. The outcome depends on the condition of each baby. Babies born following TTTS can have a honeymoon period of relative clinical stability before cardiovascular decompensation occurs.

- *Congenital diaphragmatic hernia*: survival is 50%. The dominant problems are pulmonary hypoplasia and pulmonary hypertension. These are treated with carefully titrated ventilation (frequently involving high-frequency oscillation) and inhaled nitric oxide. An operation to repair the defect is undertaken when the baby is stable. This may take days or weeks. These children can have complex needs as they grow, due to respiratory and gastrointestinal problems.

- *Gastroschisis*: the presence of uncomplicated gastroschisis does not affect the management of labour. Immediately after birth the baby's abdomen is wrapped to prevent fluid loss and trauma to the bowel. The wrapping is clear plastic so that the bowel can be visualized. Primary repair is sometimes possible (i.e. the bowel loops can be placed into the abdominal cavity and the abdominal wall can be closed in a single procedure). More frequently the abdominal cavity needs to be expanded before the bowel can fit into the cavity. In these cases, the abdominal cavity is expanded using gravity. The bowel is placed in a 'silo' that is suspended above the baby. Over a few weeks the size of the silo is progressively reduced and the bowel sinks into the peritoneal cavity.

- *Pulmonary hypoplasia*: is most frequently seen in the context of prolonged preterm premature rupture of the membranes (PPROM). PPROM before 20 weeks' gestation is associated with pulmonary hypoplasia. Neonatal management is based on titrated ventilatory support taking care not to overdistend the lungs. Mortality reflects the severity of the hypoplasia and the extent of the ventilatory support that is required.

- *Spina bifida*: the presence of spina bifida does not affect the management of labour. At birth the baby is wrapped in clear film to protect the back from trauma and infection. Following assessment on the neonatal unit an operation is performed within 48 hours to close the lesion on the back and remove any external tissue. The aim of the surgery is not to affect the neurological outcome but to prevent infection and support general care. Subsequently the baby will be seen by a large multidisciplinary team to address the problems associated with spina bifida, which include: paralysis of the lower limbs, hydrocephalus, urinary and faecal incontinence and learning disability. A large range of treatments can address these problems including medical, social, surgical, physiotherapy and other approaches.

Breastfeeding and medication

Very few medications are absolute contraindications to breastfeeding. These are cytotoxic agents and radioactive medicines. For all other medications an individualized assessment is needed. The components of the assessment are:

- Maternal need for medication.
- Likelihood of significant amounts of drug reaching the neonatal circulation. Consequences of neonatal exposure.
- Social context.
- Implications for management.

If breastfeeding needs to be interrupted because the baby is unwell, support the mother to express her milk until the baby can take mother's milk again.

Safeguarding

Maternity and neonatal services cannot operate in isolation from other elements of the health and social care system. When adults or children are at risk of harm, or come to harm, staff have a duty to meet the needs of the vulnerable person. Babies may be at risk of harm from negligence, physical abuse, sexual abuse and emotional abuse. The maternity team frequently identifies these risks during the antenatal period. When risks have been identified a plan is put in place. All staff need to work together to deliver the plan and monitor whether any new concerns arise after the baby is born. Safeguarding issues for babies and other family members may arise at any time. It is essential to maintain surveillance for any untoward events that may indicate risk to mother or baby. All maternity services need to have systems for assessments and referrals when safeguarding concerns arise. All staff need to know these systems in the work place. Staff have a responsibility to share any concerns with relevant colleagues.

Palliative care

Death before or shortly after birth is common. The perinatal team needs to develop a shared approach to this distressing circumstance. Fetal medicine services frequently identify fetuses who are likely to die shortly after birth. When the families of babies with a potentially life-limiting condition choose to continue the pregnancy, a series of discussions is convened to discuss the options. Sometimes it is possible to give a firm estimate that the baby will die within minutes of birth. More commonly, it may not be possible to be sure whether the baby will live for minutes, hours or days. The neonatal contribution is to identify the possible scenarios and outline what is likely to happen in each scenario. Short-term survival for minutes of hours is often managed on the labour suite, preferably in a dedicated area that is designed to enhance family comfort. If the baby survives for 2–3 days, management in a sensitively selected area of the postnatal or neonatal wards may be optimal. If survival for more than 2–3 days is possible, then contact can be made with a local hospice so that families can consider that option.

Parallel planning is undertaken for a number of scenarios because of the uncertainty and variability between babies. Thus, a plan is made for each of the likely scenarios. These plans provide a framework for discussion and are often changed in the light of events. Parents should be given a range of options and supported to identify the course of action that meets their preferences. Paediatric palliative care team involvement is very helpful even if the baby is not expected to travel to a hospice. The birth plan takes account of the neonatal options and the mother's obstetric needs and wishes. The trade-offs between type of birth (e.g. vaginal birth versus caesarean section) and the condition of the baby will be specific to each family. The team may need to account for the need for postnatal investigations if there is any uncertainty about the diagnosis or prognosis.

Families may wish to take a dying baby, or a baby's body, home and this should be facilitated. Organ transplant of some organs is technically possible in some cases but requires considerable planning and organization so that an efficient system is in place before an opportunity to discuss transplantation arises.

The secret to the 'perinatal hospice' is shared working, advance planning and prospective mapping of the relevant services. Once a plan (or set of parallel plans) has been agreed for a family then all members of the team need to be aware of the plan and to follow it. This requires very clear, comprehensive documentation that is immediately available to all caregivers. Unexpected events need to be escalated rapidly to the most experienced member of the team so that appropriate adaptations to the plan can be made. Palliative care services can facilitate follow-up for the family. Supporting a family before and after the death of baby is demanding work and staff should be offered debrief sessions and other support as appropriate.

Conclusion

Supporting the baby's care after birth is a rewarding part of the obstetrician's role. Colleagues from maternity services are always welcome on neonatal units to share information about babies and families, to promote team-based continuity of care and for informal team building. In busy units, regular contact (several times a day) even during quiet periods facilitates good teamwork during crisis periods, for example when there is a shortage of cots or a baby is unexpectedly sick at birth. Well-informed, sympathetic obstetricians are key members of the neonatal team and are highly valued by colleagues and families.

KEY LEARNING POINTS

- Communication between maternity and neonatal teams is essential. It is important to give families realistic expectations of how their baby will be cared for and to share with the neonatal team information that is relevant to clinical management. Good communication requires consistent discussions between individuals that supplement regular communications between teams that are embedded in well-established systems and care pathways.

- Keep families together whenever possible. If separation is required to deliver care then optimize contact between mother (and father) and baby. Move to skin-to-skin care as quickly as possible.

- Breast is best – all neonatal care must promote breast-feeding unless there is a contraindication to breastfeeding. If breastfeeding is interrupted due to problems with the baby, the mother must be supported to express her milk so that the baby can receive the milk when appropriate and the mother's supply is maintained

- Keep babies at the right temperature. Preterm babies also need to be kept at the optimal humidity.

- Premature babies have a range of outcomes. Many extremely premature babies have no or mild disability.

- Neonatal encephalopathy has a number of causes: not all encephalopathy is due to perinatal asphyxia. When dealing with an encephalopathic baby it can take 1–2 weeks to establish the importance of events before and during labour.

Global issues

- Neonates contribute disproportionately to the global burden of disease so that efforts to improve the maternal and neonatal care will be disproportionately beneficial to families and to society.

- Infection is a major cause of neonatal mortality and morbidity. Care pathways that reduce the incidence and impact of neonatal infection are essential. This includes antimicrobial stewardship.

- A systems approach is necessary for good neonatal care. Systematic care is needed to ensure that all babies have timely access to the preventive and treatment measures that they need.

- Appropriate technology has a role in neonatal care, for example using CPAP in a safe but context-specific way.

Further reading

Costeloe KL, Hennessy EM, Haider S, Stacey F, Marlow N, Draper ES (2012). Short term outcomes after extreme preterm birth in England: comparison of two birth cohorts in 1995 and 2006 (the EPICure studies). *BMJ* **345**:e7976. doi:10.1136/bmj.e7976.

Available free online at http://www.bmj.com/content/345/bmj.e7976.long.

Moore T, Hennessy EM, Myles J, *et al.* (2012). Neurological and developmental outcome in extremely preterm children born in England in 1995 and 2006: the EPICure studies. *BMJ* **345**:e7961. doi:10.1136/bmj.e7961.

Available free online at http://www.bmj.com/content/345/bmj.e7961.long.

Neonatal Life Support

https://www.resus.org.uk/information-on-courses/newborn-life-support/

Nuffield Council on Bioethics. Critical care decisions in fetal and neonatal medicine: ethical issues. http://nuffieldbioethics.org/project/neonatal-medicine/.

Self assessment

CASE HISTORY 1

A 32-year-old pharmacist is carrying a fetus found to have hypoplastic left heart with anomalous pulmonary venous drainage. The cardiologists say that they will not be able offer surgery to this baby. The family opt to continue the pregnancy

A What needs to be covered during antenatal discussions at 30 weeks?

B After a normal vaginal delivery at 38 weeks what needs to be done for the male baby?

ANSWERS

Key answers are in bold; more detail is provided for reference.

A 1 **Input from the multidisciplinary team**: fetal medicine specialists, neonatologists, paediatric palliative care team.

2 **The diagnosis and prognosis**: baby will die even with palliative surgery so that surgery is futile and not in the baby's best interests.

3 **The implications for the baby**: baby may die before or during labour; an experienced neonatal team will attend the birth; the baby may die within minutes or birth – if this is likely the baby will stay with mother immediately after birth; the baby may die within 48 hours of birth – the baby may need to move to the neonatal unit while the diagnosis is confirmed, the family may choose to avoid separation from the baby in which case she/he would not be ventilated and would die soon after birth; the baby may die more than 48 hours after birth, in which case the baby could stay in hospital, move to a hospice or move to the family home. The sequence of events may turn out to be different but an initial good response after birth does not change the prognosis.

4 **The range of options for the family**: the family can choose what to do; the family can ask the professionals to do what they think best; the family can be part of joint decision making. The family can stay together at all times (in which case the baby will not be put onto a life support machine and may die a day or two sooner) or the baby could be moved to the neonatal unit and then to a place of the parents' choosing.

5 **The extent and nature of resuscitation that is offered immediately after birth**: some families will want comfort care only, even if the baby is vigorous; other families would want resuscitation to a greater or lesser extent.

The same framework will apply to any baby with a potentially limited lifespan. A baby with a firm diagnosis of trisomy 18 or trisomy 13 would have many, but not all, of the same issues.

B 1 Paediatric team must be in attendance.

2 The baby is assessed.

3 If baby is breathing, offer skin-to-skin care.

4 If baby is not breathing, follow neonatal resuscitation to the extent agreed with the family before birth.

CASE HISTORY 2

A 24-year-old farmer is in confirmed labour at 25 weeks.

A What are the key points to make to the family antenatally?

B At the end of the discussion parents and professionals decide that full intensive care is in the baby's best interests. A different neonatal team attends the birth; what do you need to tell them?

ANSWERS

A 1 Baby may die during labour.

2 Survival is c. 70%.

3 Baby will have a long stay on the neonatal unit – usually until the expected date of delivery, or 1–2 months later.

4 Many of the survivors will go to a mainstream school and many of these will need help with reading or paying attention.

5 Some survivors will have disability that is obvious and needs help.

6 Some survivors will have profound disability.

B 1 The events leading up to the birth.

2 The obstetric assessment of fetal condition.

3 Events during labour.

4 The results of the antenatal discussions.

EMQs

1 The following conditions need postnatal treatment. For each description, choose the SINGLE most appropriate answer from the list of options. Each option may be used once, more than once or not at all.

A   At birth.

B   Within 5 minutes of birth.

C   Within 1 hour of birth.

D   Within 6 hours of birth.

E   Within 12 hours of birth.

F   Within 24 hours of birth.

G   Within 1 week of birth.

H   When the baby is stable.

I   Within 3 months of birth.

J   Between 3–6 months of birth.

K   Between 6–12 months of birth.

1   Surgery for congenital diaphragmatic hernia.

2   Cardiac catheterization for transposition of the great arteries with no interatrial or interventricular blood flow.

3   Surgery for cleft palate.

4   Prevention of hypothermia in a preterm baby with a plastic bag.

5   Airway positioning if baby is in poor condition after birth.

6   Surgery for hypospadias.

7   Surgery for NEC.

8   Ganciclovir for congenital CMV infection.

ANSWERS

1H There is no rush to surgery with congential diaphragmatic hernia. The baby can suffer from complex respiratory problems and persistent fetal circulation/pulmonary hypertension and it is best to get these under control before a major operation.

2E These babies have no way to move blood between the systemic and pulmonary circulations so become profoundly hypoxic. Urgent transfer to a paediatric cardiology unit is essential.

3K Feeding can be supported in the weeks after birth and surgical outcomes are excellent if the operation is done between 6 and 12 months.

4A An extremely preterm baby needs to be placed in a plastic bag at birth in order to optimize the baby's condition.

5B   After initial assessment, a baby who is not adapting quickly needs to have the airway positioned appropriately (i.e. in a neutral position). Flexion or hyperextension will not open the airway. This is different from the 'sniffing the morning air' used in adults.

6K   Delay leads to better results. Advise the parents that the foreskin is used in the repair so it is important to advise against circumcision.

7H   Even a critically ill baby needs a to be stabilized before a general anaesthetic and laparotomy.

8F   In babies with systemic CMV ganciclovir reduces some, but not all, of the neonatal disease burden. Treatment can be started within 24 hours of birth.

---

2   The neonatal management of the conditions below requires information from the obstetric team. For each neonatal description, choose the SINGLE most appropriate answer from the list of maternal information options. Each option may be used once, more than once or not at all.

A   Social history.
B   Cervical examination.
C   High vaginal swab.
D   Maternal renal status.
E   Cardiothoracic ratio.
F   Booking blood serology.
G   Estimated fetal weight.
H   Avidity of anti-CMV antibodies.
I   Maternal thyroid status.
J   Family or personal history of haemolytic anaemia.
K   Duration of rupture of membranes.

1   High creatinine in the days after birth.
2   Suspected syphilis.
3   Suspected HSV infection.
4   Neonatal hypothyroidism.
5   Visible jaundice within 24 hours of birth.
6   Respiratory distress.

ANSWERS

1D   Some babies have high creatinine if the mother has some renal impairment.

2F   If a baby has suspected syphilis it is important to know the booking blood serology. Conversely, if the mother develops syphilis or any other infection that can be vertically transmitted, it is essential to tell the neonatal team as soon as possible. Some of the medications used to treat congenital infection are not immediately available and pharmacy departments need several days to obtain the medicines.

3B   If there is evidence of active herpetic infection in the mother, it is essential to tell the neonatal team.

4I   Maternal thyroid status can affect neonates in a number of ways. It is essential to have a system in place to transfer information about maternal thyroid status to the neonatal team, particularly if the maternal disease has been treated and the baby is still at risk (e.g. Grave's disease).

5J   Some causes of haemolytic anaemia can cause severe, early jaundice.

6K   The duration of membrane rupture can be relevant if it can give rise to pulmonary hypoplasia (i.e. before 20 weeks) or infection (and gestational age). Neonatal staff are not skilled at interpreting labour records so if the baby is sick and the maternal notes are not clear the neonatal team needs a definitive estimate of duration of membrane rupture

SBA QUESTIONS

Choose the single best answer.

1 A male baby born at 37 weeks' gestation is 2 minutes old. He is floppy and blue with a heart rate of 80 beats per minute. The first step to take to help him is:

A External cardiac massage.

B Airway positioning: 'sniffing the morning air'.

C Put him in a plastic bag.

D Position the airway in a neutral position.

E Intubate.

ANSWER

D Neonatal anatomy is different to anatomy at other ages so an age-specific approach to the airway is needed.

- External cardiac massage is indicated if the heart rate is less than 60 beats per minute. The airway is the priority and the heart rate will pick up when a good airway is established.
- A baby born at 37 weeks is not usually put in a plastic bag – the bags are for premature babies.
- This baby does not need to be intubated at this point. Intubation is only done if other approaches are not successful or the baby is very sick (no heart rate, pale, no movements).

2 A female baby born at 38 weeks weighing 3.4 kg is 6 hours old. The approach to assessment of her blood glucose is:

A Prefeed blood measurement of blood glucose.

B Postfeed blood measurement of blood glucose.

C No assessment of blood glucose.

D Pre- and postfeed measurement of blood glucose.

E Random measurement of blood glucose.

ANSWER

C This baby has no risk factors and will be able to use alternative sources of energy so measurement of blood glucose is not required.

- Prefeed blood glucose would be indicated as a screen for hypoglycaemia in babies with risk factors.
- Postfeed blood glucose measurements have no value as a screen.
- Pre- and postfeed assessments may be required in some complex cases of hypoglycaemia.
- Random samples are not informative.

3 A male baby born at 39 weeks 3 days ago weighing 3.6 kg with no maternal antibodies and a bilirubin of 320 µmol/l 8 hours ago that prompted phototherapy with blue light. A repeat bilirubin of 330 µmol/l has just been reported. What treatment is required?

A Continue phototherapy with blue or green light.

B Start phototherapy with ultraviolet light.

C Organize exchange transfusion.

D Administer Ig.

E Place on the window sill.

ANSWER

A Phototherapy with blue or green light will reduce the amount of bilirubin that can cross the blood–brain barrier.

- Ultraviolet light is not used.
- This baby does not need an exchange transfusion because the bilirubin is not rising into the zone of a bilirubin chart that prompts an exchange.
- Ig is given if an alloimmune cause of the jaundice is likely (e.g. because of a strong or very strong response on a DAT (formerly known as a Coombs test).
- The window sill has no place in UK management of jaundice.

In this case there is no need to interrupt breastfeeding during phototherapy.

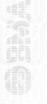

⊕BMA

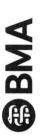

BMA Library

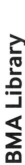

Freepost RTKJ-RKSZ-JGHG
British Medical Association
PO Box 291
LONDON
WC1H 9TG

FREE RETURN POSTAGE FOR STUDENTS, FY DOCTORS & REFUGEE DOCTORS

Use this label for the **FREE** return of books to the BMA Library

Index

Note: Page numbers in **bold** refer to figures; those in *italic* refer to tables or boxes

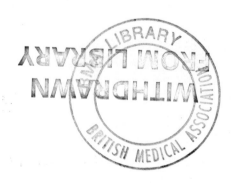